PRAISE FOR
Robert Kowalski's
8 STEPS TO A HEALTHY HEART

"A POSITIVE APPROACH AND OPTIMISTIC
OUTLOOK FOR HEART PATIENTS AND
FORMER PATIENTS."
—*Publishers Weekly*

■

"*EIGHT STEPS* SHOULD BE REQUIRED READING
FOR ALL HEART PATIENTS. . . . It is enjoyable
and provides the motivation and information
needed for a successful recovery."
—Jack Sternlieb, M.D., Heart Institute of the Desert,
Rancho Mirage, California

■

"A COMPLETE GUIDE TO PREVENT
HEART DISEASE AND RECOVER FROM
HEART ATTACKS."
—*Florida Times-Union*

■

more . . .

Other Books by Robert E. Kowalski:

The 8-Week Cholesterol Cure
Cholesterol & Children
The 8-Week Cholesterol Cure Cookbook
The Endocrine Control Diet (with Calvin Ezrin, M.D.)

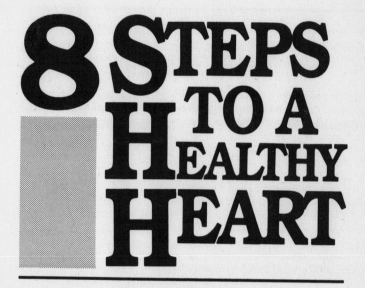

8 STEPS TO A HEALTHY HEART

THE COMPLETE GUIDE TO HEART DISEASE PREVENTION AND RECOVERY FROM HEART ATTACK AND BYPASS SURGERY

ROBERT E. KOWALSKI

Forewords by heart surgeon Jack Sternlieb, M.D., and other leading physicians

WARNER BOOKS

A Time Warner Company

To my wife, Dawn, and my children, Ross and Jenny—
the best motivation a man ever had to maintain
a heart-healthy lifestyle.

This book has been written to serve as a bridge between doctor and patient. The information in the book reflects the author's experiences and is not intended to replace medical advice. Any questions regarding your individual health, general or specific, should be addressed to your physician.

Before beginning this or any other medical or nutritional regimen, consult your physician to be sure it is appropriate for you.

Copyright © 1992 by Robert E. Kowalski
All rights reserved.

Warner Books, Inc., 1271 Ave. of the Americas, New York, NY 10020

W A Time Warner Company

Printed in the United States of America
Originally published in hardcover by Warner Books
First trade printing: January 1994
10 9 8 7 6 5 4 3 2 1

Library of Congress Cataloging-in-Publication Data

Kowalski, Robert E.
     Eight steps to a healthy heart : the complete guide to
heart disease prevention and recovery from heart attack and
bypass surgery / by Robert E. Kowalski.
         p.   cm.
     ISBN 0-446-39458-0
     1. Heart—Diseases—Popular works.   2. Heart—Dis-
eases—Patients—Rehabilitation.   I. Title.   II. Title: 8 steps
to a healthy heart.
     RC672.K69   1992
     616.1'2—dc20   91-50082
                                                          CIP

Book design by Giorgetta Bell McRee
Cover design by Mike Stromberg

ACKNOWLEDGMENTS

This book really began way back in 1978 when I had my heart attack and first bypass surgery. My first thanks, therefore, go to those who worked so diligently through the years to keep me alive in order to write the book in the first place! I can't possibly acknowledge each and every doctor, nurse, technician, and assistant for their care and kindness individually, so I must do so with one sweeping gesture. My most heartfelt thanks to one and all.

Next I'd like to thank all those who have had faith in me and my books through the years and who've been essential in bringing these pages to reality: Clyde Taylor at Curtis Brown Ltd.; Rick Hersh of the William Morris Agency; and editors at Warner Books who've made the final product better than the manuscript that first came out of the typewriter.

To help me gather all my facts and figures and sift through the mountains of data and information in the huge arena of heart health, I turned to Rick McGuire, one of the best medical writers it's been my privilege to meet. His efforts went far beyond the call of duty and made the process a pleasure. I hope we'll work together again soon.

Then there were all the wonderful people who provided all the assistance I ever requested from the American Heart Association, the Amer-

viii • ACKNOWLEDGMENTS

ican Medical Association, Mended Hearts, and many governmental
agencies. Too often such individuals remain nameless and faceless, but
their efforts benefit us all in so many ways.

For input I went to many hospitals and medical centers, and received
the insights and wisdom collected through years of professional experi-
ence. At the Heart Institute of the Desert I thank Jack Sternlieb, M.D.,
Bruce Underwood, D.H.Sc., Michael Lawlor, Ph.D., and Bonnie Farrell,
R.N. At Daniel Freeman Heart Center I thank Julia Kuwada, M.S.,
Bettey Anne Pavlik, R.N., Linda Pelletier, R.N., and Hiro Nishi,
Pharm.D. At Cedars-Sinai Medical Center I thank Harvey Alpern,
M.D., Barbara Else, R.N., and Arna Munford, Ph.D. And at Cleveland
Clinic I thank Fredric Pashkow, M.D.

After months of writing it was time to review my words. Asking people
to take their time to critically review nearly 700 typewritten pages of
manuscript walks the fine line between favor and imposition. But everyone I asked responded wonderfully. My thanks, then, to my reviewers
in alphabetical order: Willard Forney, M.D., Antonio Gotto, M.D.,
Ph.D., Jennifer Jensen, R.D., M.S., Joseph Keenan, M.D., Charles
Keenan, M.D., Julia Kuwada, M.S., Arna Munford, Ph.D., Carter Newton, M.D., Dean Ornish, M.D., and Jack Sternlieb, M.D.

Finally, my thanks to the dozens of patients who shared their feelings
and concerns with me so that I could share them with my readers who
will benefit from their experiences.

I pray that patients and professionals alike will benefit from this book,
thus repaying all those who provided their assistance so unfalteringly.

CONTENTS

FOREWORDS

JACK J. STERNLIEB, M.D.

Founder & Chairman
Heart Institute of the Desert;
Director, Cardiac Surgery Eisenhower Medical Center
Rancho Mirage, California

Bob Kowalski has, no doubt, achieved another success with the publication of *Eight Steps to a Healthy Heart*. Now, in addition to *The 8-Week Cholesterol Cure* my patients have as required reading, this informative book should help them recover from heart disease. This text is a natural progression from *The 8-Week Cholesterol Cure* and covers the A through Z of mending a broken heart. Not only should patients and "former heart patients" add this book to their library, but so should the rest of us who can do something positive towards achieving primary prevention.

Bob shares my positive approach and optimistic outlook for most heart patients, which leads them to a more rapid and complete recovery. I have repeatedly witnessed the profound effects of a pessimistic attitude that some *health care givers* project onto their patients. This attitude can lead to an overdependence on medical staff, unwarranted fear, disability out of proportion to the illness and even premature death from just giving up hope. Fortunately, we are all born with hearts that are much stronger than needed to perform most daily tasks, including many recreational athletics. A normal heart is incredibly overdesigned and, for the sake of comparison, has the potential power of a 12-cylinder engine. Therefore, should it be reduced to even half its strength following a severe heart attack, the resultant 6-cylinder engine, with some fine tuning, can allow most of us to have a reasonable lifestyle with few restrictions.

The locale of my medical practice—namely, the southern California desert—has exposed me to a unique group of heart patients who will be exceedingly receptive to Bob's recovery program. These elderly patients have retired to a resort community to enjoy their well-deserved remaining years, free of most stress and responsibilities. Suddenly, their dream is shattered by the onset of heart disease. The majority accept this *temporary* setback as inevitable since they have witnessed heart attacks among their peers. They generally get good family support since their children are now adults. Just as important perhaps, their newfound friends in retirement have the time and maturity to render emotional support needed for recovery. These patients attack the recovery program, as outlined in *Eight Steps to a Healthy Heart*, with a sense of urgency since they value their remaining years and want to be more physically fit than before. Perhaps, due to their experience with life's battles, they are better prepared to cope with heart disease and only need professional guidance to help them get back to enjoying life. The lesson I learned from my patients is that it is never too late to take charge of your recovery and adopt a healthy lifestyle.

Being a busy cardiac surgeon I don't have adequate time to address all the areas of concern that my heart patients have. Therefore, I rely on cardiologists and my paramedical staff consisting of nurses, dieticians, and exercise physiologists to help me educate the patients and their families to bring about modifications in lifestyle that will assure a speedy recovery. Interestingly, in an era when "self-help" and "how-to" books abound, there has been no comprehensive text to supplement the piecemeal advice and literature we can offer our heart patients. *Eight Steps to a Healthy Heart* fulfills this need. It should be kept at the bedside for repeated reading and for quick reference by those interested in recovering from heart disease as well as those who belong to the silent majority wishing to decrease the likelihood of gaining first-hand experience with America's number-one 1 killer.

Bob has brought a new dimension to an old cliché. He not only practices what he preaches, but has made it easier for the rest of us to adopt a healthy lifestyle. He has had a profound effect on the public's awareness of diet and its relationship to heart disease. He has pursued his goals with tireless effort and has not limited his communication to the written word, but has endeavored to educate as many people as possible through a variety of public seminars and the media. A measure of his success is that now most of my patients understand the difference between soluble and insoluble fiber and monounsaturated versus poly-unsaturated fats, a distinction that, no doubt, would have been foreign to them years ago.

One controversial area of this book, which I feel qualified to expand on, concerns the section dealing with selecting a physician. Too often, the public relies on chance in finding a physician in a hospital. More often than not, an institution is selected because it's the closest facility and a physician is chosen for them by an emergency room using a roster of on-call specialists.

I believe most patients spend more time and effort deciding on which restaurant to go to on a Saturday evening than they do choosing a practitioner who may have a serious impact on their longevity or quality of life. Even business executives, who would never purchase stocks from a company they hadn't thoroughly investigated, submit to an unknown heart surgery team for a life-threatening procedure. There are now mortality statistics, however, to help patients make a more educated choice in selecting a heart center. They chart volume of cases, length of stay, and the average cost of procedures. Ask your hospital for this data before you decide to undergo treatment. Don't be misled by hospital administrators and physicians stating that their mortality is high because they operate on only sick patients and their neighbors have better results because they handle easy cases. They would like you to believe that all hospitals and doctors possess equal skills and the only difference between them is the type of patient they treat.

Another interesting aspect of patients' tolerance for less than ideal treatment is the common statement, "He has no bedside manner and I can't communicate with him, but he is supposed to be a good technician." To return to my restaurant analogy, how many of us would patronize a restaurant that prepared good food, but treated its customers with indifference or rudeness? Only by asking hard, scientific questions of hospitals and practitioners and demanding logical responses will the quality of medical care improve.

To prove that it's possible to alter the kind of unhealthy behavior outlined in the first of Bob Kowalski's eight "steps," I recently tested Bob's Type A personality on two occasions. First, I was given a week to read the manuscript for *Eight Steps to a Healthy Heart*, but since I couldn't put the book down and read a few chapters twice, it took longer for me to submit my comments. I received no threatening phone calls. Then my foreword was one month late and I expected a chastising, but instead I received words of comfort from the author: "Thank God you're a surgeon." If this book has a significant impact on primary prevention, which I trust it will, then in years to come my fellow heart surgeons and I will have more time to write forewords and learn to play golf.

DEAN ORNISH, M.D.

President & Director
Preventive Medicine Research Institute
Sausalito, CA

Although coronary heart disease still kills more Americans each year than all other illnesses combined (including cancer and AIDS), it can be prevented in the vast majority of us if we are willing to make different choices in diet and lifestyle. In Chinese, the word "crisis" comes from characters that include the words both "crisis" and "opportunity." In *Eight Steps to a Healthy Heart*, Robert Kowalski can show you how to turn the crisis of heart disease into an opportunity for transformation.

No one understands the experience of having a heart attack as someone else who has suffered one. Robert Kowalski writes both from his own personal experience and with a comprehensive understanding of the medical and scientific literature. He acts as a personal guide through the recovery process, providing both the encouragement and the knowledge that are essential for self-healing. *Eight Steps to a Healthy Heart* can act as an important bridge between you and your doctor. I recommend it for anyone who has a heart.

ANTONIO M. GOTTO, JR., M.D., D.PHIL.

Chairman, Department of Medicine
Baylor College of Medicine;
Chief, Internal Medicine Service
The Methodist Hospital
Houston, TX

Eight Steps to a Healthy Heart by Bob Kowalski will be inspirational to patients who are emotionally crippled by coronary heart disease. The chapter on motivation is particularly good. The post-coronary bypass patient is reminiscent of the reborn central figure in *Lazarus*, the recent novel by Morris West about a pope who underwent bypass surgery.

Mr. Kowalski has had the book carefully critiqued by various experts in the cardiovascular field. The book is highly accurate and has the ring of authority.

The publication of this book is a great service to the emotionally stressed patient with coronary heart disease. I shall gladly recommend *Eight Steps* to my patients, and I congratulate Mr. Kowalski on a fine contribution to patients and public education.

JOSEPH M. KEENAN, M.D.

University of Minnesota School of Medicine
Department of Family Practice
Minneapolis, MN

This book is obviously targeted at the millions of persons who are at risk for or have already acquired heart disease. Yet, I could easily recommend it as a sound guide for anyone interested in healthy living.

This volume is unquestionably the most comprehensive informational discussion of heart disease ever assembled for the lay reader. It includes an extensive review of risk factors, cardiac physiology and testing, and common medications. Even more commendable is Kowalski's ability to present this sometimes frightening or confusing information in an easily understood and reassuring fashion. He effectively draws on his own experience as a heart patient and his extensive personal research to both motivate the reader and provide practical applications of the heart-healthy lifestyle. Kowalski demonstrates a special sensitivity to those difficult areas of cardiac recovery such as dealing with stress, sex after heart attack, family relationships and support, and returning to work. He candidly reveals his own mistakes as well as successes, and with this self-disclosure he builds a therapeutic relationship with the reader. Through the course of the book he becomes a teacher, an experienced guide, and a friend extending a helping hand and an encouraging word.

The book is upbeat and optimistic about cardiac recovery and the positive rewards of a healthy lifestyle, almost to a fault. Kowalski has a genius for empowering readers with a sound scientific basis for their optimism and helping them to internalize this into a motivation to take control of their lives. The eight steps to a healthy heart are cleverly laid out in an integrated fashion so that the reader comes to appreciate them as related parts of a holistic lifestyle. Each rationale, whether for stress reduction, exercise, proper diet or smoking cessation not only reinforces specific health goals but also buttresses one another in a matrix fashion. Thus, the reader is presented with a clear picture of how to get to a healthy goal and is challenged to provide the only missing piece—personal commitment to change.

The book will retain value for most as a handy reference. It is a veritable trove of tips and suggestions including brands of healthy foods, pros and cons of various exercise equipment, and a useful medication chart. Physicians and cardiac rehabilitation professionals will welcome this as a valuable educational complement to their efforts to manage patients with cardiovascular risk.

PREFACE

Certain thought leaders in the medical community are wakening to the realization that heart disease, even after a heart attack or bypass surgery, need not be a death sentence. The reality is that heart disease can be effectively and completely controlled, allowing the patient to live an unrestricted lifestyle.

Unfortunately, that kind of progressive thinking has not filtered down to the typical practicing physician, much less to the patients who desperately need to know that there is a way to make a spectacular recovery. Most patients received outmoded information and treatment that limits their recovery and actually leads to a worsening of the disease.

A veil of ignorance continues to prevent patients from taking the steps that could enable them to live a more vibrant, dynamic lifestyle than they ever did before encountering heart disease.

An article appearing in *Circulation*, the official publication of the American Heart Association, in 1992 reviewed the statistics of heart patients following bypass surgery. The authors concluded that five or six years post-bypass, symptoms began to reappear. And nine to ten years after the operations, vessels were reclogged and the benefits of the bypass were typically completely gone. One would need repeated surgeries because the disease just naturally progresses, getting worse and worse.

The mass media reported those conclusions without the proper interpretations, and the result was that the public—and their physicians—was led to believe, quite erroneously, that fighting heart disease is a losing battle, even with such heroic measures as bypass surgery. Why bother trying?

Well, that would be like concluding that aspirin does not cure headaches if one continues to hit himself in the head with a hammer! First put down that hammer, and let the aspirin work.

By taking certain steps, the eight steps described in this book, one can *expect* to stop the deadly progression of heart disease. One should *not* expect the disease to get worse, requiring additional bypass surgeries or leading to another heart attack.

The steps I refer to are termed "aggressive secondary prevention" in the medical community. They work. At the time of this writing, I am ten years post-bypass, and, as you'll read in the coming pages, I have completely stopped the progression of the disease. My vessels have *not* clogged up again. And I have unequivocal proof.

In the years to come, aggressive secondary prevention will become the norm in medical practice. An important step in that direction came in June of 1993, in Washington, D.C. There a panel of experts convened to issue the latest guidelines for patients and physicians regarding cholesterol control. They met under the aegis of the National Cholesterol Education Program, a cooperative effort of the nation's medical organizations in concert with the federal government.

While a cholesterol level of 200 is acceptable for the general population, the panel urged, those with existing heart disease should have a target of no more than 160. Such aggressive treatment and control was needed, they said, to stop the progression of the disease.

Theirs was not an idle conclusion. It was backed up by years of research showing that such efforts have huge payoffs.

Unfortunately, such information was not loudly trumpeted by the mass media. Fortunately, you have all the information in your hands at this very moment. Read the coming pages and chapters knowing that they contain the truths that can set you free from the clutches of the nation's number-one killer.

Introduction: A Happy Ending, A New Beginning

Two men went into the hospital to have coronary bypass surgery. Both were in the hands of competent cardiologists and cardiac surgeons. Each had excellent prospects for recovery and return to a very normal, healthy life. Yet one went on to six years of depression, anxiety, and ultimate worsening of heart disease while the other experienced a speedy recovery, complete mental and physical health, and, six years later, clear heart vessels.

Now here's the real paradox: both of those men were me!

Actually the situation is not as impossible as it first appears to be. At the age of 35 in 1978 I had bypass surgery following a heart attack. I lived the life of a cardiac cripple for the next six years, making myself and those around me quite miserable. Then, in 1984, at age 41, I had a second operation which turned my life around and started me on a path to total recovery and happiness.

The news that I have to share with you is that heart disease can be beaten. You will recover. You can lead a completely normal life. The arterial blockage that causes the disease can be reversed. I even have the photographs showing my own heart's blood vessels; they're in Figure 1 on page 2.

While every disease is different, and every patient is an individual

1

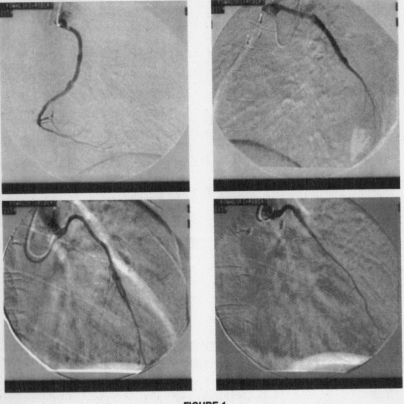

FIGURE 1

case, recovery from heart disease is, in a very real way, no different from recovery from, say, an auto accident. It's too bad it happened, you'll have to spend some time in the hospital, you'll need to work at recovery and rehabilitation, but you will get over it. As hard as it is to accept this right now, you'll be all the better for it.

Today I no longer even consider myself to be a cardiac patient. I'm a former patient who went through the hell of heart disease until I finally took charge of my own destiny and was ultimately rewarded with the heaven of optimal health. My personal physicians, as well as many others

THE ULTIMATE PROOF OF RECOVERY

I can tell you how terrific I feel, with my cholesterol level under control and all the other vital statistics. But, as they say, a picture is worth a thousand words. So I asked Dr. Jack Sternlieb to provide laser prints from my digital coronary angiogram done at the Heart Institute of the Desert five years after my second bypass operation, and to comment on these glimpses into my heart's vessels. The following are Dr. Sternlieb's words:

1. The vein bypass graft to the right coronary artery appears patent (open) with good flow to the distal portion of the coronary artery.
2. The vein graft to the obtuse marginal from the circumflex coronary artery appears free of atherosclerosis as does the native coronary artery.
3. The vein graft to the left anterior descending artery appears entirely normal as does the native coronary artery.
4. The vein graft to the anterior diagonal artery has no evidence of atherosclerosis and the native coronary artery looks excellent as well.

All four vein bypasses were constructed in 1984, and have no evidence of developing new disease, namely atherosclerosis. There has been no progression of disease in the native coronary arteries. Patent or open saphenous vein bypasses without luminal irregularities or suggestion of atherosclerosis at five years carries a good prognosis for the future.

who have reviewed my case, agree that there's no reason to expect that I'll ever die of heart disease. "We'll have to run you over with a truck," one of them told me after seeing those pictures of my arteries.

What were the differences between the "two" men who faced heart disease and bypass surgery? Why did I do so poorly after the first surgery and so well after the second? Today we have knowledge and tools that were not available years ago and that can make possible this type of spectacular recovery. The shame is that the information seldom trickles down to patients who desperately need it.

Several studies have shown that patients leave the hospital confused and afraid. I know that was true for me the first time around. Patients get sketchy information while lying in their beds, when they're more concerned about whether they're going to live or die in the next 24 hours than what to do and what not to do in the next 24 or more years. Many, if not most, feel they're being pushed into a cold world they're not likely to survive and which will be impossible to enjoy. And their spouses and families are drawn into the horror along with them.

You're not alone in suffering from heart disease. It remains the number one killer in America and throughout the western world. In the past the prognosis was gradual worsening of the disease and ultimate death. Today thousands of patients are living testimonials to the fact that heart disease can have a happy ending. I'll share many of their stories with you in this book so that you can learn from their experiences as well as from mine. Now let me tell you how I got into this.

For openers, I never expected to live to a ripe old age. My father died of a heart attack at the age of 57 in 1969. His sister also had a fatal attack in her fifties, and his brother had a heart attack and bypass surgery. I automatically assumed that I would follow in my family's footsteps. In fact, when interviewing for jobs after college, I ignored information about retirement plans, figuring I wouldn't survive into my sixties.

In a perverse and oddly cavalier way, I told friends and acquaintances that I'd "live fast, die young, and leave a good-looking corpse." That's the kind of bravado attitude only one in his twenties can muster. Actually it was, in retrospect, a stupid mental set and one I now regret, especially when you consider my education and background.

I attended Iowa State University, where I took two degrees in science journalism with dual majors in biology and physiology, and then went on to additional graduate study in physiology. For about 25 years I've written exclusively about health and medical matters. It's been my job to convey to others the best medical advice for living a healthy life. Yet for many years I ignored that very same advice. I smoked two packs of Marlboros daily, got very little exercise, was very stressed, and ate all the rich foods I wanted.

The Surgeon General had made it quite clear in 1964 that smoking was hazardous to one's health. But the association with other risk factors wasn't as clear at the time. I learned early on that my cholesterol level was high. Attending a medical convention, I took advantage of a free blood test. All the readings were normal, but my cholesterol level was

250 mg/dl, at that time termed "high normal." No one really knew what to make of it, and I chose to ignore this bit of information.

Ironically, I joined the National Dairy Council in 1973 as a science writer, and found myself involved in what was then called the "diet–heart debate." Simply enough, there was a real controversy in the scientific and medical communities as to whether the cholesterol in the diet had anything to do with the cholesterol in the blood which was associated with an elevated risk of heart attack. There were some good arguments that diet had little or no impact on one's cholesterol level in the blood, and many respected researchers whose offices and laboratories I visited said there was no reason to change one's diet as long as one maintained ideal weight and got the proper nutrients. I'll get into the details of diet, cholesterol, and heart disease later in this book. Suffice it to say for now that I was on the wrong side of the argument back then in the '70s, and my personal diet remained rich in butter, cheese, and prime steaks.

Attending a food writers' convention, the journalists and I were asked to take a kind of test. The speaker, a researcher from Vanderbilt University, had developed a way to determine the number of years of life one had left, based on medical history and current lifestyle. Add so many points for regular exercise, subtract so many points for each cigarette smoked daily, and so forth. The resulting number reflected one's life expectancy. My number was zero.

I actually turned to the writers on both sides of me and laughed. "Look," I said, "I'm dead!" Well, I guess I shouldn't have laughed so hard. I was 35 years of age, and within months I'd have a heart attack that would nearly kill me.

My introduction to the gray and shadowy world of heart disease came on a warm, late spring night in Chicago. Returning from a drive-in theater, about to pull into the driveway of my apartment building, I began to have a dull, throbbing sensation in my left arm, radiating down from my shoulder. There was also a tightening in my jaw and a vague feeling of gastrointestinal disturbance. Moreover, I felt oddly uneasy, aware that something was very wrong.

Yet my first reaction was to dismiss it all as the result of working too hard, smoking too much, and being under a lot of both personal and professional stress. "Go to bed and sleep it off," I thought. Then a wiser inner voice reminded me that I'd read and written about those symptoms before. They were the warning signs of a heart attack. So I drove to the nearest emergency room which, on the near-north side of Chicago, wasn't too far away.

There I was told that I was experiencing angina pectoris, the pain of oxygen insufficiency to my heart. It wasn't a heart attack, I was reassured, but a warning that shouldn't be ignored. Released with a bottle of nitroglycerin tablets, I returned to my apartment, where I spent the better part of the night in desperate anxiety.

The next day I asked a physician friend for a referral to a good cardiologist. After reading my ECG (electrocardiogram also abbreviated as EKG) from the night before and another taken that day, that cardiologist put me on a combination of potent drugs designed to keep the coronary arteries open and flowing. Considering my age and the poor ECG, he scheduled me to have an angiogram performed in three days, the first available time slot open at Michael Reese Hospital. Those three days were filled with fear and anxiety. Like so many others before and countless others after, I asked the eternal question, "Why me, God, why is this happening to me?"

The night before entering the hospital I began to have the same symptoms that had first taken me to the emergency room. But this time they didn't go away. Filled with dread and fear, I paced my apartment from 2:00 A.M. until about two hours later. Why didn't I go immediately to the hospital? Granted, it was a terrible, potentially fatal mistake. But at the time I just kept praying that the feelings would pass. And they finally did.

With the sun shining, I checked into the hospital for my scheduled angiogram to find out just what was going on in my chest. Later that morning, having gone through some tests and examinations, I lay on a table being prepped for the procedure. Literally minutes before the incision would have been made in my arm to introduce the catheter into my coronary arteries, a laboratory technician hurried into the room to stop the angiogram. Enzymes had been discovered in my blood. I had had a heart attack the night before. A tear fell from my eye and down my cheek. Life as I had known it came to an abrupt end.

Wheeled to a room in the CCU (coronary care unit), I learned that I was lucky to be alive. If it hadn't been for the drugs I was taking, the heart attack might have been fatal. Looking back, I realize that I got very little more information or understanding regarding my condition. For the next 10 days I remained in the hospital and was released. Then came two months of recovery, mostly resting, before they could do the angiogram.

Again, this was 1978. Much has changed for the better and the scenario today would be quite different. Medical developments have facilitated patient care and far less is left to chance.

The eventual angiogram revealed blockages in three vessels. Coronary bypass surgery was indicated. My reaction? Good, let's get this over with so I can get on with my life; I'd much rather have the surgery to "cure" my problem than to put up with the disease. I still denied that I could have anything to do with the disease's development, that the way I was living was the reason for the way I was dying.

The medical community at the time fostered that erroneous train of thought. Checking me out of the hospital, my surgeon in a good-natured manner put his arm around my shoulder and said, "Bob, let me give you some advice. You had something wrong. We fixed it. Now forget this ever happened and go out and enjoy your life."

My cardiologist concurred. Of course, he said, smoking was bad for me. But then again, if I smoked just a few, he thought, I'd probably get some benefit from the relaxation. As to exercise, just walk a bit. Diet? Some people have a genetically elevated cholesterol level. Men with my condition were known to live for decades. Don't worry about it.

But worry I did. I received no real sense of direction, and was left floundering. Despite the encouraging words, I couldn't help but realize that this disease was killing me. I didn't know what to do. No cardiac rehabilitation was offered. No counseling helped me through the anxiety and depression that followed.

Shortly after the bypass surgery I returned for an exercise stress test on the treadmill. The findings weren't good. At a moderate level of effort I began to show what is termed "ST segment depression," signaling oxygen insufficiency to the heart. The bypass hadn't been completely effective; it now appears that at least one, and probably two of the bypassed vessels closed down shortly after the surgery. Even following the operation, then, I was in jeopardy of a heart attack.

I felt I was living under the Sword of Damocles. I refer to the Greek myth of the man who was seated before a marvelous feast, but had a sword hanging above him, suspended by only a hair. How could he enjoy that feast knowing that the sword could end his life at any moment?

Each day, literally every day, every time I felt a twinge in the left arm, or a pressure in the jaw, or a wave of indigestion, I wondered whether the next heart attack was on its way. It's difficult to live, much less enjoy, life that way.

I didn't make things easier for those around me, either. I yelled at people, complained about everything, demanded this and that. I never smiled, never felt gratitude or joy.

Rather than making improvements in my lifestyle, I actually allowed my bad habits to get worse. I drank quite a bit and smoked some marijuana along with my cigarettes in the evening. Now I recognize that I was trying to anesthetize myself from my psychological pain.

I knew that I was supposed to exercise, but how much was too much? I was told it was all right to have sex, but could too much excitement kill me? At work, were the tensions and pressures and politics going to be the death of me? Not knowing the answers to any of those questions, and not knowing where to turn to get help, my natural tendency was to live to much less than my fullest potential.

I was miserable. I looked in the mirror each morning and saw the scar on my chest, reminding me that another day of anxiety and anger and grief was about to begin. I was single at the time. Would any woman want a "diseased and flawed" man? If so, would I die in the throes of passion? Could I get another job, since my current one had long ceased to offer fulfillment? What about insurance? And paying the bills? Moreover, did any of it really matter? Was life worth living? I began to wish that the heart attack had just finished me off. And I swore that I'd never have another surgery.

Was I alone in such feelings? Actually millions of others experience similar misgivings and pain. They get to the point where they refuse sex, work, or virtually any physical exertion. They become cardiac cripples.

President Dwight Eisenhower was one of the most famous cardiac cripples. He was filled with depression and remorse after his heart attack, fearing even his beloved game of golf. There are many other famous examples. But before you get depressed, let me hasten to say that there is no reason today to suffer as I did, as others in the past have done. Let me offer a parallel.

As a child, I lived in fear of polio, especially during the summer months when it appeared that more cases developed than at any other time of the year. I had to avoid swimming pools and indoor activities, according to my father, so that I wouldn't contract the disease that could cripple me for life. Today, of course, we have the wonderful vaccine developed by Drs. Salk and Sabin which effectively removed this curse. My children don't fear polio, and I doubt they even know what it is. The polio era is dead and gone.

Similarly, though not so dramatically, we have learned a great deal about heart disease and how to come to grips with it. One can not only expect to recover from a heart attack, bypass surgery, or other heart-associated problems but to attain a rich, full, and vibrant life of good health. The era of the cardiac cripple is—or at least should be—over.

How did my thinking change so radically? What happened to me that could turn me around 180 degrees? To explain, let me return to my story.

In 1980 I moved from Chicago to Los Angeles so that I could pursue a career as a freelance medical writer. I had had it with office politics, endless meetings, conflicts and budget problems and wanted to spend more time doing what I knew I was best at, writing about medical and health matters. The geographic move also got me away from some domestic difficulties. Moreover, I had always wanted to live in California and I felt I had nothing more to lose. As they say, when you hit the bottom, there's no where to go but up.

Slowly but surely my life began to improve. I loved living in California, My career was starting to bloom. I married and had two terrific children. Even my health habits improved. I was eating "California healthy" with more fruits and vegetables and fresh seafood and poultry, and I was swimming up to a mile of laps five days a week in my apartment pool. Still, fears related to my heart remained, and far too often I thought a sudden attack could end it all.

In 1984 my worst fears were realized. During an annual exercise stress test, my cardiologist spotted a worsening in my ST depression and suggested having another angiogram. That test showed that two of my bypass vessels had shut down and two more areas of my native arteries were blocked. I needed another bypass, this time a quadruple.

I was in the hands of a marvelous cardiologist, Dr. Albert Kattus, who recommended a cardiac surgeon at Santa Monica Hospital Medical Center. Dr. Bill Plestead pulled no punches in his pre-surgical conference with me. The risk of a first-time bypass surgery is very low, about one percent mortality in good centers such as SMHMC. But for "re-dos" it was another story, he told me. The mortality rate jumps to between five and six percent.

My reaction, at first, was denial. He couldn't mean that to apply to me. He meant it for older people, those who were out of shape physically, those who continued to smoke cigarettes. Not me, not a 41-year-old man in good physical condition who had long since quit the cigarettes. Sorry, he said, the risk applied across the board. There was a five to six percent chance that I wouldn't get off the table. I could seek another opinion, but that's what the rates were at all the good centers. And if

I didn't have the second surgery, my condition indicated that I could have another heart attack at any time.

I went home that day feeling numb. My wife was at work teaching. Jenny, my three-year-old, was in preschool. And my son Ross, six at the time, was in his first-grade classroom. The apartment was empty. I thought about the kids, how much I loved them and enjoyed them, and how my wife would have to explain to them, perhaps, that Dad had gone into the hospital to have surgery but he'd never come home again. They'd have to grow up without their Daddy. I'll admit it. I lay across the bed that day and cried openly. Life had finally started to look up, and now I just might die, leaving my wife and the two kids that really made life worth living. But I knew I had to have the surgery or I'd turn into even more of a cardiac cripple than I'd ever been before.

And I swore that if I came out of the bypass surgery I'd make sure that it would never happen again, that I'd find some way to take charge of my own destiny and turn my own health around.

With the help of some really terrific and dedicated doctors and nurses, that's just what I did.

My new life really began even before I went into the hospital for that "re-do." During the time before the operation I got really serious about lowering my cholesterol level. I'll go into the details of that in Chapter 13, but for now I'll just say that I managed to get it down from a dangerously high 284 mg/dl (milligrams/deciliter) to a nice, comfortable 169 mg/dl in just eight weeks with a program I developed and later called "The 8-Week Cholesterol Cure."

After the surgery my surgeon ordered a regular diet for me. "I want you to eat anything that tastes good to you," he said, "so you can get the nutrition you need to heal quickly." I asked about the need for a low-fat, low-cholesterol diet. He replied that I could do that once I left the hospital. Well, no way was I going to do that. It was the only medical advice I blatantly disregarded. I had my wife smuggle oat bran muffins into the hospital so I wouldn't have to eat the bacon and eggs. And I ordered foods from the daily menu which were acceptably low in fat and cholesterol.

Somehow I knew that I was on the right track. I wanted to go as fast as I could toward attaining my goal of complete and thorough recovery and good health.

When Dr. Kattus prescribed a course of cardiac rehabilitation I agreed to do it. But to tell the truth I didn't really welcome the idea. I didn't understand why I couldn't just get back to swimming my laps in the pool once my chest incision healed.

And when I entered the rehab center at SMHMC I was put off more than a little. I was only 41 years old, and the other patients were, for the most part, old and gray. How could I relate to them? Then I saw them performing on treadmills, bicycles, rowing machines, wall pulleys, and other apparatus in ways that I couldn't match. I thought to myself, well, there might be something to this, after all. Give it a chance, I thought, it's only for 12 weeks.

Again, I'll go into a lot more detail in the chapters on cardiac rehabilitation and exercise. But here's the bottom line: In a very short period of time, I found myself getting stronger and better than I would ever have expected, based on my prior post-op experience. Just when I thought I was doing as much as I should, one of the nurses would ask that I step it up a bit. Soon I was doing far more on those machines than I would ever have done on my own. And I realized that if I could do *that*, I could do *anything* on the outside. For the first time in years I began to feel like a whole person again, without fears of another heart attack.

After finishing the formal period of cardiac rehabilitation, I signed up for an unmonitored program at the hospital. By that time Dr. Kattus was grinning over my recovery. And I was becoming more and more confident in my health.

I don't recall exactly when it happened. It could have been after the first three months, or perhaps longer, but I came to a realization, a revelation if you would, that changed my life forever. It centered around a simple question that came to mind: If I feel this good now, just a short time after major surgery, how good could I feel if I really worked at it in the coming months and years? I decided that it was worth putting to the test. Since that time I've never quit my workouts and I now feel better than I did 20 years ago. In fact, I don't recall *ever* having felt this fantastic!

It didn't happen over night, of course. But it did happen, and it can happen for you, too, whether you've had a heart attack or bypass surgery or your doctor simply has said you have heart disease.

A sound program of cardiac rehabilitation was just one of the elements in my formula for a complete recovery. The dietary changes I made not only lowered my cholesterol, but also gave me the means to permanently control my weight. And I was lucky enough to be in the hands of some really wonderful doctors and nurses. We'll talk about the need for establishing a strong support group later on. It's really essential to have people to rely on, a way to get the answers to your questions. Unlike my earlier, horrible experience, this second time around I had that support. I learned what I needed to do to recover, I received the encouragement we all require, and got answers to my questions.

But more than anything else, my attitude changed. This time I realized that I was in control. I could decide whether I was going to continue a downward spiral of heart disease that ultimately would take me away from my kids and the life I enjoyed or whether I was going to take charge of my own destiny and achieve the happiness that had been so elusive for so many years.

When it comes right down to it, so many things in life depend on one's mental outlook. The right attitude can make the world of difference in business, in sports, and in one's personal relationships with others. This book stresses the importance of a good mental attitude and shows you ways to achieve the outlook that can help you make it through the night and ultimately out of the darkness and into the bright daylight of vibrant good health.

Don't get me wrong. It's not going to be easy. You have a lot to deal with, both mentally and physically. Even now I remember some of the terrible moments. I'd like to share my experiences with you so that it'll be easier for you to deal with them as they happen to you. It'll be tough, but you can do it.

Like me, and many others, you can become a *former* heart patient. Let me tell you how that final transformation took place in my own life.

Following the second bypass, the benefits of my changed lifestyle were dramatic. My cholesterol was down to between 150 and 160 routinely; my blood pressure was absolutely normal; my resting heart rate was showing the benefits of extensive exercise, beating at about 50 per minute; and I was learning to control the stresses in my life, to alter some of my Type-A behaviors; annual treadmill tests proclaimed me to be in excellent health.

Yes, all seemed to be in order. But was the disease re-clogging my arteries and bypass vessels? My book, *The 8-Week Cholesterol Cure*, had become an international best-seller. But that success meant an unbelievable schedule of travel and interviews across the country and around the world. I was working harder than ever before, burning the candle at both ends. While I loved every minute of it, I couldn't help but wonder how my heart was dealing with the pressures.

I actually thought about going into semiretirement so that I could spend the rest of my years with my children. After all, it had been five years at the time since my second bypass, and it was only six years after my first one that I needed a "re-do." Perhaps I should chuck it all and move to a quieter place in the country if I had only a limited amount of time left. In fact, my wife and I actually began house-hunting in a quieter, slower community.

Then I decided to find out, once and for all, just how I was doing. In the intervening years I had met Dr. Jack Sternlieb at the Heart Institute of the Desert in Rancho Mirage, just outside of Palm Springs. He and I had worked on some programs of community education together, and we had gotten to know each other well. At one point I mentioned my concerns to him, and he suggested having an angiogram done to see just how well my rehabilitation program was working.

It was one of the better decisions of my life. I went for the angiogram with the expected anxiety; after all, it is a major, invasive method of testing, not to be taken lightly. But all went well, and the results were spectacular.

In Dr. Sternlieb's words, my bypass vessels look today as if they were put in last week. Completely clear. The cardiologist who performed the procedure was equally delighted. He said that in his 10 years of experience, doing up to 20 angiograms each month, he had come to expect that an angiogram done five years post-bypass would show significant blockage. He had rarely seen a case in which the vessels were 100 percent open and flowing, with no clogging at all. Take a look yourself. The pictures are right there on page 2.

(In May of 1993 I returned to the Heart Institute for another angiogram. It was then nine years since my second bypass. Once again the doctors found that my bypass vessels were free and flowing. "Widely patent" is the term officially used in the report. And my native arteries remain free of any disease progression. So much for the dire predictions of those who claim that the benefits of bypass surgery "wear off" and that another bypass is inevitable.)

As we'll see in a later chapter, we now have significant clinical evidence that *one can not only stop the progress of atherosclerosis, one can actually reverse the disease.* A number of studies bear this out in documented research. But, for me, the best proof of all came that day out in the desert.

My reaction was predictable. I was elated. I knew that my lifestyle changes had paid off in spades, and that if I continued to follow my own regimen I'd be forever free of heart disease. And, you guessed it, that was the end of my plans to slow down! I knew that I needed to share the benefits of what I had learned with the millions of men and women who are now fighting their own battles against heart disease. I had already written the book on cholesterol and dietary changes, but there was a lot more to total cardiac recovery.

So back I went to the medical literature, to meetings at which top researchers share their latest findings, and to the clinics at which cardiac rehabilitation has been taken to a fine art and science. I wanted my personal views and experiences backed up by unshakable science.

One of the places I visited, not surprisingly, was the Heart Institute of the Desert. I got more than I had bargained for. Dr. Sternlieb invited me to observe a bypass surgery. Part of me was journalistically and scientifically excited by the prospect of watching one of the world's top heart surgeons perform the operation, and to learn the nuances of the surgery which one could never get from merely reading about it. But part of me was terrified. I remembered my reaction to seeing a bypass done in the movie *All That Jazz*. What would it be like to see it in person, just inches from a heart being mended? How would I cope with the idea that I had been a patient lying on a table with my own heart exposed and vulnerable?

Well, that experience was a real milestone. I observed the surgery no differently than I would have if it had been a gallbladder removal or some other procedure. I didn't identify with the patient on the table at all. That was then and this is now, I realized. I was no longer a heart patient, but rather a former heart patient.

I can't begin to express the way my life has changed in the past few years, the way I feel about myself, my children, others around me, and life itself. Life is to be enjoyed, and the best way to do that is to be in spectacular good health.

The process really begins in your own mind, even more than in your heart. As in tennis, it's the inner, mental game that really makes a winner. That's why I've devoted so much of this book to the psychological aspects of recovery and rehabilitation. I know the fears, the anxiety, and concerns you have, because I've been there.

I think the psychological aspects of heart disease have been tremendously underrated. Your doctors and all your friends have been smiling and telling you how lucky you are that you're alive, that you survived the heart attack, that you had the life-giving surgery. Yet you feel that more than a little part of you has, in fact, died, and you wonder whether it wouldn't have been better if you had actually died rather than lived. Those around you are doing their best to help, yet you feel smothered by them. You feel envy at the young and healthy, resenting those who have what you don't. You feel alternately sad and angry, with unjustified or at least unexplainable mood swings, and you experience emotional outbursts as never before.

At the same time you feel your body has let you down, that life will never be the same, that you'll never be the same. Your doctors and loved ones are telling you to give up everything in life that seems to give you any pleasure at all. Stop smoking. Don't eat those foods anymore. Calm down. Exercise. Take your pills. Go to one medical appointment after another. This is living? You may have actually wondered about ending it all. Don't feel alone.

I experienced all those emotions and more. But I'm more than just a former patient. My background and experience in journalism and science provide excellent credentials and capability to guide you through this experience.

As the title of this book states, there are eight steps for you to take on the road to total recovery and rehabilitation. Each one is important, and you'll want to read each section carefully to follow the suggestions provided. You may also wish to skip around a bit to get to those aspects for which you need immediate information.

In the *first step*, you'll learn to deal with the depression and anxiety that invariably accompanies heart disease. And you'll develop coping strategies to help you relax not only now, but in the many years to come.

The *second step* in recovery is to understand your own heart and how it got sick in the first place. When your car or your dishwasher breaks down you might not need all the details; you just trust the repairman to get the job done well. But this is too important for you to remain a passive recipient of care. You can benefit enormously from getting involved in your own care, and that means you need to learn how your heart and your cardiovascular system work and what you can do to get them back to superior working condition.

As your *third step*, you need to get back into the swing of life as quickly as possible. But you have a million questions. One of the biggest, and yet most embarrassing for many heart patients, deals with sex after heart attack and surgery. Seldom is this issue discussed to patients' satisfaction by doctors and nurses.

You also want to know about returning to work. Many have unfounded fears about working, and some people cut productive careers short. I'll deal not only with the physical aspects of working, but also with strategies for coping with work-related stresses.

At the same time, you'll need a solid support base. When you have heart disease it affects the entire family. Your spouse will experience significant stress. Your children, relatives, and friends are affected too. All of you need to work together as part of your recovery. You might also like to know about various groups that have formed to help heart patients.

Moreover, you'll need to work as part of a total health care team with your physicians, nurses, pharmacist, and therapists. How can you be sure you're getting the best care? What's the best way to establish a nurturing relationship with a doctor for long-term treatment?

Your *fourth step* will be to follow a long-term prescription for cardiac rehabilitation and future exercise to build strength, stamina, and confidence. Exercise needn't mean drudgery. Even if you haven't been physically active in years, you'll be able to achieve cardiovascular fitness in short order. You'll revel in the confidence and dynamism that comes from knowing that your body has been turned into a well-tuned machine.

If you've already quit smoking, you've come a long way. If you haven't, you'll need the assistance offered in *step five*. No question about it, quitting the cigarette habit can be difficult. You know that because you've probably tried to do so many times before. There are techniques and strategies that have worked for millions of others, and we'll discuss a wide variety of approaches, one of which will be best for you. I never thought I could live without my cigarettes; now I'm amazed that it took so long to get rid of them.

In *step six* you'll get your cholesterol in control, lose those extra pounds you've been carrying, and learn to enjoy a whole world of heart-healthy foods. I'll guide you through the confusing issues of fat, saturated fat, cholesterol (both good and bad), shopping and label reading, restaurant fare, and everything you need to know to enjoy delicious and healthful foods. You'll do it all without deprivation or hunger.

Controlling hypertension, a major risk factor in heart disease, is our *seventh step*. Bringing high blood pressure down to normal can be accomplished very often with just diet and exercise. But we'll also cover the drugs your physician may see fit to prescribe, and how to take those medications without adverse reactions. You'll develop a complete understanding of just what blood pressure means and how you can control it.

Finally, in *step eight* you'll learn about the full array of medications that exist to help you enjoy life to its fullest. Your doctor may prescribe a variety of drugs for various indications. You should understand those drugs, how they work, and what possible interactions and side effects they may have. I've asked a top hospital-based pharmacist to work with me in providing a breakdown of the most commonly prescribed medications and their side effects.

But life is far more than regaining and maintaining your health. Life is to be enjoyed! That's why I've provided an appendix containing a raft of suggestions for taking your heart-healthy program on the road. You'll learn how to obtain heart-healthy foods in restaurants, travel on airlines that cater to your needs, stay in hotels that have heart-healthy menus and exercise facilities, and vacation at resorts and on cruises with the heart-smart man and woman in mind.

If a doctor told me that he had an injection that could render me completely immune to the ravages of heart disease, and that it would eliminate the need for the exercise, diet, and relaxation methods I've been using since the time of my second bypass, I'd certainly take that shot. It would be nice to have that kind of insurance. But I'd continue to stick with this program's eight steps, because they've made me feel so good! I'd never go back to feeling tired and run-down the way I did when I was eating the wrong foods, smoking cigarettes, and getting no exercise and no proper relaxation.

This is a book for those who have suffered and are suffering from heart disease. It's about recovering from a life-threatening illness and putting that disease in your past. Yet ultimately it's about learning to live life with a gusto you've never experienced before.

I know you're still feeling down. It'll take quite a while for you to have your spirits lifted. Right now you view just about everything in a negative light, and you have a right to be more than a little angry about it all. I just wish I could be with you right now to look you straight in the eye, shake your hand, and welcome you to the growing number of us who have beaten heart disease.

Take it one day at a time. Take those eight steps to cardiac recovery and a healthy heart. The light at the end of the tunnel is glowing!

THE FIRST STEP:

Playing the Inner Game of Cardiac Recovery

*Anger is the cholesterol of the soul,
hostility is the saturated fat!*

CHAPTER 1

Getting the Psychological Advantage over Heart Disease

Which organ of your body do you suppose is most affected by heart disease? It's not your heart, or your coronary arteries, or any other part of the cardiovascular system. The organ most likely to affect your life and to determine the success of your recovery and ultimate return to vibrant good health is that bit of gray matter between your ears.

Most of the disability patients experience comes from anxiety, depression, and distress. Those problems are the rule, not the exception, so don't feel that you're all alone out there. In fact, anxiety and distress are virtually universal. Young or old, rich or poor, educated or not, male or female, we all go through a period of mental disturbance.

When patients suffer from other kinds of illnesses and disease, even those which are life-threatening, they typically get involved in the battle against the disease. This helps them to remain in control. Not so with a heart attack, which is most often followed by feelings of helplessness.

The psychological toll of a heart attack, or other events including surgery, cannot and should not be overestimated. According to Dr. Paul Thompson, medical director of cardiac rehabilitation at Brown University, "Even among patients who outwardly function well and appear to do just fine, they too may have a lot of psychological problems."

In two reports of the *Journal of Psychosomatic Research*, 23 percent of

21

post-heart attack patients showed mild psychological distress and 30 percent had moderate and severe symptoms, with depression and anxiety being the most common. Worse yet, researchers noted little change in these statistics even a year after the heart attack.

Dr. Thompson notes that in his own practice a large number of the men and women he sees report sleeping problems once they return home from the hospital. Many also go through a period of depression. The limitations on activity, chest pains, the family's overprotectiveness, fear of another attack, and the sick role in general are all new and discouraging experiences for previously well individuals.

"After a heart attack there is a lot of grief, a feeling of loss. It's as if a part of that person has died. They lose a part of their self-image," Dr. Thompson explains. He says that men are, in effect, emasculated by a heart attack. Physicians tell patients to be careful, to avoid arguments, and pretty soon wives won't even let their husbands sign any checks.

He says, "Look, if I tell you I'm going to help you live ten years longer, but I'm going to make you miserable and frightened for every one of those years, nobody would accept that. But all of us (physicians) who have not had heart attacks have neglected the quality of life issues with these patients."

I couldn't agree more. My own first experience in release from the hospital was a horror. I felt totally out of control, filled with fear, anger, anxiety, and an overriding feeling of depression. Of course that was many years ago. But for many people, things haven't changed. Even when patients receive a briefing before leaving the hospital, many if not most of their questions remain unanswered.

I've accompanied nurses and doctors on their rounds as patients were getting ready to return home. They seldom get down to practical issues such as sex and work. Instead, they typically give patients a few brochures and a photocopied list of do's and don'ts.

It's no wonder patients and their spouses have a lot of fear. And fear leads to unwarranted anxiety and distress. If the doctor didn't feel a patient was perfectly capable of living quite well at home, with no particular danger, he or she simply wouldn't be released. Moreover, no doctor expects spouses to be qualified 24-hour nurses.

Most patients are remarkably capable of a wide range of activities, right from the start. Unless there are particular complications to be considered, the majority of men and women can carry on without fear of relapse. Probably 80 percent can expect a completely uneventful recovery, perhaps even more.

Yes, there are patients who have suffered irreparable damage to the heart muscle and will have a degree of debilitation. Most don't. Talk turkey with your doctor. If he or she tells you that your case is uncomplicated, you really have nothing to fear. And, in all cases, listen to your physician's recommendations.

For most of us, successful recovery will hinge more on how much you do rather than how little. As we'll see in chapter 7, most patients could have sex the very day they return home. And they can enter a program of physical activity from the very beginning. That's particularly true for surgery patients.

If nothing is done to curtail fears, they'll continue for years. Los Angeles psychologist Herb Budnick has spent 12 years specializing in counseling patients with heart disease. "When I was growing up, my dad suffered four heart attacks," he recalls. "That was back in the '50s when treatment was a lot different. He was laid up by that first heart attack for about a year. I watched a really nice guy turn into one big bundle of anger which generally got more directed toward my mother. He eventually just isolated himself emotionally. He died of his fourth attack when I was 15."

Today almost all people experience many of the same things Dr. Budnick's father went through after a heart attack. He says most people could benefit from some basic insights into how to cope with this traumatic period of recovery.

"That's where cardiac rehabilitation comes in handy," Dr. Peterson at Brown says, "because it lets you know you're not going to die. It lets you know you can exert yourself and the quicker you do the better." We're going to get into the details of a solid cardiac rehabilitation program in the coming chapters.

But to make the most of cardiac rehabilitation, and to ensure the success of other lifestyle modifications which can result in long-term health for your heart, you must first come to grips with the psychological distress that's keeping you in a vise-like grasp. Dr. Budnick points out that "when people become emotionally overwrought they begin to feel overwhelmed and helpless. That leads to hopelessness. Life after heart problems can be rich and fulfilling, but only if the patient and his family take the steps needed to assure that recovery includes treatment of both the mind and body."

Psychological recovery from a cardiac event is more a family matter than strictly an individual one. A spouse's notions about the patient's physical capabilities can either assist or impede the recovery process.

Even in low-risk patients whose potential for recovery is greatest, medically unwarranted fears and concerns from the spouse may seriously impede functional recovery.

In a hospital-based cardiac rehabilitation program, wives were invited to take a walk on the treadmill at the same level of exertion their husbands were doing. They were amazed at just how much physical ability their spouses actually had. So much so that they stopped treating their men like fragile china dolls.

DEALING WITH PSYCHOLOGICAL SYMPTOMS

What are we really talking about when we use terms like anxiety and depression? While most of us experience distinct psychological distress, patients don't "go crazy" in any way. In fact, when given standard psychological tests to measure behavior, they are diagnosed as normal. That is to say, the symptoms associated with heart problems are not in the realm of illness. Rather, we're talking about distress. After heart attack, bypass, angioplasty, valve replacement, or a physician's diagnosis of existing heart disease, we're placed in a state of mental unrest, of unease. Let's look at some parallels.

Remember back when you were a student and had an exam coming up. You were anxious, and that anxiety was normal. If you didn't do very well on the exam, you became depressed. But neither that anxiety nor depression was expected to last. Only rarely do students enter a malignant state of mental disorder. They go on and eventually get their degree or diploma.

The important thing to remember is that the kind of anxiety and distress associated with heart events should be temporary. I sincerely believe that overcoming those psychological states quickly can facilitate recovery and speed us along the path toward good health and well being. You *know* you're going to get better.

Here's an interesting statistic on the power of knowledge. In a study looking at altering preoperative anxiety and assisting postoperative recovery, researchers at the University of Wisconsin found that bypass patients who failed to read an educational booklet on the surgery were in the intensive care unit (ICU) approximately two days longer than those who did read it. Patients who read the material had lower post-operative anxiety scores and they experienced a faster recovery. Other studies similarly suggest that better informed patients recover more quickly. And that's what you want, right?

Certain characteristics appear in patients who become overly anxious and distressed. Here are some things to look out for.

* Low energy levels. Every task becomes monumental.
* Lack of interest in personal appearance and grooming.
* Changes in physical appearance, gait, and posture.
* Failure to make eye contact with others.
* Withdrawal from family and friends.
* Refusal to assume responsibility owing to feelings of powerlessness and worthlessness.
* Increased dependency on others.
* Trivialization of past accomplishments.
* Magnification of negative events; minimizing of positive ones.
* Resentment of those who are well.
* Refusal of rehabilitation efforts.
* Continued bad moods from day to day.
* Crying spells.
* Intense guilt.

One must deal with psychological distress before the very things that can improve health can be effective. At the very outset, you, yourself, have to make the decision to go on to a healthy outlook and outcome. So how do you come to grips with the problems of denial, anxiety, distress, and depression?

DEALING WITH DENIAL

Many of us deny the very existence of a heart problem. We do that either directly or indirectly. Some people refuse to admit that their arteries are clogged even when shown their own angiograms. One man said that he would probably get a different opinion if he showed the pictures to other physicians; he turned down the opportunity to do so, however.

Other patients, rather like whistling in a cemetery, say there never was a heart attack in the first place. Those symptoms must have been something else, since they feel perfectly fine later on. Of course, the longer the time lag after the heart attack or surgery, the more likely that kind of denial will make sense to the patient, as recovery takes place naturally.

Can you imagine denying the problem in other situations or diseases? Picture a man being bitten by a rattlesnake saying, "Oh, it probably was just a little garter snake. I really don't need treatment." Or the woman who has accidentally swallowed poison saying, "Come on now, that was just soda pop. Why should I take an antidote?"

Those who deny they have heart disease are unlikely to adopt the long-term strategies that will enable them to remain well. I suppose I was one of those deniers, but of a different stripe. I was fully aware that I had heart disease, and never denied the fact. But I denied that I had to do anything about it. Yet as much as I denied the reality in terms of preventive behavior, I remained virtually paralyzed, fearing the next heart attack.

It's time to accept and overcome!

"Ah," it's been said so often, "if I only had known then what I know today." Things, perhaps, would have been different. Maybe I wouldn't have needed that second bypass. But that's water under the bridge. There's no point in dwelling on what might have been. All of us have to learn to let go of the past and go on to the future. That's never been more true than in the case of heart disease.

Without having to be a mind reader, I can tell you that right now you'd like to somehow turn the clock back, to the time before the heart attack or before the bypass. You'd like to live the way you lived before heart disease entered your life. Right? Of course that's right, because virtually everyone has those same thoughts.

But let me ask you this: Was life really that terrific before heart disease? Were you living every day to its fullest, thinking about the present moment? Or were you really living without thinking much about it at all, always saying that you'd get around to this or that tomorrow or next year? You need to forget about that way of thinking and focus on the present. Live for today.

OVERCOMING ANXIETY AND DISTRESS

Certainly you're having some bad times right now and it may be almost comforting to deny the reality of heart disease and the impact it has had and will have on your life. Yet the best way to deal with almost anything is to get on with your life rather than to avoid it.

You must have had some other experiences in the past. When you think about them, they all had one thing in common: they all passed. No matter how horrible something appears to be at the moment, the tincture of time heals all wounds.

What were some of your most dreadful incidents? The loss of a job? A divorce? A financial setback? None of these things simply "went away." You didn't wish them out of your life or deny their reality. You took action. The same must apply to heart disease.

The Chinese have a wonderful saying, that a journey of a thousand miles begins with a single step. If you're a lawyer, think how hard you worked to get that law degree and how long it took to achieve your goal. But you did it. One day at a time, one examination at a time, one course at a time. The same can be said for virtually any accomplishment. Recovery from heart disease will be your next major achievement, and, as is true with all landmark accomplishments, it will change your life for the better.

The first step for you to take is to accept that heart disease can be completely controlled in the vast majority of cases. No, it cannot be cured in the sense of curing pneumonia or mending a broken bone. It is more like one's efforts to control alcoholism. The disease will always be there, ready to become acute again if the person falters in his or her resolve, but it can be controlled and kept from doing further damage for the rest of one's life. And, in many cases, as we'll see, heart disease can be reversed. I did it, and you can too.

LOOK TO THE FUTURE

The next step in coming to psychological grips with this disease is to ask yourself what you really want. Of course, you say, you want the disease to simply go away. But what does that mean? Is what you want a return to the past, a return to the dissipating habits that led to the problems, such as cigarette smoking, poor eating habits, and a wanton disregard for your health? Or is what you *really* want a chance to live a marvelously healthy life in which you wake up each day ready for the challenges and opportunities that come your way? If that's what you want, and you're willing to work for it, you've got it!

You can't get hung up on negatives along the way. This is the time to get the word "can't" out of your vocabulary. Here we come to the philosophical difference between those who view the glass as half full as opposed to half empty. Don't say "I can't smoke cigarettes anymore." Instead, say "It's about time I got rid of that habit as I've been meaning to do for years." Don't say "I can't have the steak and bearnaise sauce on the menu." Instead say "I really enjoy salmon (or pasta, or crab legs, or roast chicken) and I feel so much better after eating a lighter meal."

At first you might just mean those words half-heartedly. As time goes on, you'll come to believe them with all your heart. And your heart will thank you for it.

It will take time to achieve every step on the way to recovery. Go with the flow, knowing that there will be some tough times along the way. Don't try too hard or attempt to rush the process. If you were in a cast with a broken leg, you'd know it would take a long time for the bone to mend and then a longer time for physical rehabilitation.

Every illness and injury has its own peculiar and particular way of healing, with unique pains and problems. Heart disease is no different. Sure, you're going to feel tired. You'll get exhausted from doing things that you never even thought about before. Like taking a shower. Or doing some small task around the house. The natural reaction is to get distressed, even angry, about yourself.

Depression is really nothing more than an extreme case of destructive self-absorption. Everyone feels sorry for himself now and then. That's natural. But it's self-defeating to dwell on the negative.

When we are feeling depressed, life seems to be so complex that it defies simple solutions. We can all make our lives seem more or less complex by the way we view our situation. That's our choice. Break down any complex problem, though, and you have simple, or at least simpler, problems that can be handled one at a time.

GET MOVING!

The worst part of depression is that it tends to feed upon itself and grow out of control. The more we think about whatever it is that's making us depressed, the more depressed we get. The solution is to take action, any action, to get yourself moving.

But it's not always so easy to get moving. Your mind starts to play tricks on you. You come up with a long, circuitous thinking process that convinces you that no movement is possible. "I can't do this because . . ." "I can't do that because . . ." The solution is to *just do it.*

Consider a new way of looking at your life. Psychologists call it "values clarification." As usual, they make it sound a lot more complicated than it actually is. Here's the bottom line: What's really important to you? What do you really enjoy in life?

Your assignment for today is to make a list of all the things that are important in your life and the things you enjoy doing. You might want to rank them according to priority. Then take a look at your list. You'll probably come up with some surprises, as most people do.

My own list included fishing and golf. But when I asked myself when I had last done either of those, I began to wonder whether fishing and golf really were important to me or whether I'd allowed other things to get in the way. The latter was true. I'd guess that making your boss happy is *not* on your list. Yet you probably spend much more time and effort trying to make your boss happy than you do your spouse and children. Sure, your job or career is important to you and, in the best of worlds, is also enjoyable. But have you allowed it to dominate your life?

Examine your own list and ask yourself whether you've really been living in close accord with your priorities. That's the clarification part of it. If the answer is no, it's time to put things into proper perspective. Some of the things on your list might have to wait awhile, maybe even a long while. You're not going to be up to climbing Mt. Everest in the next month or two. On the other hand, you can start making some definite plans as to how you're going to spend the rest of your life.

That gets us back to the notion of movement. The best way to get rid of momentary depression is to do something, anything, to get moving. Do something you've wanted to do but never had time to do. Maybe you'd like to read a history book (rather than business journals), or do some painting or sculpting, or write some letters, or perhaps sort out those boxes of photographs that tend to pile up in everyone's closet. When you start feeling blue, pick up one of those things and do it. You may even have to force yourself to get started, but once you're into it, you'll soon lose the blues. Sound simplistic? Just try it.

Take another look at your list of priorities. Have you written down smoking two packs of cigarettes a day, or eating high-fat foods, or watching hours of television, or getting into stressful situations? Probably not. And yet an analysis of your behavior might lead an objective observer to conclude that those are the most important things in your life.

It's time to get a clearer vision of life's pleasures and the prices one has to pay for them. Currently you're feeling sorry for yourself. You therefore want to give yourself some comfort and so you say "I deserve a big dish of ice cream." That kind of thinking is obviously destructive. Moreover, momentary pleasures never give one a true sense of satisfaction. Think about it. You keep on indulging, chasing after satisfaction, until guilt instead sets in.

A man with heart disease who continues to smoke cigarettes is saying unequivocally that tobacco means more to him than his family, his career, his hobbies or sports, the sunrise and sunset, and everything else in life. Because that behavior will, very certainly, end his life.

SHAPE YOUR OWN DESTINY

Now that you have a lot of time on your hands, use some of it to put your life into proper perspective. Let me share with you an insight I gained in reading a wonderful book, *Rapid Relief From Emotional Distress*, by Drs. Gary Emery and James Campbell. They put the whole matter into a clear perspective in what they call the ACT formula. One, you

Accept the present reality. In this case, it is the fact that you have heart disease. Two, you choose to *Create your own vision* for your life. Here it's a matter of the ultimate goal of vibrant good health. And three, you *Take action* to make that vision a reality.

The ACT formula is but one expression of the approach many psychologists agree is particularly effective in dealing with health issues such as heart disease. They call this method "cognitive therapy." It simply means that you critically analyze your situation, think about your options, and do something about it.

Once you accept the challenge to defeat heart disease, to realize that new vision of yourself, let nothing stand in your way. Knock down the barriers that could keep you from achieving your goal, much as a runner fights the wind and rain, ignoring everything but the final goal.

BECOMING OPTIMISTIC

You have the ability to succeed. But will you? There are optimists and pessimists in the world. Which are you? For some people, optimism comes naturally. I love the story about the two boys who are brought into separate rooms to receive their birthday gifts. One boy sees a room filled with toys and games, but simply sits in a corner with a frown on his face. Asked why, he explains that there's no use in getting excited about the toys, since someone will probably take them away. Told that, no, they're really his, the boy still is glum, saying he probably wouldn't have fun anyway, and maybe he'd hurt himself. The other boy enters another room and finds it filled with horse manure. Immediately his face breaks into a broad smile. Why? "There must be a pony in here someplace!"

Which boy are you more like? Even if you're naturally pessimistic, you can work at being more optimistic. In a very real way, you can "psych" yourself into a more positive way of thinking. Virtually any doctor will agree that the patients who fully recover are those who believe they will from the very start. There are a few steps you can take to start you off on a lifetime of optimistic outlook.

Optimism will not just come to you overnight, and it won't become a trait without some definite effort on your part. Like virtually every good habit, becoming optimistic requires a commitment. Promise yourself that from this very moment you will try to view things in the most positive light.

Start listening to your own train of thought as you run things through your mind. You'll probably hear quite a few negatives. Start substituting some positives.

Remember back to your school days again. If an exam was coming up, you had two ways to view it. First you could have told yourself that if you flunked the exam you'd be kicked out of the program. That's pretty negative. Or you could have thought in a very positive sense about what it would be like to succeed in your field, to work on the kinds of projects that would inspire you and live the lifestyle to which you aspired. Going into that exam with that positive outlook would certainly provide a big advantage.

By all means don't put off your good intentions until tomorrow. Start today. Get rid of those high-fat foods in the kitchen and replace them with heart-healthy alternatives. Accept no excuse to not exercise. Take some time to relax. All the while, keep that vision of your healthy self clearly in mind.

There's a fine line between love and hate, and sometimes we can't see the distinction. Currently you're filled with a lot of hate, a lot of very negative mental energy. You hate your heart disease, you hate the scar if you had bypass surgery, you hate the events or persons you believe may have precipitated the event. Cross the line and replace that hate with love, love of yourself. Don't *you* deserve more attention than the disease you fully intend to get rid of?

Today you have a more distinct fear of death than you ever had before. Ironically, you wonder if it wouldn't have been easier if you *had* died. Well, yes, it would have been easier. But our survival instinct is stronger than any other drive. You always knew you were going to die. Today you simply have a greater sense of your own mortality—far more so than others, because you came so close to the edge. You can put this to your advantage. You can take the opportunity to recover and to get healthy. I certainly don't want you to start thinking about death and dying all the time. That's morbid. Instead think in a positive way about the joys of living. What are the things you enjoyed today and this week? A visit from your children or grandchildren? A videotaped movie that you've been putting off until now? Watching the rain fall or the sun set or the clouds drift by?

Don't be afraid of death. After all, if you die you'll either go to your reward or you'll cease to think and exist. The far greater fear, I think, should be the thought of a compromised life. The notion of living as a cardiac cripple, to my way of thinking, is about as horrible as it gets. I've lived that way. I know what it's like to be totally out of control, with the Sword of Damocles hovering over my head.

You have the ability to respond. That means you have the ability to get better. To coin a use of the word, you have the ability to get "best." Give it a chance. I'll bet that if you give yourself that chance you won't even be tempted to go back to those old ways.

RECORDING YOUR PROGRESS

As I've said before, you can't rush it. Heart disease, like any other major injury or illness, takes time to control. Most authorities concur that full recovery takes up to a year. Unlike someone who's sustained major injuries, let's say in an auto accident, you're not going to lie in a hospital bed for months and months. You'll get better day by day. You're getting better even as you read these pages. Within a very short period of time you'll be back to work, playing golf, going out to movies and to dinner, and doing everything that makes your life worth living. And, assuming you follow the steps to recovery in this book, you'll enjoy those things more than you ever have before. But it all happens so gradually that you don't notice the day-by-day differences and improvements.

That's why I'd like you to start keeping a journal of your progress. This is one of the best ways possible to show yourself how well you're doing, and just how far you've really come along in a relatively short period of time.

Buy a spiral-ring binder with at least 150 lined pages. Set aside a few minutes daily to make your entries, no matter whether you're feeling good, bad, or indifferent. As time goes on, you'll be extremely happy you took the time to do this. And you'll also need the journal to keep track of all the steps in my recovery program. Here are the items to be recorded daily.

Date and Day. Be sure to include the day of the week as well as the date. Then you'll be able to compare one Thursday with another; you may find you feel different on Mondays, for example, than you do on

Fridays. That bit of information in itself may help you to determine what it was that made the difference. It also will help you plan your week's activities.

Exercise. We'll get into a lot more detail on this in the coming chapters on cardiac rehabilitation and physical activity. But even now you'll want to note how much you're doing. Record not only the formal exercise periods at the hospital, but also your daily walks and other strenuous activity. Be as specific as you can, so you can compare details in the weeks and months to come.

Be sure to include a subjective evaluation of your activity as well. Note whether you were tired or exhilarated after your walk. Did you need to nap afterward? Did it feel particularly good that day? Did you dread your walk at the beginning and then come to enjoy it by the end?

Diet. Most people eat and drink without giving it much thought. Your journal can help you realize just how much you're eating. Moreover, it will help you see how you can make some substitutions to make the transition from a high-fat, artery-clogging diet to a heart-healthy one.

In the coming weeks please keep track of literally everything you eat and drink. List even the glasses of water and cups of coffee you drink. If you eat away from home, jot down what you had when you return.

You'll have to take my word for it: This will make things *much* easier for you. The more detailed you make this part of your journal, the better you will succeed, and you'll be amazed at how rapid your progress will be.

Most people find that they lose weight as they cut back on fat. At least once a week, mark your weight in your journal. This will be a satisfying "fringe benefit" of your efforts.

As you get into the chapter on dietary modification, you will want to make this part of your log more detailed. But don't put it off until then. Start today.

Smoking. Did you quit long ago? If so, enter a remembrance of how you did it, how long it took to be completely free of the cravings, and how you feel now. This will remind you that you can very effectively change your behavior.

If you just quit following your heart attack or bypass, record your daily feelings. You're not completely out of the woods yet, and your cravings will come and go. The important thing to remember is that those cravings will diminish in intensity and will come less frequently as time goes on.

Still smoking? I completely understand. Those cigarettes seem to be your link to a more desirable past. You know you should quit, but it's tough. And hearing everyone around you nagging doesn't help a bit. You probably are smoking less, though, than you did before. Record your feelings, and list the cigarettes you smoke through the day. We'll get into more detail as to how to help you get rid of nicotine in chapter 12.

Feelings. Especially during the first couple of months following your heart attack or bypass, this should be the section of your journal you'll want to write in the most. You have an enormous jumble of feelings right now. It's a mixture of denial that this ever happened to you, anger that it did, anxiety that it might happen again, and depression that a part of you has died and that it seems life will never be the same again. That's all very natural, and it happens to all of us. The only really important thing to realize right now is that these feelings will pass, as long as you take some steps to get yourself through these tough times.

Record your feelings in whatever detail you wish, but don't turn your journal into a voluminous tome. If you do want to really purge your soul, do so in a separate diary. That could, indeed, be very valuable for you. But the purpose of this particular journal is to give an overview of your day-to-day progress.

Assign a ratings system of one to ten, with ten noting the most intense feelings. Then, on a daily basis, rate your feelings in terms of anger, depression, anxiety, sadness, and hostility. Very briefly state the situation that may have precipitated the feelings, or note if they simply came out of the blue.

Don't fail to record any of your feelings in your journal. Each situation is important.

Medications. If you're like most of us, right now you're keeping track of more different medicines than you've taken in the past few years put together. In many cases, those medicines will only be temporary and soon you won't have so many to worry about.

But medications pose a number of questions for patients. You may wonder whether it's this pill or that tablet that's making you tired, or causing you to lose your appetite, or what have you. Use your journal to record your reactions to your medications, so that you can discuss them with your doctor.

Symptoms. Let's face it, you've gone through a major, life-threatening event. It's not all over yet. You're going to have some aches, pains, and symptoms. Use your journal to keep track of them. You'll accomplish two things. First, it's a good way to discuss the matters with your physician; you'll be able to report with precision and accuracy how often you felt that way, what the circumstances were, and how severe the feelings were. Second, you'll start to see rather quickly that your symptoms are diminishing.

That brings us back to the purpose of this journal keeping in the long run. Even after a week, you can look back at those pages and start to see your progress. Moreover, as we go through your steps to recovery, the journal will become an integral tool.

Recalling that Chinese proverb, you're taking that first step in the journey of a thousand miles. Many others have walked that path before you and have succeeded in reaching their goal. I'll share many of their stories with you as we go along. Very soon you will be added to the list of those voyagers to good health.

CHAPTER 2

Stressed to the Breaking Point: The Mental Link to Heart Disease

S tress. The very word is enough to make the muscles tighten and the jaws clench. Most of us who have had a heart attack can point to mental conditions which we believe precipitated the event. As much as cholesterol, the term Type-A behavior has come to be a household word. While the whole issue of a direct link between mental stress and heart disease has been hotly debated in medical and scientific circles, no one doubts that where there's smoke there's likely to be fire.

Actually, interest in the emotional factors supposedly associated with health and disease is nothing new. For about three centuries, those who have forged medical history have thought, taught, and written about the ties between emotional well-being and health. Hippocrates told his students that state of mind influenced state of health. In the 1920s and 1930s it was popular to link emotions with illness. High blood pressure, also termed hypertension, it was said, resulted from suppressing anger.

With the advent of the hard-nosed scientific method, ideas about anything other than the purely physical were given short shrift. Then, starting in the 1960s and getting more attention in the 1970s, Drs. Meyer Friedman and Ray H. Rosenman put forth the idea that the individual with the Type-A behavior was prone to coronary disease. Their book, *Type-A Behavior and Your Heart,* became a best-seller. It was soon fashionable, even in certain medical circles, to believe this personality trait was as important as other major risk factors in heart disease. The dairy industry, among others, spent a lot of money promoting this view, hoping it would obscure the role of cholesterol in the diet.

Friedman and Rosenman described the Type-A personality as a syndrome with three predominating characteristics. First was a sense of time urgency. Time schedules, appointments, and deadlines were ever-present considerations for the Type-A man or woman. Second was an extreme degree of competitiveness. Winning wasn't everything, it was the *only* thing. Third, these people were quick to get angry and displayed openly hostile and aggressive feelings.

Dr. Friedman believed from the very start that the best way to identify Type-A, coronary-prone patients was to spend a little time in a one-on-one interview. Their eyes darted around the room, fingers drummed on the table, knees jerked nervously, and they were quick to finish a sentence for you or to fill in a word you couldn't come up with right off the bat. As you spoke, they didn't really listen; rather they'd be formulating their responses.

But subjective evaluations were difficult to quantify in research, and the National Institutes of Health were starting to show interest in funding major projects to demonstrate the actual role Type-A behavior played in heart disease. So researchers needed a way to measure personality uniformly. Two methods were developed. One was the Jenkins Activity Survey, basically a self-assessment approach with paper and pencil. The other was a structured interview conducted by a trained individual. Results of various studies have been defended or attacked in the research community, depending on the kind of assessment used.

Throughout all of this, cardiologists in general paid little or no attention to the theory. Most of the research was done by people with Ph.D. degrees in psychology and social sciences, whereas physicians often don't trust the work of those without medical degrees. They tend to scoff at data that cannot be measured in the blood or seen under a microscope.

To make matters worse, studies in different research centers came up with radically opposite conclusions. Certainly this was an area of controversy in that one could very well argue either side of the debate, armed with seemingly ironclad scientific data.

Regardless of arguments, however, there appears to be far more than a coincidental association between personality and heart attacks and death. A major, often quoted, project from the 1970s called the Western Collaborative Group Study had shown that Type-A patients had double the chances of coronary disease when compared to their easier-going, Type-B counterparts. Moreover, Type A patients were more likely to suffer more than one heart attack.

Other convincing evidence came from studies of risk factors in patients having an angiogram. Three separate research groups found that patients with Type-A behavior had more extensive coronary artery disease; two of those studies showed that the relationship was clear even when one considered the effects of other risk factors such as cigarette smoking.

Virtually everyone experiences a certain amount of stress, almost from birth, and even in the most primitive societies. It would be practically impossible to earn a university degree without the stress of taking an examination. One could hardly win a race without pre-competition jitters. And no teenager has ever asked for a special date without heart pounding. But, largely owing to societal influences, stress becomes uncontrollable for many people.

When the student has taken his examination, or the athlete has run his race, or the teenager's invitation for a date has been accepted, the stress quickly diminishes. One has time to recover, perhaps to get ready for the next mental challenge. But what happens when stress is unrelenting, when there's no time to recuperate, and when the individual loses all control over circumstances and over his or her emotions?

As Rod Serling would say in introducing the evening's episode of the Twilight Zone: "Imagine if you will," . . . John Public is roused by a jangling alarm clock from a fitful sleep in which he was dreaming about his mortgage and unpaid bills. He turns on the radio to hear that traffic is building up on the interstate highway he travels to work. Having rushed through his shower, John cuts himself shaving while hearing his wife Joan yelling at the kids. Arriving at work, he finds that an extra meeting has been scheduled, his boss is angry that he's ten minutes late, and a pile of mail and telephone messages is thrust in his hand by the secretary even before John can put down his attaché case. The day at the office is a series of crises with a liberal sprinkling of internal politics. Lunch and coffee breaks are devoted to a continuation of work discussions, laced with colleagues' complaints about this and that. Arriving home, he learns that the washing machine has broken down, one of the kids is flunking in school, and the other is dating someone best described as a Hell's Angel. There was no time to prepare dinner, and the decision is whether to order sausage or pepperoni on the pizza. John's mother calls and can't understand why he's not happy to hear from her, since he never bothers to telephone. Two martinis later the pizza arrives, and

John washes it down with a couple of beers while watching television. Exhausted from the day, he never leaves the couch. Yet when it's time for bed, John has difficulty falling asleep and finally resorts to a pill that leads to another drug-forced unconsciousness, which ends as the alarm signals another day just like the one that preceded it. The Twilight Zone? No, for far too many Johns and Joans in the world, this is Reality. John will quickly point to his lifestyle as responsible for his heart attack when it happens.

Many men and women live just as hectic a lifestyle and they do not have the heart attack. Why then do some suffer an attack? Certainly other risk factors besides stress must be taken into consideration. Those pizzas are loaded with saturated fat; lack of exercise is considered an independent hazard. John in our scenario might have had hypertension along with a family history of heart disease. But even so, a number of studies have shown an indisputable link with the stress in life, especially for the driven, Type-A individual, and heart disease. For years we seemed to have been overlooking some sort of missing element.

It now appears that rather than having something missing, researchers were looking at too much. The net, as it were, was made with too small a gauge, thus too many individuals were clumped together. The broad listing of personality traits that made up the Type-A syndrome included patients who were not at all at risk.

This makes logical sense, remembering that one of the criticisms of the Type-A theory was that virtually everyone who is at all successful has a high degree of competitiveness. Dr. Redford Williams, a professor of psychiatry at Duke University, concludes that of all the aspects originally described as making up the Type-A syndrome, only those related to hostility and anger make one prone to coronary disease. He has also pointed to recent laboratory research of biological characteristics of hostile Type-A persons that may account for their increased risk of developing coronary disease.

You may wish to make a more comprehensive examination of Dr. Williams' work in his 1989 book *The Trusting Heart: Great News About Type A Behavior.* In the meantime, you'll be interested in an overview of his work.

In 1980 Dr. Williams published a paper showing that high scores on a hostility scale from a psychological test widely used by psychologists related more closely than Type-A behavior itself to severity of arteriosclerotic blockages in the coronary arteries of patients being treated at Duke. The test used was the Minnesota Multiphasic Personality Inventory (MMPI), which is often used by corporations in making employment decisions. One particular trait the test measures very well is hostility, scored on the so-called "Ho" scale.

The "Ho" scores were very accurate in predicting increased coronary disease rates, as well as death from all causes. The more hostile men and women were, the more likely they were to have heart disease. Dr. Williams tested a group of 255 male doctors and 1,877 employees of a large Chicago industrial firm. The doctors had taken the MMPI test while in medical school. Over a 25-year period, 14 percent of those with a high "Ho" score had died. This compares with a mortality rate of only two percent for those with low "Ho" scores. Almost incredibly, those displaying anger and hostility were seven times more likely to die than their more relaxed counterparts. The Chicago participants showed a similar tendency.

In his most recent study, Dr. Williams followed a group of 118 lawyers who had taken the MMPI while in law school 25 years earlier. Those with high "Ho" scores had died at a rate 4.2 times higher than that of lawyers with a lower score.

Then Dr. Williams began to dig deeper into the data to determine which specific traits were the best predictors. He found that men displaying a cynical mistrust regarding the motives of people in general, who frequently experience anger, and who openly express their anger toward others are most likely to die. The questions reflecting those anger-prone characteristics accounted for only half of the 50 questions on the "Ho" scale. But they reflected virtually all of the increased mortality associated with high "Ho" scores. Men with high scores on the questions depicting these traits had a 25-year death rate 5.5 times higher than those with low scores. The same conclusions hold true when one reviews the hostility/anger components of a structured interview intended to identify the classic syndrome of Type-A behavior. Only those involving anger and hostility independently predict increased coronary disease rates.

If you're the kind of person who asks hard questions, you might now be wondering what in the world one's personality has to do with dying of heart disease or other causes? How does the psychology influence the physiology?

When persons with high "Ho" scores are placed in experiments that bring out their mistrust of others and that anger them, they show larger blood pressure responses than those with low "Ho" scores. In Dr. Williams' research at Duke, when patients were harassed while performing a mental task, men with high "Ho" scores displayed much larger blood pressure increases than those with low scores. The anger and irritation brought on by the harassment leads to larger blood pressure reactions, but only in the more hostile patients.

How does that relate to real-life situations? Think about your own life. The list of factors that cause stress can be almost endless, and any of the factors is likely to elicit an angry, hostile response. In the past, researchers believed the link was time urgency and competitiveness. In reality, it's not so much a matter of time, but rather of becoming more than mildly annoyed.

When Dr. Meyer Friedman tried to work with Type-A individuals, hoping to slow them down to a Type-B pace, he told them to read the complete work of Proust. Even English teachers might find that chore to be more than a little boring. Imagine the reaction of highly driven executives! They rebelled, not so much because they resented the time it took to read the books, but because they perceived the assignment as senseless, totally meaningless in their lives. Dr. Friedman no longer makes the assignment.

When the hostility and anger components of a patient's personality are brought into play, the patient displays a number of biological reactions. The body's chemistry actually changes. And those chemical reactions can damage the heart and its vessels.

I spoke earlier of the effects of mental tasks and the stress they can invoke. Dr. Alan Rozanski, formerly at the University of California at Los Angeles, now at St. Luke's Roosevelt Center in New York, studied the cause-and-effect relation between acute mental stress and oxygen insufficiency to the heart. He evaluated cardiac function in patients given a series of mental tasks including arithmetic, simulated public speaking, and reading.

Of the patients with heart disease, 59 percent had distinct cardiac abnormalities on an electrocardiogram when given stress-inducing tasks. Nearly half of the patients experienced no symptoms. Cardiac dysfunction brought on by public speaking was similar to that induced by exercise.

We've all experienced the unpleasant physical reactions to pressure situations. We feel sweaty palms, beating heart, and sometimes even light-headedness. As Dr. Rozanski showed, mental stress can also have significant effects on how well our hearts function.

If normal mental stress puts Type-As in danger, imagine what happens when one deliberately invokes anger and hostility. When New York researcher Dr. David Glass asked Type-As and Type-Bs to play a video game, both groups showed similar patterns of increased reactions as long as the opponent kept quiet. But when he began to irritate them with comments such as "Can't you keep your eye on the ball" and "Christ, you're not even trying," the Type-As' heart rate, blood pressure, and levels of adrenaline all went up higher than those in Type-Bs.

Adrenaline, also termed epinephrine, is the hormone produced by stimulation of the sympathetic nervous system. We know the unpleasant sensations it can evoke, such as trembling hands and irritability. But what about long-term effects? Adrenaline releases fats into the blood which may end up in the plaques that block the coronary arteries. Another hormone, noradrenaline, also causes blood platelets to clump together, increasing the chance of a blood clot which could precipitate a heart attack. Moreover, noradrenaline passes the signal from the sympathetic nervous system for the heart muscle to contract. In normal circumstances, this maintains a normal heart rhythm. But when released in large quantities, as is the case in hostile encounters, noradrenaline can lead to heart rhythm disturbances which can be at the least uncomfortable and at the worst fatal.

The link between stress and cholesterol levels in the blood has been well documented. Two classic studies provide the evidence. In one, cholesterol levels of accountants were measured before and after the April 15 tax deadline. In the other, medical students' levels were tested before and after a major examination. In both cases, cholesterol levels rose before and fell after the deadlines.

Just how dramatically stress can affect the heart was reported by Dr. Williams in the *New England Journal of Medicine*. His report involved the case of Mary Smith, who nearly died after experiencing profound emotional arousal. The patient had felt a "severe, crushing pain" with radiation to the left shoulder after learning that her 17-year-old son had committed suicide. Rushed to a major medical center in Boston, she was given extensive tests, all of which showed her heart to be normal. Yet there was heart damage as shown by the elevation of enzymes in the blood. No blood clot could be detected, and her arteries appeared to be free of blockage. Further tests showed inflammation of the heart muscle itself, which responded to drug therapy. Attending physicians concluded that the event was, indeed, precipitated by the tragic news of her son's death.

Dr. Larry Scherwitz, a psychologist at the San Francisco campus of the University of California, confirmed his hypothesis that Type-A individuals who are most prone to heart disease are those who become totally self-absorbed. Listen for the use of the pronouns "I," "my," "me," and "mine." Such individuals, says Dr. Scherwitz, are twice as likely to have heart attacks.

Conversely, Dr. Kenneth Pelletier finds that those showing a deeper spiritual dimension, believing in a higher power, have significant protection from heart disease. The psychologist, also at the University of California, studied corporate executives and found that those with spiritual beliefs experienced fewer cardiac events than those without such support.

There seems to be little doubt that there is a psychological component to heart disease. Dr. Arna Munford, at Cedars-Sinai Hospital in Los Angeles, has worked to determine the effects of rehabilitating those debilitating traits. She believes that it is just a matter of time before the psychological elements will receive as much "credit" for heart disease as elevated cholesterol levels and hypertension.

There is an increasing consensus that the angry, hostile Type-A individual is more likely to have a heart attack. But what can make an individual more angry and more hostile than the reality of having that heart attack? Think about it yourself, you're now experiencing a great deal of anger and hostility. You're blaming anything and everything for your attack, lashing out mentally in every direction. You'll not be pleased to hear, then, that those exhibiting the traits of anger and hostility are far more likely to have another heart attack and that their chances of survival are far less than those of calmer Type-Bs who manage to accept heart disease and go on to control it.

But how can one change one's emotional responses? Moreover, do you really want to change? You can be sure that those around you would welcome the change, not only to ensure your greater odds of survival but also so that they can enjoy your company more.

The important thing to remember here is that one does not have to go from being a classic Type-A to the serene, becalmed image of the Type-B. You can still expect to be competitive in your business dealings. You can still seek to be punctual in your meetings. You can still be driven to achieve your goals, whatever they might be.

I must put in my own personal endorsement at this point. I've always been a Type-A. Anyone who's ever known me can attest to that fact. Most of those traits haven't changed since the heart attack and two bypass surgeries. Actually, I've been working harder than I ever have in my life. I face deadlines for magazine articles. My schedule of media appearances and lectures around the world puts me at odds with airline schedules, hotel reservations, rude cab drivers, and on and on. It's all been quite unrelenting. Am I still a classic Type-A? You bet, and I'm proud of it, in typical Type-A fashion. But the difference is that I've learned to control my previous tendencies toward anger and hostility. I recognized those characteristics in myself, and I've worked at taking off the sharp edges. My angiogram has shown that I've been thriving on my current lifestyle. And believe me, I don't miss getting almost violently angry when things wouldn't go my way. I feel much better and sleep much more soundly these days.

But you needn't trust just one isolated and obviously biased opinion. The medical literature is crammed with success stories of how one's psychologically detrimental tendencies can be tempered. Real benefits have been derived.

Reporting in the *European Heart Journal,* researchers have found that relaxation therapy combined with exercise reduces the occurrence of both cardiac events and hospital readmissions in patients following heart attack. The investigators felt one reason was that patients who learned to relax were better able to cope with anginal pain. They also noted that patients with reduced Type-A behavior had a far lower recurrence rate than those whose behavior remained unchanged. They noted that individuals especially at risk for angina or those who might be candidates for bypass surgery are particularly suited for this combined effort.

Studies suggest that modifying Type-A behavior, and here we're really focusing on the anger/hostility components, is possible. And when it is modified, rates of future heart attacks are reduced. Dr. Meyer Friedman reported that 44 percent of nearly 600 patients studied had lower heart attack rates after three years during which they followed programs of behavior modification. After the three-year study, the experimental group had 7.2 percent occurrence of nonfatal heart attack; those getting only medical attention experienced a 13 percent rate of another heart attack. In another study, 900 patients were followed for 54 months after their heart attacks. Those receiving counseling to modify Type A behavior had a 2.5 percent rate of future heart attacks, while controls had a recurrence rate of more than 5 percent. Simply stated, one can cut one's risk of future heart attack in half by making an effort to change behavior.

Everyone is different and our problems and difficulties appear to be almost insurmountable at times. Before starting the next chapter, I'd like to give you an assignment. Make a list of all the things that really make you stressed out, angry and hostile, and just plain unhappy. Write down all that you can, and, as time goes on, expand the list as various events bring on a stressful reaction.

Then, at a time when you're really calm and relaxed, take a few moments to review your list. Look at those situations which are stressful and judge them as objectively as you possibly can. Next, think if there might not be a way to deal with them effectively.

Only you can assess your own situation and try to deal with it. Let me share with you one aspect of my personal assessment.

Before writing *The 8-Week Cholesterol Cure*, I made my living as a freelance medical writer and consultant. Many of my clients were in Orange County, which was a one-hour drive from my home in normal traffic. But, Southern California freeways being what they are, often there would be a snarl caused by construction, an accident, or a gawkers' block. Not having a car phone, I'd start to get white-knuckled on the steering wheel, concerned that I'd be late for my appointment. Being very time-conscious, this was a frequent source of anger and anxiety for me. Actually, I must admit that at the time I didn't realize the anger component: I was hostile at the idea that the traffic was keeping me from being relaxed and ready to do business at my appointment.

Next on my list of annoyances was the fact that I was never able to keep up with my reading of scientific, medical, and trade journals. It seemed that I was always behind. Again, this led to anger since I actually enjoyed the reading, but felt that "unseen forces" were somehow keeping me from it.

Looking at my own list of stressors, I realized that I could take those two lemons and make a nice batch of lemonade. From that moment on, I began putting a few magazines and journals into my attaché case and leaving 30 minutes early for all my appointments. If I hit a traffic delay, it wasn't a problem, since I had the extra half hour. If I encountered no traffic problems and arrived early, I'd use that time to sit and catch up on my reading. After a while, I wondered why I hadn't thought of this earlier. It made my life much more pleasant.

Another man I spoke with had a similar problem with L.A. traffic. He solved his anger by stocking his car with various tapes that he could listen to during those long drives and delays. He told me that having started this practice, he was actually sorry when trips went more quickly than anticipated and he was unable to listen to all his tapes.

Now that we're on the subject of traffic, let me tell you a great story about how one man dealt with the problem in New York City. Perhaps the most difficult thing to accomplish in Manhattan is to find a parking place. This man was a liquor salesman who had to carry samples, order forms, and all sorts of things. Carrying all that from a parking lot took a lot of time and made him mad as hell, because he knew he'd never get to all his stops for the day.

His solution not only got rid of his hostility but actually made him the top NYC salesman, the envy of his peers. He hired a limousine! That way he rode in style, felt good about himself, got to more appointments than any other salesman, delivered more goods, and very quickly made lots more money than the limo cost. Now that's creative stress management!

You're not going to be able to get rid of every stressful element in your life. But you can shoot for three approaches to management. First, reduce the number of stressful incidents. Only you can determine which ones on your list can be eliminated. I'm reminded of the story of the man who told his doctor, "It hurts when I do this." To which the physician replied, "Don't do that!" Simple but effective. If you can possibly walk away from stress, by all means do so. Second, reduce the intensity of those stressful episodes. If an encounter with an individual with whom you don't get along can't be avoided, you can at least limit the amount of time you must be exposed to him or her. Third, find ways to rest and relax between stressful incidents. We'll discuss some ways to ease stress in the next chapter. The important thing is to not go from one stress right into another one without a moment of respite.

There's one cold, hard fact that none of us should ever lose track of: our days on this earth are limited. I say that in a positive, joyous way, not at all as a negative. We all have known for many years that we'd never get off this planet alive. Now that we've had our heart attacks we're simply more aware of our own personal mortality. That should make us even more receptive to doing the things that are necessary to prolong life as much as we can.

When you were in the hospital, life went on without you. All those stressors at the office, at home, and elsewhere suddenly were unimportant and forgotten. Many patients in the CCU have said that in a weird way they almost welcomed their heart attacks since they had provided the first moment's rest in years. Now that you're recovering, it's up to you to get more control over your life. Don't get trapped into the wrong thinking that you "can't" change the things that cause you stress and make you angry and hostile. And don't think you can't change the way you react to those stressors. You can and you must.

Being angry and hostile, exposing oneself constantly and continuously to terrible stresses, is like hitting yourself in the head with a hammer. It sure feels good when you stop. Not only will you live longer, you'll enjoy your life a lot more. Take that on faith from one who's done it.

CHAPTER 3

Successful Strategies for Easing Stress and Distress

This very possibly is the most important chapter in the book. It can help you live longer and love living. And it will make all the other steps to a spectacular recovery much easier to follow. Most of all, it can make you much happier. Quickly.

Let's face it, right now you're not at all happy. And you've got every reason in the world to feel pretty damn mad and miserable. You've probably said a number of times that no one understands what you're going through. You're right, no one does who hasn't gone through the same problems. Not your spouse, not your doctors, not anyone.

But as much as you have a right to be angry at what's happened to you—and this has probably made your Type-A inclinations a lot stronger—you can't allow yourself to wallow in self-pity. In a perverse kind of way, you'll start to become addicted to your own suffering. In so doing, you'll limit your chances of making a good recovery and living a healthy, normal life.

Yes, it's too bad you had that heart attack or the surgery. It's not fair. But no one said life was fair. On the other hand, you're in the company of millions and millions of us who have gone down the same road. It's not a very exclusive club at all. But what *can* make your membership exclusive is your complete recovery and your ultimate victory over heart disease.

In the past, having a heart attack meant that you were doomed. Maybe sooner, maybe later, but as sure as the tide comes in every evening, heart attack victims were virtually certain to eventually die of the disease. Recovery from the first attack was dreary, most became cardiac cripples to one degree or another, and medical care was a matter of putting off the inevitable.

Today's prognosis is totally different. Look how quickly you got out of the hospital! And before you ever left you were out in the halls starting to walk. By the time your doctor released you, he knew that you were going to be just fine. Except that you still don't believe it. And you keep letting the reality of your heart get you down.

It's important to realize, right off the bat, that, given half a chance, your mental anguish will pass. Right now it's as natural for you to be angry and depressed as it is to be easily tired. Both will pass, and you can make that passage quicker on both counts. Let's look at one extreme example.

If you had bypass surgery, you might have experienced a state known as ICU psychosis. While in the intensive care unit soon after surgery, some patients enter a really scary condition in which they feel paranoid, disoriented, and sometimes wildly anxious. I was one of those patients.

I had my second bypass on July 3, 1984. On the Fourth of July my family came to visit me in the ICU. I had no idea where I was, what I was doing there, or what was going on. Suddenly I was actually mentally off-balance, in a true state of delirium, trying to pull the tubes from my body. Needless to say my family was horrified. But it passed. I returned to normal.

Right now you're probably experiencing significant mood swings. One moment you're smiling, the next you're crying. It doesn't take much to set you off. Virtually every emotion is intensified. A sad movie on the one hand, or a particularly uplifting and touching one on the other, can fill your eyes with tears. You're not alone. We all go through this, and, as with other aspects of mental distress, it will pass.

Arna Munford, at Cedars-Sinai Hospital in Los Angeles, told me that it might be a matter of an intensified feeling of vulnerability. She explained that mood swings are very common, if not universal, and may be the result of the tremendous mental jolt heart patients receive. One day you're totally in control of your universe, the next you almost die. That swing in realities sets the stage for swings in mood.

Frankly, many of us carry some of those tendencies toward mood swings for years to come. I still find myself more likely to cry at a poignant film than I would have previously. And other heart patients have confided that they experience similar swings. It's not so bad: I think it means that I and others have simply gotten closer in touch with our feelings. Importantly, though, you must realize that the unpleasant, rather wildly erratic mood swings you now may be going through will diminish with time.

You'll probably notice that your moods are most likely to swing when you're feeling tired. You just don't have the energy to overcome the emotions. I found that the best thing to do in such cases was to take a little nap. Nothing major, just lie down on the couch or the bed for a few minutes, close your eyes, and relax. That'll be even more efficient when you master the relaxation techniques we'll discuss in the coming pages.

Another way of dealing with the kind of mood swing brought on by moments of anger or other kind of stress is to do some gentle stretching exercises. I do some kind of stretching at least a couple of times daily.

Finally, you can control your emotions very effectively by recognizing the fact that you can't be in two mental places at one time any more than you can be in two physical places at once. Does that sound like gobbledy-gook? Here's what I mean.

If you're thinking about something that's making you angry or stressful, think about something else. Don't allow yourself to stay in that mental place. Two techniques can make this easier to do.

First, develop a little collection of things that can get you into a good mental mood. A photo album reminding you of wonderful experiences in the past, of those you love, of a quieter place and time. Silly as it sounds, one of my favorites is a yo-yo. I can pick it up and concentrate on doing various tricks like "walk the dog" or "rock the cradle" and I get out of thinking about the negatives in life. I keep one of those yo-yos in my office and another in the house.

Second, just *do* something. Get moving. Don't just sit there and stew. Get up, put on a jacket or sweater and go out for a walk. Pick up the telephone and call someone you haven't visited with for a while. But *don't* talk about what was troubling you; keep it on the light and pleasant side.

There are times when it's perfectly justifiable to be angry. If you've had surgery, for example, you're probably not terribly happy about your scars. Especially if you're a woman. In fact, you're damned mad about those disfiguring "zippers" running down your chest and legs. It's absolutely natural to feel that way. But the scars are a fact of your life. They're not going to go away entirely, though they will fade with time. Realize that you're far more conscious of the scars than others are. Many patients go to ridiculous extremes to cover their scars and to not let others, even their spouses, see them. Your physical attractiveness will not be hampered, and your sexual activities should not be altered one iota.

Regardless of those rationalizations, however, you're going to be angry now and then. Let yourself go. But make a deal with your emotions. Set a discrete time limit to allow yourself to rage. You might even go so far as to set a kitchen timer for five minutes. Yell and rant and rave, and when the buzzer goes off, stop and go on with your life. I think you'll find that your rages are shorter and of less intensity as time goes on.

Have you ever played a musical instrument? Piano? Guitar? This is the perfect time to polish some of those forgotten skills. Bring out some sheet music, find some tunes that will put you into a good mood, and keep your music handy for those moments when you need a lift.

Even if you don't have special musical skills, you can sing. Or whistle. Or play the kazoo. As they say, music can soothe the savage beast. For those of us in the cardiac club, those early emotions can be beastly.

Make a conscious effort to make music daily. Sing in the shower. Hum a tune while you walk. Whistle while you work. It can make a huge difference in your life.

When was the last time you had a good belly laugh? If you're like I was after my heart attack, you can't even remember. Moreover, you probably sneer at the thought. Well, the best thing you can do is to go out of your way to put some humor in your life. Not once in a while, but routinely.

Actually there's a physiological basis for the healing and calming effects of laughter. Heartfelt belly laughs can set off the release of the body's beta-endorphins, which are chemically similar to morphine. That's an addiction you can live with!

Where can you go for a good laugh? Start with your TV listings for late-night reruns of classic programs. Everyone has his or her own favorites. I happen to love old episodes of "Bob Newhart," "Green Acres," "Barney Miller," "Cheers," and "Night Court." They're always good for a laugh. I program my VCR for a few of those reruns, which usually come on in the middle of the night. Then I always have a nice file to choose from when I need a lift.

Next, head off for your video rental outlet. Here, too, you'll find some classics that are sure to get you into a good mood. Woody Allen alone has a veritable library of tapes; I especially like his earlier, funnier works. The *Pink Panther* series is another personal favorite. Many places now have midweek specials so you can keep the costs down to a minimum.

Don't forget the bookstore and library. You'll find a wealth of comic genius in those pages. Jean Shepard. Max Shulman. Erma Bombeck. And don't forget the wonderful cartoonists such as Gahan Wilson and Jules Feiffer and Gary Larson. Whenever possible, I prefer to buy such books rather than borrowing them from the library so that I have them on my shelves when I want them. I've spent many a wonderful hour smiling and laughing as I reread those pages. The power of humor is strong, and it has absolutely no adverse reactions or side effects.

Children spend a lot of their time laughing. As parents we would wonder whether a child were normal if he or she didn't laugh often. Why not revert just a bit to childhood?

At first you might think that the suggestions that follow are more than a little strange, and you might feel embarrassed. But trust me. Buy a coloring book and a box of crayons. Try to stay in the lines! Remember how that was so difficult way back when? Use all the different colors. Maybe you like to outline your colors; I know I do. You'll be amazed at just how soothing this can be. Want to get goofy? Color the hair green and the sky purple.

Don't stop at coloring. Try your skills at shooting marbles and playing tiddlywinks. Those games are very inexpensive and can provide many hours of pleasure. Buy a yo-yo and try to master some tricks. Rent the Smothers Brothers video tape to really learn to be the envy of the yo-yo crowd.

Did you enjoy reading comic books as a child? My favorites were Uncle Scrooge and Donald Duck, but I also liked Superman. Archie and his Riverdale buddies Jughead, Moose, Reggie, Betty, and Veronica weren't too bad either. You'll be shocked at how the cost of those comics has escalated, but pick up a few of them when you're at a newsstand. If you're embarrassed, tell the clerk they're for your grandchildren. Better yet, admit they're for yourself and give the clerk a big smile.

Now how about the books you read as a kid? Were you a fan of the Hardy Boys mysteries? Did you like nature stories? Tales of sporting heroes? I was a real fan of Tarzan and Bomba the Jungle Boy. Recently I went to a used book store and found some out-of-print Bomba books. I bought them for my son Ross and wound up rereading them myself. I must say I enjoyed them even more than he did. I find it tough to worry about anything in my own life when I'm wondering how Bomba will manage to escape the coils of a 15-foot anaconda.

Now don't get me wrong. I'm not saying that you should become an escapist and ignore the real, adult world around you. Of course you'll continue to read some best-sellers and professional journals and the *Wall Street Journal*. Just give yourself permission to have fun now and then.

The fact of the matter is that most adults don't have much fun. Ask any kid and he or she will tell you that adults are boring. Why not schedule fun on a regular basis just like you schedule everything else in your life?

Ask yourself what you do for fun. Watch television? That really doesn't count, since you probably just plop down in front of the tube and watch whatever happens to be on. Making the effort to rent and watch a classic comedy is a different matter. Most adults don't go out to the movies very often. Pick up the newspaper and plan to see a film some time this week. How about a midday matinee?

Mark another category in your daily journal. Write down what you do every day for fun. Not just what happened to be fun, but something you planned in advance to do and enjoy. That's another nice habit to get into.

If you're up to it in the coming weeks, seek out one of the local comedy clubs. They're opening in virtually every major city. Get a reservation for the evening and for a couple of hours allow some stand-up comics to entertain you. It's a lot of fun.

Arthur Murray actually made an advertising phrase out of it: "Put some fun in your life, try dancing." When have you and your spouse gone out for an evening of dancing? I'll bet you haven't danced for years, other than at a wedding. You may not be ready for it for a while, but when your doctor gives the all-clear signal, head off for the dance floor. You might even decide to take a few lessons. And dancing can be terrific exercise.

I've been discussing and suggesting some things that you probably haven't thought much about in years. All of them have one thing in common. They get your mind off the negative thoughts that can come to roost in your mind, replacing them with positive fun and laughter and entertainment.

Promise yourself that you'll not allow yourself to stew. Instead, have some things in mind that you'll be able to use to get yourself moving in a positive direction. The time to make this promise to yourself is before you get into a stew. Then when it happens, *move!*

Get out of bed or out of your chair. Pick up that comic book, or yo-yo, or cartoon collection and focus on it for a while. Or take a walk, or sharpen some knives in the kitchen, or replace that burned out light bulb in the closet. Just *do* something positive and productive. At first this may be difficult. But it can make all the difference in the world for your recovery, both long-term and short-term.

You're bombarded daily by messages coming from every direction. Newspapers, TV, radio, magazines: all relate information and communicate a wide variety of messages. You're also the recipient of your own messages, originating from Broadcast Central in your own mind. Unfortunately, many if not most of those messages are quite negative: "I wish I were . . ." "I wish I had . . ." "I'm sorry I can't . . ."

Psychologists have found that most people have mostly negative thoughts. In fact, most people originate five to six times more negative ideas than positive ones. You're the Program Director of your mind's Broadcast Central. It's time to make a programming change. It's time to start originating positive ideas and thoughts on a regular basis.

Here are some positive thoughts for you to consider: My body is getting healthier and stronger. Each day I get a new start. I love myself and deserve the best attention. I'm going to feel better than I have in years. Today is the first day of the rest of my life. I'm going to enjoy life to its fullest. I'm in control of my own destiny.

Now pick one or two of those, and add one or two of your own. You might even want to jot them down on little cards or Post-it stickers and leave them around the house to remind yourself. Several times during the day, say those words either to yourself in your mind or, if you're alone, out loud. Of all those affirmations, those positive thoughts, the most important is that you love yourself and that you accept the present knowing you're going to get better.

The concept of affirmations is an ancient one, used widely in many religions. In the Catholic Church, the devout are urged to frequently recite what are called ejaculations throughout the day. These ejaculations are merely affirmations of one's faith: Our father who art in Heaven; Hail Mary, full of grace; Jesus, save me. The more often one makes such an act of faith, the stronger one's faith becomes. So it is with the affirmations of one's health and well-being. Frequent recitations will, indeed, put a focus on the positive act of getting better, one day at a time.

Don't get discouraged by what seems to be a slow progress. Make your daily entries into your journal; after just two or three weeks you'll be able to review your own progressive recovery.

Keep in mind that it took literally decades for your arteries to become clogged, leading up to your cardiac event. Don't expect that your recovery will take place overnight. But you *can* expect that you'll get better a lot faster than it took to get sick!

Concentrate on taking it all one day at a time. That applies to every aspect of your recovery. As we'll see in chapter 12, it's important not to think about quitting smoking, for example, for the rest of your life; just try to make it through one day without a cigarette. If you have 50 pounds to lose, or you have to greatly reduce your cholesterol level, those dietary changes must come one day at a time.

COPING WITH ANGER

The mere fact that you've had a heart attack or surgery has made you angry. In that state of mind you're ripe for getting angry at others. The littlest thing, though it may not appear insignificant at the moment, is likely to set you off on a tirade. To make matters worse, you're actually afraid of getting angry since you fear that anger might set off another event.

A waiter brings the wrong dish and you're too much in a hurry to wait for the kitchen to prepare what you ordered. A police officer is writing a parking ticket for your car just as you walk out from an appointment that ran a little late. Your spouse forgets to pick up an item from the store. Your children play music too loud, interfering with your reading. You react in one of two ways.

First, you might explode and yell, venting your spleen and blowing the event out of all proportion. You find your heart beating and your hands tremble. Now you're angry that you got angry and you further blame the waiter/cop/spouse/children. "Don't they understand what I'm going through? Don't they know their behavior can kill me?" No, they don't understand at all. But then, you don't understand your own anger, either.

Or, you might keep your anger bottled up inside. You're afraid to explode. Instead you have an internal argument. You rage in your mind against the waiter/cop/spouse/children. You go through a whole litany of arguments, as though there were some arbiter inside your head who will judge you to be in the right and somehow punish the wrong-doer. In this instance, that internal rage may go on and on, and it may well be repeated over and over, as you add even better arguments to justify your anger. Do you recognize yourself here?

Let's face it, getting violently angry doesn't make you happy. Sure, there are some mean-spirited folks out there who take pleasure in arguing and yelling and screaming. But you're probably not one of them. The fact is that for most of us, getting angry is one of the most effective ways of wrecking the whole day. It can take away the pleasures of anything else that's happening.

On the other hand, you can't expect to be able to simply walk away from an injustice meekly, without giving it another thought. Even if you avoid direct confrontation, you're likely to retreat to internal rage. So what can one do?

Dr. Arna Munford at Cedars-Sinai Hospital in Los Angeles is an expert in this very area. She believes that virtually anyone and everyone can effectively modify the way he or she thinks about things so that anger is not the result.

The first step, she says, is to focus on your goals, to determine what it is that you want to be doing, and work to achieve those goals. Your ultimate goal is obvious: you want to fully recover, to have a healthy heart, and to have a vibrant, productive, and happy life. No matter what, you must not lose track of that long-term goal. At the same time, your short-term goals should also remain clear in your mind. You want to feel better as quickly as possible, and you're starting on that path by enjoying your life as much as you can. Getting angry is not compatible with that short-term goal, either.

As we begin to modify the thinking process that leads to harmful anger, it's nearly impossible to objectively view a current difficulty or seeming impasse with others. So we must learn to practice on things that have happened in the past. We have to review things that have happened, think about how we reacted and how the thinking that led to that reaction may have been illogical. Then we can restructure the process, and come up with a more logical approach. The next time a similar situation arises, we hope, we'll be able to react in a manner that's not as self-destructive.

Take an example from my own experience. Recently, I was out for a walk/jog one morning when I didn't have time to get to the gym for my routine workout. A patrol car came up alongside me and the officer explained that I'd jogged through a red light. "Don't you look at the lights?" the officer asked as he started writing a jaywalking ticket. I was furious. "Doesn't he have better things to do than hassle me?" I thought.

As it turned out, I was out without any identification. He could have taken me to the station until someone could come to identify me. Fortunately I'd gone through a reevaluation of my typical responses to such situations, and was able to see that by simply going with the flow I could avoid a lot of potential trouble. I took my ticket and managed to laugh about the incident later.

I've thought about that incident a number of times. There's no doubt in my mind that just a few years ago it would have spoiled my day. I had a choice. I could make a big fuss about the ticket, get upset, and risk getting into more trouble. Or I could accept the reality and choose to not let it bother me. I chose the latter, and I'm glad I did.

It's been well documented that the rate of divorce goes up when one spouse begins to get fitness conscious and the other does not. At the very least, the situation can lead to stress and friction between mates.

Picture this: the heart attack victim sees that he or she must make some lifestyle changes in order to attain optimal health status. Regular exercise and dietary discretion become a way of life. Soon the person begins to not only feel but look better. A look in the mirror reveals toned muscles and a more youthful appearance. A glance at the spouse shows a still-overweight, paunchy, and generally frumpy individual.

Dr. Meyer Friedman of Type-A behavior fame has had patients who become enraged when they view their spouses. They go into internal dialogs decrying "the fat pig" and wondering "can't she see how she looks?"

Once again, you have a choice. Actually at least two choices. One would be to simply accept the situation, enjoy your own state of good health, and try to ignore perceived flaws, balancing them with your spouse's good points. Another would be to invite your spouse, gradually, into a shared lifestyle. Begin, perhaps, with an evening stroll. Suggest a weekend away at a health-spa resort. Select restaurants that serve low-fat cuisine. Compliment a new hairstyle or some clothing. Buy a family membership at a health club. Let her know how much you enjoy exercising together. Invite your spouse to join you in your healthier way of life.

BE NICE TO YOURSELF

Not only don't most people in our society today have much fun, but seldom are they really nice to themselves. It's no wonder they're not too nice to others, either. Promise yourself to be nicer to yourself. Start doing some special things, just for yourself.

Do you have a hobby? Have you ever wanted to have one? This might be the time to do something about that. Maybe you'd enjoy photography or oil painting. Perhaps you'd like to try your hand at sculpture. My wife loves to take out a jigsaw puzzle with about a million pieces, working at it for days, a little bit at a time. Dawn finds it very relaxing, I find it tedious and boring; everyone has his or her own tastes. We both really enjoy working crossword puzzles, especially together.

The list of hobbies can go on and on almost indefinitely. But all have one thing in common: they help to keep one relaxed and give one something to look forward to in a very active way. People with a hobby are far more content than those who have no hobby.

Don't be the kind of person who says "My work is my vocation and my avocation." As much as you might enjoy your career, it's not right to make it the only thing in your life. A true avocation of some sort can deeply enrich your existence.

But being nice to yourself doesn't end there. Think about how often you do things for others. You buy them gifts, you take them out for meals, and so forth. You schedule their needs into your calendar. Why not do the same for yourself?

One of my special treats is going on a regular basis to have a massage. The person who does my massage has a nicely appointed room with lots of plants. She plays some wonderfully relaxing music, the kind of tapes that feature soft instrumentation and the sounds of gurgling brooks and chirping birds. She has really turned me on to yet another way of relaxing. I soon bought one of the tapes to use at home, and I relax almost instantly whenever I play it.

You mark your calendar with doctors' appointments, deadlines in your work, birthdays and other special occasions for others, and varied and assorted commitments you have. Why not pencil in a few ideas for doing something nice for yourself?

You may not have time to do something today, or even this week, but surely somewhere down the line you'll see an empty slot. Before someone else beats you to it, make an appointment to do something for yourself. Maybe it'll be a trip to the museum or to the zoo. Maybe it'll be that massage. How about a whole day to go fishing?

I've been self-employed since coming out to California in 1980. It's very easy to say "I'll wait until there's an opening on my calendar" to take even a few days off. Soon I found myself never taking any time. That's when I began to mark time on my own calendar for myself.

In my own case, I ask my wife when she and the children have vacation time from school. Then I block out some of those days so we can spend them together. And sometimes we plan to send the kids away to relatives so we can have a little time on our own, just the two of us. When was the last time that you and your spouse went away together for a day or two? It doesn't have to be a major vacation. Try getting a hotel room even on the other side of town, make reservations for dinner, and bring along something you like to do together. For Dawn and me it's a Scrabble game and a crossword puzzle or two. Special rates on weekends can make some time away a real bargain.

The more you get into your new lifestyle of heart-healthy living, the better you'll feel, and the more you'll want to do for yourself. You'll find that many of those things will tie right into that new lifestyle, like spending a little more time at the gym, going to a fruit stand to buy some particularly nice produce, buying some new clothes to show off your newly fit physique. Your self-esteem will escalate considerably, and that's good.

Researchers at the University of Texas found that people who were the least hostile and angry were also the ones with the best sense of self-esteem. Those who were angered easily, on the other hand, were likely to have less-than-terrific self-esteem. They concluded that angry, hostile responses to situations and others are actually a reflection of the way you feel about yourself.

Escalating self-esteem and being nice to yourself becomes rather like the endless debate about the chicken and the egg. Which really comes first? Actually it doesn't matter. The two feed each other. The more you do for yourself, the better you'll feel about yourself, and vice versa.

There's a very important aspect of recovery from heart disease to consider here. I believe that the reason most men and women do not fully recover from a heart attack or bypass surgery is that they're angry at themselves, and that they never forgive themselves for having that heart condition. The rest of life becomes a punishment, a self-imposed punishment.

Recognize self-destructive behavior and do something about it.

CAFFEINE AND ALCOHOL

If one were to ask the average middle-aged man or woman, heart disease notwithstanding, whether he or she uses recreational drugs, the answer would be a resounding "No!" But if you clarified your question to include caffeine and alcohol, the response would be quite different. In fact, the respondent might even be indignant that you'd call caffeine and alcohol drugs at all.

That cup of coffee in the morning as an eye-opener must be viewed as a stimulant drug. Yes, it's pleasant to sip a hot beverage with breakfast and to savor the aromas. But one can achieve those benefits by drinking decaf. And when consumption goes over two cups daily, regular caffeinated coffee can lead to jangled nerves and sleep disturbances, especially for one recovering from a heart attack or bypass surgery.

The best bet for the first several weeks after heart attack or bypass, I believe, is to stay away from caffeine in all forms. That includes coffee, tea, iced tea, and colas. Later on, limit your consumption to no more than one or two cups of coffee or glasses of iced tea or cola per day. Better yet, after you break the habit, why not stay away permanently?

We all become tolerant of caffeine, to the point where it takes more and more to achieve the "lift" we're looking for. In the meantime, the intake of caffeine results in irritability during the day and restlessness and disturbed sleep by night. Do you really need one more problem in your life? This is the time to learn to relax, to calm down, not to consume something that, by its chemical nature, can make you and everyone jumpy.

I really enjoy coffee, so when I made the switch to decaf, I made a point of getting the best I could find. Try some of the coffees sold in speciality shops. Make it a bit stronger than you normally would, and you really won't be able to notice much of a difference in taste. And the difference in your temperament will be worth the effort.

You might have heard that decaf coffee raises cholesterol levels. That research came out of Stanford University. They found that drinking several cups of inexpensive decaf coffee made with robusta beans did raise the levels of cholesterol. But the better coffees, using arabica beans, had no such effect. Check to see that the decaf you're buying uses arabica beans, not the robusta varieties.

While society sanctions the use of caffeine as a pick-me-up, it seemingly also blesses consuming alcohol as a calmative. In moderation, alcohol appears to actually give one a bit of an advantage over teetotalers when it comes to longevity. That protection appears to come from alcohol's ability to raise levels of the so-called "good" cholesterol, the HDL, in the blood. But there's a significant downside to alcohol, especially during the recovery period.

First, data from the famous Framingham study has shown that, for middle-aged men with slightly to moderately enlarged hearts, alcohol can lead to arrhythmias. Such men probably should drink no alcoholic beverages whatsoever. Talk with your physician about this.

Second, during recovery from either heart attack or bypass, alcohol can result in temporary heartbeat disturbances. Some find that either red wine or straight alcohol such as gin or scotch are particularly troublesome, while a glass or two of white wine or beer with meals will pose no problems.

Third, that alcoholic nightcap might actually result in sleep problems. Sure, a drink or two might make you sleepy and help you to fall asleep. But when the immediate effect wears off, at say 4:00 A.M., you might wake up feeling irritable and be unable to fall back asleep, and your heart might be pounding slightly. You need a good night's sleep to keep you feeling rested the next day and up to doing your exercise and taking your other steps to recovery. Alcohol might interfere, especially if taken beyond moderation. Again, during the immediate period of recovery, it's probably best to stay away altogether.

After several weeks of recovery, you may wish to return to moderate alcohol consumption. Here moderation is defined as one to two alcoholic beverages daily, no more: a six-ounce glass of wine or 12 ounces of beer with a meal or mixed drinks with a one-ounce shot of liquor. The principal problem with straight drinks is that they're consumed rapidly, leading to excess. Moreover, they pose the hazard of arrhythmias for some patients. Discuss alcohol use with your doctor.

SEEKING PROFESSIONAL COUNSELING

While our society condones the use of alcohol and other mind-altering chemicals, it typically frowns on those who seek professional assistance in dealing with mental disturbances. That's really a shame, and there's no reason for it.

Virtually everyone who has had a heart attack or bypass surgery will suffer depression to one degree or another. Certainly the strategies we've been discussing can help pour oil on those troubled waters. But often a helping hand can be of enormous benefit.

We turn to professionals in virtually every other aspect of our lives, so why not in the important arena of our mental well-being? Professionals can help with some temporary problems that face so many heart patients, including marital adjustments, depression and anxiety, and anger management. This does *not* mean long-term, expensive therapy. Often just two or three sessions can help put things into perspective, allow us to voice our concerns, and help prepare us for the future. Studies have shown repeatedly that those who take advantage of such counseling do much better in their recovery efforts than those who flounder on their own.

Many physicians and hospitals now routinely screen patients and refer those who need it to professional assistance. If those services are offered to you, by all means take advantage of them. And most cardiac rehabilitation programs include some sort of behavioral modification and relaxation programs. Again, don't pass them by. If those services are not offered, you might want to ask your doctor or nurse for a suggestion of someone to talk with. There's no need for any embarrassment

What about fees? Certainly you're already deluged with medical bills, and you're concerned about them. This is not a good time to incur more bills. Your health insurance may very well cover these services as part of your total cardiac recovery. Many, if not most, therapists will vary their fees according to one's ability to pay. And there are community services available at no charge at all.

Probably the best source of therapist referral will come from your physician. Or you might know a friend who has used someone in the community successfully. Finally you can call your state psychological association or the national group, the American Psychological Association, in Washington, D.C., at (202) 833-7600. Their address is 1200 17th Street, N.W., Washington, D.C., 20036. Ask for a listing of professionals in your area, especially those with experience in helping recovering heart patients.

Most people with depression never see a mental health professional either because they can't afford it or because they view their condition as a sign of personal or moral weakness. For those with a personal computer at home, a new program offers affordable therapy, allowing the user to work at one's own pace whenever needed. For additional information, write or call Malibu Artifactural Intelligence Works: 25307 Malibu Road, Malibu, CA 90265; (310) 456-7787.

PUTTING IT TO WORK FOR YOU

The strategies I've discussed in this chapter can help you ease the stress and distress so common for those men and women on the road to cardiac recovery. They've worked for me and for many others. But to make them work, you've got to use them. And like any other skill, practice makes perfect.

Make daily notes and comments in your recovery journal. Remember that you always have choices in how you react to any given situation. It's truly a marvelous skill to make those choices which will help rather than hinder recovery. From time to time you will want to refer back to this chapter to refresh your memory and to sharpen those skills.

But we're not quite finished with our discussion of mastering the "inner game" of beating heart disease. Certain relaxation techniques have been developed which have proven particularly useful to those of us looking not only for recovery but total cardiac rehabilitation. Those techniques are so important that I've devoted an entire chapter to them. You'll start to learn how they can revolutionize your life and health and well-being as you go to the next page. . . .

CHAPTER 4

Tried and True Relaxation Techniques

Why do we need to learn techniques to relax? Can't everyone do that quite naturally? Well, the Food and Drug Administration tells us that in 1988 60 million prescriptions for tranquilizers such as Valium were gobbled up by anxiety- and stress-ridden men and women in the United States. There's definitely a problem in our society, and I hope you agree that drugs aren't the best way to handle it.

In a way, it's quite sad that we really don't know how to relax. Sure, we plunk ourselves in front of the TV set in the evening, but is that really relaxing? Even more active diversions such as going to the races or playing a game of cards may not afford the stress-reducing benefits of truly profound relaxation.

As you can see, I'm not talking about what most of us would consider to be relaxation. It's not a matter of doing nothing, but, rather, of doing something. It's a positive rather than negative concept. Relaxation is a skill that can be learned, and it can invoke a strong and beneficial physiological response for the recovering heart patient.

The mountain of data documenting the benefits of active relaxation techniques has grown considerably during the past few years alone. One such study sought to determine if a program of relaxation and behavioral modification could affect rates of repeat heart attack, termed reinfarction.

At three years into their five-year project, subjects in the experimental group show a reinfarction rate half that of a control group receiving only cardiologic counseling. Not a bad start!

Relaxation combined with an exercise program in post-heart attack patients improved the outcome of exercise training in patients participating in a study done in the Netherlands. Investigators found that training failures, that is to say individuals who got no benefit from exercise, made up about half their patient population. By adding relaxation techniques to exercise, the number of such failures was cut in half. The researchers conclude that relaxation may calm the overzealous and anxious patient, providing a more solid framework for exercise to work its beneficial effects.

The same Dutch researchers, in an earlier study, termed relaxation a treatment in its own right for heart attack patients. That study showed that Type-A individuals got the most benefit from relaxation.

A number of different, yet similar, relaxation techniques provide those benefits. Deep breathing, progressive relaxation, yoga, meditation, prayer, and biofeedback all invoke a remarkably strong curative response. All enable patients to take the other steps needed for a complete cardiac recovery. And all share a power to strengthen the body while soothing the mind, providing an overall improvement in well-being which can be tested on both objective and subjective planes.

You're already an expert in the basic principle of all stress management and relaxation. From the moment the doctor, nurse, or midwife gave you that first swat on the bottom and you started breathing, you've never stopped. And you've been breathing without even thinking about it ever since. Scientists call us involuntary breathers; that compares us with other animals such as the dolphins of the sea who are voluntary breathers: they must not sleep lest they stop breathing. We breathe no matter what.

Now it's time to start thinking about that breathing. It's time to be a bit more like the dolphins.

BREATHING

As a first step, think about this: When you're about to do something special, you take a deep breath. When you finish a major task, you take a deep breath. When you feel a bit of anxiety, you sigh, that is, you take a deep breath. All that proves that your body automatically takes advantage of such breathing. Now it's a matter of taking this natural activity to its ultimate benefit.

I was first introduced to the idea of deep breathing as a specific relaxation technique in 1971 when I took a course in yoga at a Chicago YMCA. I must admit that back then I did it really as a lark, and taking courses like that was a good way to meet women. But I soon learned that I'd stumbled onto something quite valuable.

The instructor, who had traveled a number of times to India to become expert in yoga, tried to explain how this ancient discipline was not only another way of getting exercise and increasing flexibility, although it was quite effective in that vein as well. Yoga, she maintained, was able to effect significant changes in the body's physiologic functioning. "Sure," I thought, "and next you'll tell us about levitating." I didn't take it very seriously at all. Yet I did begin to feel the benefits.

Interestingly, as I've looked at some of the hand-out materials she gave us, I'm amazed at how on-target that yoga instructor was. She wrote, for example, about how yoga could diminish the activity of the sympathetic nervous system. At the time, I dismissed such claims out of hand, thinking that the only "truth" possible came out of a scientific laboratory. Well, two decades later we're getting affirmation of what she knew to be true and, Doubting Thomas that I am, I'm accepting the research data coming from prestigious universities and medical centers showing the benefits of yoga and other relaxation techniques which utilize deep breathing.

Don't jump to the conclusion that I've become some sort of swami or a zealot chanting in the streets. Far from it, I remain a hard-nosed science writer, quite conservative in my professional and personal life. But when someone gives you a valuable gift, the best thing you can do is accept it and say thank you.

Let me share with you, now, how you can start to immediately benefit from deep breathing therapy. There are five different methods of breathing, each with its own advantages. Try them all.

Alternate Breathing allows you to learn to concentrate on your breathing. Sit in a comfortable position with your eyes closed and rolled slightly upward. Close your right nostril with the right thumb, and inhale slowly, very slowly, through the left nostril. Do so noiselessly and in a relaxed manner. Now close the left nostril with the index finger of the right hand and exhale slowly through the right nostril. Keeping the index finger pressed to the left nostril, inhale, again very slowly, through the right nostril; close with the thumb and exhale through the left nostril. Continue for 12 breathing cycles. Don't hold your breath between inhalations and exhalations. Try to balance by keeping a slow count as you breathe in and out.

The main purpose of this exercise is to make you become aware of your breathing. You've taken it for granted until now. Concentrate on that breathing and feel the relaxation spreading through your body. After a few sessions the matter of closing off the nostrils will become second nature and you won't have to pay as much attention to it.

Diaphragmatic Breathing is a great way to relax and take a break during a hectic day. You'll want to take advantage of this soothing exercise when you return to work. In the meantime, try to practice a few times each day.

Lie on the floor with your hand on your abdomen. Feel the stomach muscles lift as you inhale and fall as you exhale. Try to keep your shoulders and chest still. This is actually the reverse of the high, shallow chest breathing most adults use. Using the abdominal muscles helps us fully expand the lungs. You may find this feels strange at first because we have to relearn a process we've performed unconsciously for many years. Watch a very young child breathe and you'll notice how the tummy rises and falls. Perhaps adults breathe the way we do because we want to keep our stomachs flat. Try as much as possible to breathe using the abdominal muscles. By all means, practice this technique a few times daily. It's the basis of breathing exercises to come.

Three-part Breathing builds on diaphragmatic breathing, and is the first step in this complete breathing cycle. First inhale as fully as possible via the abdominal muscles. Next expand your rib cage to further fill your lungs. Finally take a few "sips" of air through your nose, feeling the throat area fill with air. Practice following those three steps in a smooth, unrushed fashion.

Exhale in the same, not the reverse, order. First depress the abdominal muscles, next deflate the lungs by pressing down on the rib cage, and finally feel the air leave the throat through the nostrils. To fully expel all the air, do three reverse sniffs through the nose, pushing the very last bit of air from the body.

This, I think, is one of the easiest and best ways to relax. You can do it anytime and anyplace. It should be a part of your routine day.

At the beginning it's best to do this while lying on the floor with your back firmly pressed down. Try to imagine that gravity is pulling your body, especially the buttocks and lower back, down. After you master the process, and it does take some practice to perfect, you can try it while in a seated position. I personally don't like to sit in a chair; I prefer to sit cross-legged with my back as straight as possible, hands on the tops of my thighs.

Concentrate on the process. Breathe the air in slowly and fully, then release the air in a similarly slow fashion. Be sure to "sniff" that last bit of air out. Think of nothing but your breathing, putting all your attention on the air rhythmically entering and leaving your body.

I know that you're reading all this with your eyebrows lifted in skepticism. You can't picture yourself doing anything like this, so foreign to your normal way of thinking. But I can assure you that this breathing exercise can work for anyone.

Everyone has a favorite trick for getting rid of hiccups. But none of them works for everyone all the time. At parties, I've encountered many a person with hiccups that just won't go away. I invite them into a darkened room away from the hustle and bustle of the party, instruct them to take a seated position on the floor, and talk them through the breathing exercise I just gave you.

With a gentle, muted voice I walk them through their inhalations and exhalations. As they fill their lungs with air, I ask them to hold their breath for a few seconds, remaining conscious of the air in their bodies, and then instruct them to slowly release that air, down to the last few sniffs. After just a few minutes, I ask them if their hiccups are gone. Amazingly most have forgotten they ever had the hiccups at all. Many have elected to remain in the room for a few minutes more, so they could fully relax because the breathing made them feel so good.

When my son Ross was just eight years old, he got a nasty case of the hiccups. I took him into a room, just as I've done so many times with adults, and walked him through the procedure. Sure enough, the hiccups were soon gone. Moreover, Ross discovered a great way to relax. Now, when he's having some particularly tough times in school he'll go off to do his breathing because, in Ross's own words, it makes him feel as though he'd had a nap.

Rapid Abdominal Exhalation is the fourth type of deep breathing, and is particularly suited for dealing with those moments of stress and anger. To start, inhale and exhale rapidly, forcing in the abdominal muscles vigorously on the exhalation. Then relax the abdominals, letting the air rush in. Continue, stressing the exhalation. As compared with the breathing exercise with three parts, here we concentrate on the abdominals.

Think about it this way. If you normally take a deep breath and blow it out when under stress, think how much more effective a series of rapid breaths would be.

After the initial series of rapid breathing through the abdominals, switch to a more relaxing three-part breathing. Continue that relaxing breathing until you're calm and feeling refreshed.

I must caution you here not to do that rapid breathing while standing up and inhaling and exhaling through your nose. That might result in a state of hyperventilation and cause you to feel a bit dizzy.

Instead of getting angry at your spouse or boss, do some breathing. When the IRS wants its pound of flesh at tax time, do some breathing. When someone cuts you off in traffic or a cop writes a ticket, do some breathing. There are numerous provocations in everyone's life. You'll find that deep breathing is as addictive, and a lot more healthful, than drugs such as Valium.

Cooling Breath is the fifth yoga deep breathing technique. It's not one of my favorites, but I pass it along as some people find it very rewarding.

Protrude your tongue beyond the lips and curl it upward. Inhale through the mouth along the path of the curled tongue. Feel the coolness in your mouth. Hold the breath for a few seconds, and slowly exhale through the nostrils. Repeat six to fifteen times.

Deep breathing is a basic concept of yoga. If you were to take a course at the YMCA or elsewhere as I did, you'd no doubt get a lot of the mystical jargon thrown into the bargain. I don't take that very seriously, but I do enjoy the rather rhythmic cadences of the instructor as he or she soothingly goes through the instructions of the breathing and the various stretching poses. Of course you'll need to be a bit further along in your recovery before then, especially if you've had surgery.

One of the first poses you'd learn is called the "savasna" or the corpse pose. This is one way to get really relaxed, back to life as it were, by playing dead. Here's how it goes.

Lie flat on your back, relaxing the arms at your sides but not touching the body, with your palms up, the fingers curled slightly, naturally. Separate the legs a bit, and consciously relax the knees. Let your feet fall away from each other. Unclench your teeth, and let the tongue and jaw relax. Close your eyes, but lightly so, with the gaze through the lids slightly upward.

Feel your body becoming very relaxed, with the entire length of the spine on the floor. You feel the weight of your body pressing into the floor as gravity pulls you down. Give no resistance, allowing yourself to fall, as it were, toward the center of the earth.

Begin to consciously relax your body by concentrating on one part at a time. Give your feet the command to relax, relax, relax. Notice how your feet, first the right, then the left, begin to feel heavier and heavier as you tell them to relax. Work your way up the body to your calves, your knees, your thighs, and on and on. All the while, breathe slowly through the mouth and exhale through the nose.

As you feel yourself approaching total relaxation and contentment, begin to concentrate more completely on your breathing. Perform the three-part breathing, but don't push the last "sniffs" too hard.

Certainly you can achieve relaxation all by yourself in this way. To assist yourself you might want to make a tape of instructions. Play some soft music as a background and soothingly give yourself instructions, using the paragraphs above as a guide. There are also tapes on the market which can assist you in your deep breathing exercises.

VISUALIZATION/IMAGERY

Imagine a cool, refreshing drink you enjoyed on a hot, muggy day last summer. Picture the glass in your mind's eye. See the condensation on the glass, feel the coolness in your hand, taste the first drenching sensations on your parched tongue as you drink that delicious liquid refreshment. As the image fades, what remains? The inside of your mouth is probably primed with saliva and you may even be wondering what's in the refrigerator that you could drink.

This is a simple demonstration of the powers of visualization. Some people get so good at such imagery that they can tell their minds that they are seeing one thing when in fact they're looking at another. In cancer wards, professionals guide patients as they visualize wonderful scenes and experiences while undergoing chemotherapy. Incidence of side effects plunges. The mind is a wonderful thing.

One way to use visualization in relaxation is to imagine a moment in time when you were absolutely at ease. Recall that experience with as much detail as you can. Were you in sunlight or shade? Inside or out?

Alone or with someone else? Was there grass, blue sky, furniture, or carpeting? Were you inside with a fire blazing in the fireplace while it rained outside? Were any sounds associated with your memory? The soothing rhythms of breaking ocean waves, perhaps, or the distant sounds of children laughing? What did your body feel like? Could you touch anything, or was anything touching you? Recall every sensation associated with this relaxed moment. If it wasn't perfect, make it so. If you were walking along a beach in full dress, imagine yourself barefoot in the most comfortable attire. If the sky was a bit overcast, make it sunny. You're the author of that moment in time.

The approach isn't limited to cancer or heart patients. Psychologists working in human performance laboratories use visualization with athletes who want to improve their performance. They've been able to measure changes in breathing patterns and lessened muscle tension.

How can you apply those techniques to your personal recovery efforts? I remember very well the images I brought to mind during the years following my second bypass. I pictured my cholesterol going down, visualizing the numbers like degress of temperature on a thermometer. I saw myself running through a field, without strain, effort, or pain. And ultimately I visualized myself getting that momentous angiogram, the day I'd be told that my heart's vessels were clear as a bell. How much did such visualization contribute to the eventual reality? I really can't say. But I can tell you with no hesitation that every time I brought one of those thoughts to mind, it made me feel better. Give it a try yourself. You have nothing to lose.

MEDITATION AND THE RELAXATION RESPONSE

People have been meditating for centuries, possibly all the way back to the dawn of man as a thinking being. Virtually every culture has some sort of meditation. For some it may be chanting. Buddhists seek a state of nirvana. In Western cultures, monks have long cloistered themselves in much the same way as their Eastern counterparts do. And in both societies those with lesser callings content themselves with a diluted contemplation. Many call it prayer.

Scientific recognition of the enormous benefits of meditation began in the 1960s. A pioneer in the field is Herbert Benson, M.D., the author of *The Relaxation Response,* a book I heartily recommend for your heart-smart library. At first, he admits, he was a conservative academic who refused to even listen to a group of students who became interested in his research on techniques for lowering blood pressure. They told him they already knew how to do just that, by way of Transcendental Meditation. They'd seen remarkable results in themselves and in others, and had heard of even more amazing case studies involving feats that bordered on the incredible. Despite Benson's initial rebuffs, the students dogged him, and the doctor finally agreed to listen.

What he heard was so striking that he continued his investigation and found that the results were not only medically thrilling but also could be duplicated again and again in any number of patients of all colors and stripes. He saw blood pressures fall, metabolic rates drop, sympathetic nervous system functioning decrease, and saw the patients achieve states of extreme relaxation. He had previously believed these changes to be possible only with potent medications.

The basic instructions for performing meditation in order to achieve the relaxation response is really quite simple. First, choose a comfortable position in a quiet place. Some people prefer a darkened room while others like to keep the lights on. You can sit in a chair, on a couch, or on the floor with your legs crossed. Disconnect the telephone. Do not use an alarm clock or timer to let you know when the meditation period is over; rather, glance at a clock or your watch.

Close your eyes and spend a few minutes concentrating on your breathing as we discussed earlier. Then proceed to the progressive relaxation of the parts of your body, commanding each in turn to relax. To help concentrate on each part of the body, tense the muscles, then relax, tense, then relax. Pull your abdominal muscles in to harden your stomach, then relax. Tense the anal sphincter as though you're trying to hold back urination, then relax. Raise your shoulders to your ears, hold, then relax. Do an exaggerated smile, hold, then relax. Raise the eyebrows as high as you can, hold, then relax.

For the next phase, you have your choice of two approaches. For one, simply concentrate on the three-part breathing method. Fill the lungs first by expanding the abdomen, then the rib cage, and finally "sniff" in more air. Expel the air in the same sequence, collapsing first the abdomen and then the rib cage, and finally forcing the remaining air out with a reverse "sniff." Your other choice, that used in traditional forms of meditation including TM, is to repeat a single word or phrase over and over, concentrating your entire consciousness on it.

The power of prayer can also be enormously powerful. Dr. Benson has written extensively about that in his follow-up book *Beyond the Relaxation Response* (1984). If you are currently religious, or once were, this is the time to bring this gift out in your life. Choose a word or a brief phrase which has great meaning for you. Examples include "Jesus saves," "My Lord," "Hallowed be Thy Name," "Hail Mary," and "Allah be praised." Every religion in the world has its own special words, prayers, and ejaculations.

Continue the meditation process for 20 minutes, each and every day. You may prefer to spend 10 minutes, doing so twice a day. If at all possible, meditate in the same place at the same time and under the same circumstances routinely. Don't think about whether you're doing it "right" since there is no right or wrong. Meditation is not competitive. There are no losers, only winners. Try not to miss a day; the more you practice, the more you'll benefit, and soon you'll actually look forward to your sessions. Don't allow yourself to make excuses; just do it.

Different people respond differently, and some may have some problems that others may not encounter. Most, however, find that the only time meditation should be postponed is one hour after eating. There will be distractions; try to eliminate as many as you can, and learn to ignore the rest. If you find you can't sit still, try doing your meditation after taking a walk or doing other exercise.

You may find that you can't stay awake during meditation, that the process relaxes you to the point that you just fall asleep. Not that that's entirely bad, since you may find that a bit of meditation is a wonderful alternative to sleeping pills, but you won't be getting meditation's full effects. To avoid this problem, choose a time of the day such as early in the morning when you're most likely to be wide awake.

The flip side of the coin is that some people find that meditating gives them a jolt of energy such that they can't fall asleep at night. The solution here would be to do one's meditation earlier in the day.

BIOFEEDBACK

Psychologist Laurence Miller provided an excellent way of explaining the concept of biofeedback in *Psychology Today*. Imagine playing a video game while blindfolded and wearing earplugs. Without some kind of feedback or guidance, you'd probably be pretty lousy and there's little chance you'd learn how to play the game well. That's similar to what happens in the human body.

The "bio" in biofeedback refers to imperceptible physiologic processes including blood pressure and heart rate. In biofeedback, special devices amplify these processes into perceptible tones that can be "fed back" to the patient. The signal can then help one detect and control the body's functions.

Typically, a sensor is fastened to a muscle and a light or buzzer goes off when the muscle is tight. The objective is for the individual to find a state of relaxation that soothes the muscle and cause the biofeedback sensor to cease registering tension.

Cues controlled by biofeedback in addition to blood pressure and heart rate are muscle tension, skin temperature, and perspiration. By signaling reductions in muscle tension, improving blood flow to the extremities, or reducing sweat gland activity, these techniques help people to relax. Certainly not everyone needs machinery to learn good relaxation techniques. But some people do find themselves caught up in it, learning relaxation faster when there is an objective clue. Engineers and others geared to mechanics and gimmicks are particularly suited to biofeedback.

A typical course of biofeedback runs 12 to 20 weeks, with a few follow-up sessions likely. After that, most can relax on their own without the machinery. Some, however, find that they want their own equipment for home use. The cost of the machinery varies. The cost of the training is similar to that of psychotherapy, $50 to $125 per session. But in many communities biofeedback courses are offered through hospitals for a fraction of that amount. If you'd like more information, you can write to the Association for Applied Psychophysiology and Biofeedback at 10200 West 44th Avenue, Unit 304, Wheat Ridge, CO 80033.

You may also be interested in a program developed by Keith Sedlacek, M.D. He has produced a book and audio cassettes for home instruction in his own version of biofeedback. Along with the book and tapes you'll get a ring or strip which changes color in the same way the mood rings of a few years ago worked. The difference is that Dr. Sedlacek's devices are accurate to 0.5°F, whereas the mood rings and common stress cards are usually only accurate to 5–6°F.

By using the tapes you'll learn to control your stress levels, thus changing the temperature of your skin. As the temperature rises, the color on the ring or fingerstrip changes. Ultimately, this is the same principle used in every biofeedback program. Using Dr. Sedlacek's program is significantly less expensive, of course. If interested, you can call his Stress Regulation Institute at 1-800-637-3529.

TUNING OUT THE NOISE

The first few times I got a massage, I found my mind wandering. Rather than enjoying the skillful ministrations of my masseuse, I kept thinking about work back at the office, bills that had to be paid, and a million and one other things.

Needless to say, that same problem affected me when I'd do some deep breathing or other techniques as well. And many others report having the same difficulty when they try to relax. The fact of the matter is that most of us just have not been conditioned to fully relax; rather, we've learned to remain alert and instantly reactive. No teacher ever rewarded a pupil for staring out the window and daydreaming during the math or spelling lesson. You don't get ahead in your career by thinking of last week's golf outing while attending a sales meeting. No wonder we can't concentrate on relaxation!

The tip I'm about to pass along to you came not from a learned university researcher or an experienced Ph.D. psychologist. I thank my masseuse for this one. Picture your mind as a radio capable of tuning in many channels. What do you want to listen to on your radio? You can twist the tuning knob to pleasant memories of a walk in the woods, or the sounds of a waterfall, the music in the room, your own deep breathing, or the sensations of your muscles as they relax. Or you can tune in to the noise, the static, of interference such as pressing business, family disturbances, and medical bills to be paid. You have control over the dial.

You really do have a choice. Your mind is not pre-programed. You don't have to listen to the noise. Tune that static out. Listen, instead, to the rhythms of your breath going in and out. Picture it as something physical that you can see and feel with each inhalation and exhalation. Allow yourself to return to that childhood innocence when daydreaming was a worthwhile activity.

GETTING A GOOD NIGHT'S SLEEP

Feeling tired lately? Well, don't be surprised, you're not alone. Having a heart attack or bypass surgery takes a lot out of the body, and getting lots of extra sleep is nature's way of helping the body to heal. You may feel the need to get quite a bit more sleep for up to a full year.

The unfortunate flipside of the sleep coin is that you may be experiencing more sleep disturbances than before. One Italian study reported in the *Archives of Internal Medicine* found that sleep disturbances significantly affected about 46 percent of the men studied one year after heart surgery. Again, don't forget that you've gone through some very real trauma, and your body is slowly adjusting and healing.

But the simple fact is that *most* people in our society today just don't get enough sleep. Back in the days of our primitive ancestors, man fell asleep when he was tired or when it was dark outside or both. There were no pressures to go to bed or to get up. Man simply followed his body's mandates naturally.

Then we entered the Era of the Alarm Clock. Suddenly there were multiple responsibilities of work and family, and we started cutting back on what appeared to be "wasted" time in bed. After a hard day's work, we feel we deserve a few minutes of pleasure, and we push the sleep hours even further back by watching "The Tonight Show" past midnight.

To make matters worse, sleep isn't considered "macho." Says Thomas Roth, Ph.D., director of the Sleep Disorders Center at Henry Ford Hospital in Detroit, nobody openly states that they need nine hours of sleep to feel good; rather, they brag about getting by on four or five.

The result is irritability, depression, lack of concentration, and loss of any sense of humor. Merrill Mitler, Ph.D., a psychiatrist at the University of California in San Diego, reports a decided increase in accidents and mistakes directly related to sleep deprivation. For those recovering from heart disease, the need for sleep becomes even more pronounced.

But why do we really need to sleep, anyway? Dr. Mitler says that we don't have a clear scientific explanation. We do know that all mammals and many other animals sleep on a regular basis. Some doctors think sleep comes in order to get rid of certain chemicals that build up in our bodies during the day's activities. Others believe we need a psychological break from the stresses of our waking hours. And, again, our bodies need rest during any healing periods. Even wounded animals slink off into the brush and sleep until they heal.

How much is normal, and how much is enough? Well, it appears that our society in general doesn't get as much as we need. American men average about 7.2 hours a night. Compare that with the 8.0 to 8.5 hours most experts recommend. Adding an hour or two of extra sleep increases productivity and decreases negative mental states. There are some guidelines to make resting more efficient and pleasant.

Try to avoid the temptation of taking sleeping pills. They produce an unnatural state of unconsciousness rather than natural slumber. You're likely to awaken with a groggy, vaguely hung-over feeling. And the ability of this pill or that tablet to get you to sleep diminishes as time goes on, requiring ever higher dosages to achieve the numbing effect.

Ultimately, the best way to get a good night's sleep is the same as the best way to have a wonderful day's activity: engage in techniques of relaxation and stress reduction that will allow you to be at peace with yourself and allow you to proceed with the period of healing that your body requires. While those relaxation techniques may appear foreign to you now, they can become a part of your lifestyle with which you'll never want to part.

THE SECOND STEP:

Getting to Know
Your Heart

CHAPTER 5

Your Heart: A User's Guide

If it's any comfort at all, you're not alone. About 66 million Americans have one or more forms of heart disease, blood vessel disease, or both. Of these, 5 million have a history of heart attack, angina pectoris, or both. Each year as many as 1.5 million Americans will have a heart attack. So far you've been lucky: more than 500,000 heart attack victims die. As to treatment, about 350,000 coronary bypass surgeries and almost as many angioplasties are done annually.

Amazingly, to me at least, most heart patients know almost nothing about their hearts, how they work, and how they got sick. Many would retort by saying that such matters are the business of doctors: just fix me. But those patients who take the bit of time needed to come to at least a basic understanding of their hearts do a lot better in terms of both short- and long-term recovery.

Your heart is an incredibly strong chunk of muscle a bit larger than a big man's fist. From the moment of birth, it has pumped blood through the circulatory system to all parts of your body, never stopping neither day nor night. It will beat about 2.5 billion times over a lifetime, pumping 4,000 gallons of blood daily.

For years scientists, physicians, and engineers have tried to build an artificial heart. Thus far they have not succeeded in creating one that

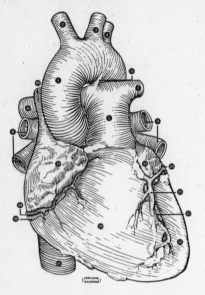

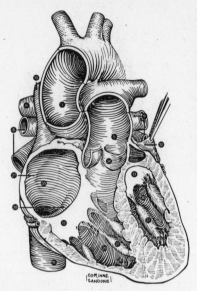

© *Illustrations and Symbols Kit*, 1987

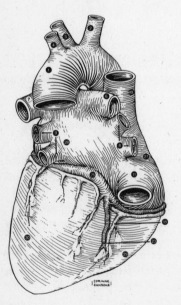

Legend

1. Aorta
2. Brachiocephalic artery
3. Left carotid artery
4. Left subclavian artery
5. Pulmonary trunk
6. Right pulmonary artery
7. Left pulmonary artery
8. Right pulmonary vein
9. Left pulmonary vein
10. Superior vena cava
11. Inferior vena cava
12. Tricuspid valve
13. Mitral valve (bicuspid)
14. Pulmonary valve (semilunar)
15. Aortic valve (semilunar)
16. Right coronary artery
17. Anterior cardiac branch of right coronary artery
18. Posterior descending branch of right coronary artery
19. Left coronary artery
20. Circumflex branch of left coronary artery
21. Anterior descending branch of left coronary artery
22. Great cardiac vein
23. Middle cardiac vein
24. Small cardiac vein
25. Coronary sinus
26. Opening of coronary sinus
27. Right atrium
28. Left atrium
29. Right ventricle
30. Left ventricle
31. Right auricular appendage
32. Left auricular appendage
33. Interatrial septum
34. Interventricular septum
35. Fossa ovalis
36. Ligamentum arteriosum
37. Papillary muscle
38. Eustachian valve

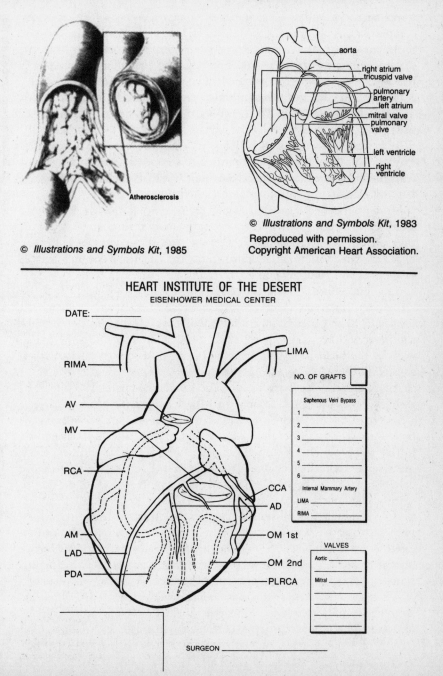

Atherosclerosis

© *Illustrations and Symbols Kit*, 1985

aorta

right atrium
tricuspid valve

pulmonary
artery
left atrium

mitral valve
pulmonary
valve

left ventricle

right
ventricle

© *Illustrations and Symbols Kit*, 1983

Reproduced with permission.
Copyright American Heart Association.

HEART INSTITUTE OF THE DESERT
EISENHOWER MEDICAL CENTER

DATE: _____

RIMA

LIMA

AV

MV

RCA

AM

LAD

PDA

CCA

AD

OM 1st

OM 2nd

PLRCA

NO. OF GRAFTS

Saphenous Vein Bypass

1 _____
2 _____
3 _____
4 _____
5 _____
6 _____

Internal Mammary Artery

LIMA _____
RIMA _____

VALVES

Aortic _____

Mitral _____

SURGEON _____

works nearly as well as the original equipment. When you think of the complexity involved you can understand why. Imagine this virtually tireless machine pulsing through every minute of life from birth to death, never stopping for rest or repair. Amazing. But even more astounding is the way it works in conjunction with the needs of the entire body, responding to complex signals through physiologic electrical circuitry.

Let's take a closer look. The heart is about five inches long, four inches wide, and 3½ inches thick. It weighs less than a can of cola, about 10 to 12 ounces in men and slightly less in women. Forget the Valentine's Day symbol. The true shape is more like a cone. The right side aligns with the breastbone in the middle of your chest. Its top angles off to the left and ends in a point or apex at the left nipple.

Most of the heart is *myocardium*, coming from the Greek *myo* for muscle and *kardia* for heart. When most muscles in your body move, they act on direct orders from the brain. Not so for the heart. Instead of getting direction from the brain, an internal electrical system regulates heart rate, the pumping action.

Your entire heart comes enveloped in a thin, silky bag called the *pericardium*. Like any piece of machinery, the heart must be kept well lubricated. The pericardium contains fluid that oils the tissue surfaces of the heart and keeps it moving easily while contracting. On the inside walls of the heart a smooth protective layer of tissue, the *endocardium*, assists in keeping the organ protected.

Arteries and veins carry blood to and from the heart. The largest of the arteries is the *aorta*, attached to the left ventricle. From there, it snakes over the top of the heart and sends oxygen-rich blood off to your body through a system of increasingly smaller arteries, ultimately ending in tiny arterioles and then microscopic capillaries whose widths are not much larger than the blood cells they transmit. For the return trip, those cells are picked up by venules, and then pass on through a branching of veins and finally back to the heart. The exchange of oxygen and carbon dioxide takes place at the level of capillaries. Ultimately that's the whole purpose: to carry oxygen to the body's cells and to remove the carbon dioxide waste products. Along the way, of course, blood also carries nutrients and a vast chemical trove of hormones, electrolytes, neurotransmitters, and other substances vital to life.

While many mysteries remain as to just how the heart works, it's basic structure is quite simple. The heart is divided into four chambers: the left and right *ventricles* on the bottom and the left and right *atriums* (*atria*), or holding areas, on the top. There are also four valves which make sure that once blood has entered a chamber it can't flow backward and cause problems. Blood is meant to flow in one direction and one direction only. In fact, the two sides of the heart are separated by a tough wall of tissue called the *septum*.

All those parts work in beautiful, orchestrated harmony. The workhorse is the left ventricle, contracting to push bright red, oxygenated blood out to the body. It's ten times thicker than the right to provide the needed musculature for sufficient contractions to get blood to all parts of the body.

Returning through the veins, or the venous system, "used" oxygen-depleted blood enters the heart through the *superior* and *inferior vena cavas*, simply the Latin words for "hollow veins." These two main veins bring all blood back for re-oxygenating to the right atrium. When filled with blood, the right atrium pushes open the *tricuspid* valve and blood flows down into the right ventricle. That chamber, in turn, pumps blood through the *pulmonary valve* and into the *pulmonary artery*. It's here that dark blood rushes into the lungs and exchanges carbon dioxide for fresh oxygen.

Blood with a full oxygen supply flows through the *pulmonary vein* into the left atrium and through the *mitral valve* into the left ventricle, where the whole cycle begins anew.

Everything works together. In fact, the complex system doesn't work at all unless everything is in harmony. While the left ventricle fills with oxygenated blood, the right ventricle receives its supply from the upper chamber. The ventricles contract together to send the blood off through the appropriate arteries.

Timing, as in all things, is critical. Your heart has its own "pacemaker," a specialized bundle of cardiac cells called the *sinoatrial node*. Located at the top of the right atrium, your natural pacemaker produces tiny electrical currents that cause the cells of the heart to contract.

Pressures within the chambers and vessels are of utmost importance, just as they would be in a boiler or your car's radiator. Blood pressure is a way to measure the force of the blood against your arteries. Needless to say, high blood pressure puts excess wear and tear on your body's "plumbing" just as it would in a boiler. We'll get into a lot more detail about blood pressure and what we can do to control it in chapter 15.

Doctors refer to blood pressure as two numbers, as in 120 over 80. The upper, larger number is the *systolic pressure* and measures the heavy work being done by your ventricles, specifically the pressure at the moment the powerful left ventricle of the heart contracts. The lower figure, the *diastolic pressure*, is a measurement taken when the ventricles are between contractions and reflects the lowest constant pressure on your arteries as blood comes rushing through.

On average, your heart beats between 60 and 80 times each minute. When exercising, that number can reach 200, depending on your age, fitness, and level of exertion. The important thing to consider is that the heart continues to function without much fanfare throughout your life. You really never notice it other than at those times when you might get a scare at a horror movie and your heart beats faster than usual.

All the heart asks in return for its efforts is the same oxygen-supplying blood it pumps to all the body's other organs. Normally that blood comes through a system of arteries that crown the heart and are thus termed the *coronary arteries*. The four coronary arteries are the *right coronary artery*, the *left main artery*, the *left anterior descending artery*, and the *circumflex artery*. But if the heart doesn't get the blood supply it needs through those vessels, problems begin.

ANGINA PECTORIS

The first inkling many patients have that something is wrong may be a pain in the chest, arms, or jaw known as *angina pectoris*, commonly referred to as *angina*. The term literally means a pain or strangling in the chest. Symptoms vary from patient to patient. I felt mine in the left arm and jaw. Others say it was the right, rather than the left, arm. I never felt any chest discomfort, but most patients do. How does the pain and discomfort originate?

The heart muscle has nerves that transmit pain signals to the brain just like any other organ, but pain fibers in the heart are sensitive only to inflammation or a lack of oxygen. The angina most of us are familiar with occurs when the myocardium doesn't get enough oxygen, usually because of an obstruction or constriction of the blood vessels. Because of the way nerves are interconnected, we might experience pain in the shoulder, arm, or jaw as well as in the chest. Angina signals that the muscle has become oxygen deficient, a state of affairs known as *ischemia*.

But ischemia can also be silent, with no painful symptoms at all. Your heart can be in trouble, and you don't know about it. The American Heart Association estimates that three to four million Americans may have these painless episodes of *silent ischemia*. Such individuals often go undiagnosed, and the first symptom may be a heart attack, sometimes a fatal one. In a way, then, angina is a valuable warning signal, one that should never be ignored.

Angina may occur during exercise, emotional stress, or excitement, or even while asleep or at rest. After a rest, the pain typically dissipates. And some patients may take nitroglycerin tablets, dissolved under the tongue, to dilate the heart's coronary arteries enough to get the blood flowing to supply the needed oxygen.

While most angina is the result of blockage within the coronary artery, some instances may result from a spasm in the artery, effectively reducing blood flow. No one is sure why such spasms occur. The phenomenon baffled physicians in the past who were able to detect no blockage sufficient to cause the angina, yet patients complained of the pain. Such patients today can be treated with a new class of drugs, the calcium channel blockers, which prevent the spasms from occuring. Details on these and other heart drugs are in chapter 16.

The decrease in blood flow to the heart during an episode of angina is usually only temporary and does not actually damage the heart. But if angina is ignored, it will get worse and may eventually cause damage. A rule of thumb states that angina usually lasts 15 to 30 seconds, not more than one minute. If pain exceeds one or two minutes and does not respond to rest or nitroglycerin, it may be owing to a heart attack. Far better to be safe than sorry, seek medical attention immediately.

For a while you're going to be overly sensitive to *any* discomfort, thinking that it's either angina or a heart attack. That's a natural reaction and all I can say, having gone through it myself, is that this, too, shall pass. You're understandably suspicious right now. But there are other reasons for the pains and discomfort. I discuss these starting on page 104, since many have nothing whatever to do with your heart and others are temporary phenomena which result from the trauma your heart has experienced. But if there's *any* doubt in your mind, call the doctor, get immediate medical attention.

HEART ATTACK

What happens if the blockage, constriction, or obstruction of blood flow to the heart doesn't let up? Obviously, the pain continues, unlike the normal episode of angina. And the heart begins to literally scream for oxygen for its depleted muscle. In a very short time after blood flow ceases to supply life-giving oxygen to part of the heart muscle, that part begins to die. We're now in the state of *heart attack*.

Doctors have given this a few different names over the years, but the meaning remains the same. Heart attack can be called *myocardial infarction*, referring to the blockage of flow of blood to the heart muscle. Another term is *coronary occlusion*, or *thrombosis*, the blockage of the coronary artery supplying the blood. Short-hand terms include an "MI" for the former, and simply "a coronary" for the latter.

Sometimes patients don't even know they've suffered a heart attack. They might pass it off as indigestion or some kind of strain. On occasion, the heart attack isn't diagnosed until years later during a cardiac examination. But more often the symptoms are more obvious, including angina, shortness of breath, clammy skin, restlessness, apprehension, nausea or vomiting, and sometimes even loss of consciousness. For me the most horribly memorable symptom was a vague sense of impending doom. Probably because I felt no more pain, especially no chest-clutching, Hollywood-style agony, I didn't recognize it as being a heart attack at the time. The diagnosis, as I mentioned earlier, was made from the presence of enzymes in my blood.

Those enzymes are released in response to the damage done to the heart muscle during the time of oxygen deprivation and signal the fact that some of that muscle tissue is, indeed, dead and will never return to normal or be replaced. The presence of an area of dead tissue in the heart will be detected on future electrocardiograms.

I was one of the lucky ones. I survived my heart attack. Too often, the first symptom of heart disease is sudden death. That was my father's fate at age 57 in 1969.

Researchers are currently exploring the role of emotions, personality, and psychological stress in triggering the *ventricular fibrillation*, whereby the heart's contractions become wildly erratic, which can result in sudden death. My father, I know, was under tremendous strain at the time of his death. And I was extremely distressed when I had my own heart attack.

Scientists are looking for what they think might be a chemical that precipitates the process. It may be that those of us who are affected may be unable to "turn off" the chemical flood as well as those do who cope with stress more effectively. This is another dramatic example of why we should all learn valuable coping strategies and relaxation techniques.

CARDIAC ARRHYTHMIAS

While ventricular fibrillation remains the most deadly of the heart's erratic beats, other abnormal beating patterns can cause anxiety, pain, and even death. Doctors refer to a faster than normal heartbeat as *tachycardia*, while an abnormally slow beat is *bradycardia*. In both instances, the rhythm of the heartbeat may be perfectly regular, with only the rate affected. Most often such *disturbances* are perfectly harmless. We call them *palpitations* when we sense them ourselves.

At other times, the rhythm of your heart is a problem as well. For example, the upper chambers of your heart may be beating at 200 to 300 beats per minute, but the electrical message might not make its way down to the lower chambers, and thus the ventricles beat at a much slower pace. This is called *atrial flutter*.

Some patients experience a phenomenon in which the top two chambers increase their rate to from 300 to 500 beats per minute while the lower chambers can't keep up and develop irregular beats. This is termed *atrial fibrillation*.

The most common, and most harmless, arrhythmia is what we commonly call a *skipped beat*, more technically termed a *premature ventricular contraction* or "PVC." Every child has experienced this while walking past a cemetery or down into a dark cellar. Occasionally PVCs are linked together. Two in a row and you have a *couplet*, three in a row are called a *triplet*. Still, in most cases, these are harmless and usually no medication is prescribed. Deep breathing exercises often are helpful in controlling PVCs, which are more worrisome than dangerous.

The harmless types of arrhythmias are called *benign* while dangerous ones are *malignant.* Fortunately most are in the first category. However, be certain to report them to your doctor along with information as to when they occurred and what the circumstances might have been.

Following bypass and other types of heart surgery, the heart's muscle is a bit irritable and jittery. That's understandable when you think of what's happened to it. So it should come as no surprise that virtually all surgery patients experience quite a few benign arrhythmias. You can view common, benign arrhythmias following surgery as muscular tics, which are annoying, but typically not harmful. Patients may experience these one or even two years following surgery.

If arrhythmias continue to be a problem, your doctor may wish to equip you with a *Holter monitor.* In this way you're wired with chest electrodes that lead to a portable electrocardiograph the size of a large personal stereo which keeps a 24-hour record of every beat your heart takes. You fill in a diary of the activities you engage in during that time, and your doctor can compare the ECG tracing with your journal.

For those arrhythmias that just don't go away on their own, especially following surgery, there are many anti-arrhytmic drugs at your doctor's disposal, including beta-blockers, calcium channel blockers, and digitalis. We discuss those drugs in detail in chapter 16.

CORONARY HEART DISEASE (CHD)

The culprit behind most heart attacks and virtually all bypass surgery is a blockage or narrowing of the coronary arteries known as *atherosclerosis,* popularly called hardening of the arteries. We get the word from the Greek *athero* meaning "gruel" and *sclerosis* meaning "hardening". The individual fatty deposits within the arteries are called *atheroma* or *plaques.*

Those plaques are a concretion of the flotsam and jetsam that flows through our bloodstreams. An analysis of a plaque reveals dead cells, blood-clotting substances, calcium, and, most notably, cholesterol. Just how those plaques begin to develop and grow within the arteries remains a bit of a mystery. Some feel that they begin with microscopic damage to the lining of the artery. Certainly there is a genetic component, with some individuals more susceptible than others owing to their family histories. Women have a great deal of protection until menopause, after which they quickly catch up with men in terms of rates of heart attack. And we know that in many populations around the world there is little or no heart disease, strongly suggesting a powerful environmental influence. Most authorities today agree that the process of atherosclerosis is slow and insidious, beginning in childhood and continuing into adulthood undetected and without symptoms until, in many cases, it is too late to treat.

We now know the factors which increase our risk of developing heart disease. Some we can do nothing about, including our genetic history and our age and sex. Others can be controlled, such as hypertension, diabetes, and thyroid abnormalities. And still others are simply a matter of lifestyle: elevated cholesterol levels owing to a diet of high-fat foods, a sedentary existence with little or no physical exercise, cigarette smoking, and obesity.

Ideally, heart disease can be avoided or at least significantly postponed by way of what are referred to as primary preventive measures. After we've developed the disease, and often after the heart attack or bypass has already happened, we start thinking about what is now called secondary prevention.

Happily we now have the proof that by implementing those secondary preventive measures and thereby changing our lifestyles we can stop the insidious progress of heart disease virtually dead in its tracks, and in many instances including my own and probably thousands of others, actually reverse the disease such that the blockage actually begins to disappear from the arteries.

HEART FAILURE

Certainly one of the scariest sounding terms in cardiology, *heart failure*, sometimes called *congestive heart failure*, conjures up images of sudden death. While serious, this illness can be treated and patients can live productive lives for years to come.

Heart failure simply means that your heart is unable to pump blood efficiently to all parts of your body. It may accompany or be the result of coronary heart disease or other conditions such as congenital or rheumatic heart disease.

The principal symptoms are shortness of breath, fatigue, weakness, fluid accumulation in the lungs or arms and legs, and increasing inability to recover from exertion. Recovery from physical effort takes longer and longer. Patients may also find they need an extra pillow at night to sleep well. Swelling of the ankles is common, especially at the end of the day. That's because the heart can't work hard enough or pump efficiently enough to get fluids out of the spaces between and within body cells. Years ago this condition was called dropsy. Blood pools in the lower extremities and this causes swelling.

While incurable, heart failure can be treated with a variety of drugs. Diuretics are particularly useful in getting the fluid out of the body. And a low-salt diet is in order to prevent additional fluid retention.

In heart failure, the heart compensates for its decreased pumping capabilities in two ways. First it enlarges by stretching its muscle fibers as well as by dilating or widening its vessels. By increasing the size of its chambers and vessels the heart can keep pumping out as much blood as possible. Of course there are limits to just how much a heart can enlarge and, once it is larger, there is increased risk of irregular rhythms. A second, potentially self-defeating, method by which the heart can boost its output is by beating faster. This brings with it a heavy toll. The faster the heart beats, the less time it has to refill with returning blood, thus ultimately pumping a smaller quantity with each beat.

The sophistication with which physicians treat heart failure today allows remarkable control and the best possible quality of life. Ultimately, however, there is no cure, and for those with a life-threatening condition the only remaining treatment is heart transplantation. While that certainly is a last-ditch effort, and a sobering prospect, transplantation becomes increasingly successful with each passing year. It can no longer be viewed as experimental. More than 90 percent of patients survive after the first year, and long-term survival is now well over 20 years.

OTHER HEART CONDITIONS

Although this book is not intended to be an encyclopedic overview of every aspect of cardiology, you might want to know a bit more about other, rather common, problems of the heart.

Aneurysm is a weakening of the wall of the heart or a blood vessel, most commonly an artery which is under pressure, with subsequent ballooning out of the vessel's wall. While some people develop aneurysms as part of their genetic history, others may find their arterial walls weakening as a result of the atherosclerotic process. Although a physician can often detect an aneurysm by listening to the heart with a stethoscope and hearing a distinctive *blowing* murmur, too often the first sign is a life-threatening internal bleeding that occurs when the aneurysm ruptures. Medications can be used to reduce blood pressure and to reduce the force of heart beats. Large aneurysms may be surgically removed.

MITRAL VALVE MATTERS

Your heart has four valves that make sure blood flows in the right direction. They open when blood pulses against them, and close immediately afterward to stop blood from flowing back. The mitral valve controls blood flow from the atrium, the upper chamber of the heart, to the ventricle, which is the lower chamber.

For a percentage of the population, however, the mitral valve poses special concerns and possible problems. Some people, twice as many women as men, are born with a congenital heart defect known as *mitral valve prolapse*. For such individuals, the leaflet or flaps which comprise the valve become enlarged and misshapen. This results in improper closing, allowing blood to regurgitate back into the atrium. When a physician listens to the heart with a stethescope, he or she can hear this regurgitation which sounds like a click or murmur.

For many patients, mitral valve prolapse presents absolutely no symptoms whatever. They may even be surprised to hear that they have the condition, which is often discovered during routine examinations.

Other individuals experience a variety of symptoms including heart palpitations or skipped beats. Some notice light-headedness, dizziness, or shortness of breath. And occasionally mild chest pain may occur. A few patients may suffer anxiety, sometimes even panic attacks, owing to the condition.

Patients diagnosed as having mitral valve prolapse (MVP) can often relieve symptoms with a program of exercise. In a study published in the

April 1991 issue of the *American Journal of Cardiology,* 32 women had frequent symptoms that had been attributed to MVP. Half of them were assigned an exercise training session three times a week; the other half did no exercise. By the end of 12 weeks, the exercisers had a significant decrease in anxiety, chest pain, fatigue, dizziness, and mood swings compared with the nonexercisers. They also had a general increase in the feeling of well-being.

For most patients, simply knowing what may have been causing their symptoms is sufficient to put their minds at ease. Most of those with this condition live a completely normal life and require no medication whatsoever.

But prolapse patients are at greater risk of infections of the valve called bacterial endocarditis. Doctors will frequently recommend as a preventive measure that such patients take antibiotics prior to undergoing any surgical or dental procedure which can introduce bacteria into the bloodstream.

Very rarely mitral valve prolapse can lead to serious heart beat disturbances which can result in stroke or even sudden death. Bear in mind, however, that such occurrences are very rare. Your doctor is in the best position to put your condition into proper perspective.

If examination with a stethoscope reveals a mitral valve problem, or, for that matter, an abnormality of any of the heart valves, you'll probably be asked to have an echocardiogram performed, a procedure by which the anatomy of the heart and its structures can be studied via sound waves. Today an echocardiogram can be conducted at the same time as a treadmill test to see how the heart and its valves perform during exercise.

Finally, about five percent of patients with mitral valve prolapse will require surgery. In some instances the valve can be repaired, and in others it will be replaced with an artificial valve.

Rheumatic Fever can damage heart valves, making them stiff and incapable of closing properly. Though the illness may occur in childhood, valvular damage isn't immediately seen and may not show up until well into adulthood.

TESTING YOUR HEART

By now you've been poked, probed, wired, monitored, measured, tested, and analyzed until you're sick of it all. Most of that testing is now in the past, but you're still in for more of the same in the months and years to come. While I hope that your doctors have informed you about these tests in general, you might still have some questions remaining.

Electrocardiogram (ECG or EKG). Your heart is driven by a mild electrical current; problems can be noted by changes in this activity. To measure your heart's electrical patterns and to diagnose heart ailments, physicians take an electrocardiogram, abbreviated ECG or EKG. This produces a detailed graph called a tracing that, with some accuracy, reveals your heart's condition.

As you no doubt know by now, ECGs are noninvasive and cause no pain. The electrical activity comes from your heart, not from the electrodes which are affixed to your chest and limbs, and is measured by the apparatus to which the wires lead.

To the casual observer, the ECG tracings look like squiggly lines. But each beat of your heart produces a specific series of waves which are designated as the P, Q, R, S, and T waves. Ventricular activity, reflecting the power of your heart, is measured by the Q, R, and S waves, which make up the spike you see on the graph. The Q begins the spike, the R is its apex, and the S, which descends a little lower than the Q, finishes it. As the ventricles relax, the T wave measures this relaxation. The P wave is the slight rise that occurs just before the spike, triggered by activity in your heart that occurs right before your heart's chambers contract. Take a look at the sample ECG tracing in Figure 2 on page 96.

Variations from the normal P, Q, R, S, and T waves indicate cardiac abnormalities. For instance, a depressed ST segment indicates that insufficient oxygen is getting to the heart's muscle. Note that the ECG does not measure or examine your arteries, but rather the heart muscle itself. One can indirectly assume that the arteries are not supplying sufficient blood, for example, if one notes the depressed ST segment.

Exercise Stress Test (Treadmill Test). While a resting ECG, taken while you lie back on a table, can give valuable information, there are

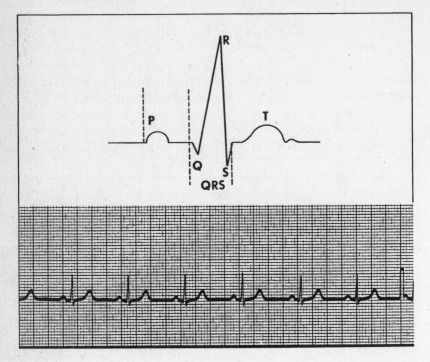

FIGURE 2

The Normal Electrocardiogram (ECG/EKG)

distinct limits to its diagnostic abilities. Most of us don't spend our days just lying down. The exercise stress test, then, can measure our heart's activity during the stress placed on it by increments of exercise, usually on a treadmill. The more the exercise, the more oxygen the heart requires, and the more blood will have to flow through the coronary arteries. On the other hand, the stress of exercise is not always responsible for oxygen deficits. Emotional stress may play a much greater role in some patients' lives. To measure such stress as it occurs throughout a normal, typical day, one might be asked to wear a Holter monitor, which, as noted earlier, is a miniaturized ECG machine.

Your doctor will want you to have regular exercise stress tests following your heart attack or bypass surgery. This will enable both you and your doctor to determine just what level of exercise you can safely reach. Such testing is quite safe. Bear in mind that your heart's activities are clearly displayed on the monitor or ECG tracing as you walk or run on the treadmill. The odds of having a heart attack at this time are really remote, as your doctor can see how well you're doing before advancing to the next level of exertion.

The test's greatest flaw lies in a rather high rate of false positives. That is to say, a patient's heart may appear to be functioning abnormally when in actuality all is well. If any abnormality shows up on the ECG, you may be asked to have further testing.

You may have had an exercise stress test in the hospital before release following your heart attack or bypass. At that time you were asked to exert yourself to an extent far below your maximum potential. From that test your doctor was able to predict that you would do well at home, and that typical physical activity would do no harm.

Eventually you're asked to take a more extensive treadmill test to determine your full physical capabilities. It is most likely that your physician will keep your level of exertion below the maximum to be expected for someone your age who has not developed heart disease. From this test he will be able to tell you, for example, that your top exercising heart rate should be in a range between 120 and 130. For you, this is a better guide than the standard heart-rate formulas. We'll talk in far greater detail about such matters in the chapters on cardiac rehabilitation and exercise.

Echocardiogram. This test, performed in a hospital or doctor's office, uses ultrasound to determine the internal size of the heart chambers, the thickness of chamber walls, any fluid buildup around the heart, contractibility of the heart muscle, and the condition of the heart valves.

With an echocardiogram, which is noninvasive, high-frequency sound waves are beamed at the heart via a transducer. Those waves are reflected back to the transducer, and are fed into an echocardiograph machine. The apparatus translates the signals to either a picture on a monitor which can be videotaped or to a graph on paper.

The echocardiogram may be performed at the same time you are given a treadmill stress test. It can detect any abnormal muscle contraction during exercise.

Thallium Stress Test. Sometimes a doctor will want to confirm a diagnosis obtained by way of a treadmill test, or he needs more precise information. Perhaps he doubts the positive treadmill results. He may, at such times, call for this type of testing, which is performed in a specially equipped hospital or outpatient facility. The thallium stress test, or scan as it is sometimes called, is highly accurate, easy to administer, and does not require a stay in the hospital. Moreover, this is a noninvasive procedure, as compared with the angiogram.

In addition to ECG electrodes, the patient receives an intravenous line in the arm. When the subject reaches peak heart rate, a small amount of the radioactive isotope thallium is injected through the IV line. At this point the patient lies down on an examining table and a scanning camera moves across him. Portions of the heart that receive inadequate blood flow and oxygen will show decreased thallium absorption. The patient and the doctor are able to look at a picture formed of the heart and actually see affected areas.

There is no need to be concerned about the radioactivity since so very little is involved. The test is extremely safe. It is far more accurate than the standard treadmill test, and very often will be reassuring to both the doctor and patient in proving that the positive result from the treadmill was false.

Angiography: Cardiac Catheterization. The most informative test available is, unfortunately, invasive. That is to say, the doctor makes a direct examination of the health of the heart and its arteries. At this time, cardiac catheterization remains the gold standard in testing. When a surgeon needs to plot and plan an upcoming bypass operation, it is mandatory to have an accurate map of the blockage of the coronary arteries and of the health of the heart. At other times it is necessary to provide a definitive diagnosis of conditions indicated by ECGs and other tests.

The term *cardiac catheterization* refers to the fact that a catheter, a long, flexible tube, is inserted through a needle in either the groin or the inside of the elbow and threaded through the arterial system on into the heart itself. Doctors view the progress of the catheter by way of a fluoroscope which provides a picture on a TV monitor. The patient remains awake and conscious throughout the procedure, though sedated.

Once in the heart, the catheter lets the doctor, usually a cardiologist, take blood samples and pressure readings. The former are analyzed for oxygen content and can point to problems such as leaks or defects in the heart walls. The latter may indicate scarred or narrowed valves as well as help to gauge the heart's ability to pump blood. The picture of the heart obtained is called the *cardiogram*.

To examine the left ventricle, the catheter is inserted into the chamber, dye is released, and a *ventriculogram* is taken. This helps determine the heart's *ejection fraction*, which is the percentage of blood the left ventricle pumps out with each beat. The normal fraction is about 60 percent; a diseased heart may pump 30 percent or less.

In some cases, *pulmonary angiography* is performed. The catheter is threaded to the right side of the heart into the pulmonary arteries. Dye is injected and X rays are taken. The resulting pictures show any abnormalities in those arteries, perhaps detecting a pulmonary embolism or blockage.

The next step is *angiography*, taking pictures of the coronary arteries called *angiograms*. The doctor threads the catheter into one artery at a time and injects a bit of dye. Blockages are immediately spotted, and the percentages of blockage can be measured very accurately.

After the catheterization has been completed, the patient is taken to a recovery area for 6 to 8 hours. If entry was through the groin, pressure is applied to the site until potential bleeding has ceased. In the case of entry through the crook of the arm, the area is sutured. Groin entry requires only a puncture. Both procedures have their distinct advantages, and your doctor will determine which is best in your case.

While in the recovery area, you'll be asked to drink a lot of water to allow your kidneys to flush the dye out of your system.

On the one hand, catheterization is quite safe; on the other hand, as with all invasive procedures, there is a degree of risk. About one in 1,000 patients suffers a heart attack during or within 24 hours of catheterization. The procedure may also produce arrhythmias or hemorrhaging. On rare occasions the patient could be allergic to the dye used. But, despite all that, the general consensus in the medical community is that the benefits far outweigh the risk when catheterization is indicated. The bottom line here is that while this method of testing should not be undertaken frivolously, just out of curiosity to take a closer look, it need not be feared.

I've had three catheterizations, two through the arm and one through the groin. While I must admit a degree of anxiety beforehand, the procedure isn't painful or difficult. Of course, the latest angiogram gave me the wonderful results indicating that my program has kept my bypass grafts and native arteries free and flowing, and that was worth any degree of anxiety. I have another scheduled in 1993, and I have no trepidation whatever.

Of course, by that time we may have other, noninvasive methods at our disposal. A new technique, magnetic resonance angiography, may eventually replace the conventional approach. Early results are extremely promising.

For more, detailed information on testing of all sorts, I recommend the book *Smart Medicine* by Dr. Bruce Hensel (Putnam, 1989).

TREATING THE HEART

An ounce of prevention is worth a pound of cure. Of course that's easy to say after the damage has been done, and in some cases dramatic measures must be taken to help a heart. Needless to say, doctors should and usually do take the most conservative approaches first. Diet, an exercise program, and medications may do the job well. But if all else fails, one can turn to today's medical innovations, approaches that were not available, unfortunately, when my father and many, many others had their heart attacks and died.

Pacemakers. Pacemakers provide a marvelous example of how a relatively simple procedure can save a life. A mechanical pacemaker can be implanted to replace or assist your natural pacemaker, the sinoatrial node, if it isn't "sparking" your heart to beat properly.

Several types of pacemakers are available. Fixed-rate pacemakers maintain a steady rate of impulses regardless of what the heart itself is doing. Demand pacemakers kick in only when the unit detects a slow heart rate or missed beats. Still others sense the start of the cardiac cycle and pass that signal on to the part of the heart with blocked circuits.

The procedure for implanting a pacemaker is done under local anesthesia. A physician makes a small incision and threads an electrode wire through a large neck vein directly into the portion of the heart that requires stimulation. A dual-chamber pacemaker sends one electrode into the atrium and another into the ventricle.

The pacemaker itself is then implanted, usually under the skin of the collarbone. Pacemakers operate without a hitch, typically, for many years. Pacemakers left outside the body are only temporary.

Angioplasty. What if you could simply push your arterial blockage out of the way so blood could flow more freely? That, indeed, is the principle behind this technique, the full name of which is *percutaneous transluminal* *coronary angioplasty,* or PTCA. The method is to thread a catheter through the arterial system to the heart, and then into the coronary arteries which are blocked. When the catheter reaches the blockage, a tiny balloon expands to squeeze the plaque into the lining of the artery.

Approximately 250,000 angioplasties are performed each year as an alternative to the more serious open-heart bypass surgery. About 30 percent of patients experience *restenosis,* or re-clogging of the artery shortly after the procedure. They require either another angioplasty or surgery.

If you might have an angioplasty in the future, you should be aware that research has shown that taking fish oil capsules prior to the procedure dramatically reduces the occurrence of restenosis. In research done at the Washington Hospital Center in Seattle, patients received nine fish oil capsules daily for a total of 4.5 grams of omega-3 fatty acids for six months before angioplasty. This was done in conjunction with a low-fat diet. Six months after the angioplasty, 35.4 percent of those who had not taken the capsules showed signs of re-narrowing of the arteries; the recurrence rate among those who had received fish oil was 19 percent.

Certainly some patients may not have six months before angioplasty. But if you do have such a waiting period, you would be wise to discuss this option with your cardiologist. Also, these findings do not justify taking fish oil for other patients.

Investigators are looking for other ways to eliminate the blockage without surgery. Doctors have begun using lasers to burn away plaques. *Laser angioplasty* doesn't just compress a blockage, it actually vaporizes it. This procedure is no longer viewed as experimental, but restenosis of 30 to 40 percent remains a problem.

Coronary Atherectomy. This is another method, by which a tiny rotating blade threaded inside a catheter is used to clean the arteries. One method involves a blade spinning at 2,500 revolutions per minute, shaving off plaque. Balloon angioplasty might be performed afterward to push any leftover debris into the vessel wall.

Coronary Artery Bypass Graft (CABG) Surgery. If medications and other treatments either fail to correct arterial blockage or appear to be inadequate for the individual case, surgery remains the principal method for repair. While still considered a major operation, CABG has become quite common and millions of us wear the telltale scar on our chests. About 350,000 men and women join our ranks each year, more than half under the age of 65.

The name tells it all. This is a procedure by which blood flow is shunted around portions of blocked arteries in the same way that traffic might be detoured around a construction zone. The surgeon will choose either the saphenous veins from the legs or the internal mammary arteries (also termed the internal thoracic arteries) in the chest to make the bypasses needed; sometimes a combination of the two will be needed.

The procedure, with two surgeons in attendance, is performed under general anesthetic and can take five hours or longer, depending on the number of grafts and any special circumstances. As the operation begins, one surgeon opens the chest, spreads the rib cage after cutting through the breast bone or sternum, seals bleeding vessels, and cuts through the pericardium, while the second surgeon harvests veins for the grafts.

Next, the patient is put on a heart-lung machine, which completely takes over for his own heart and lungs. This permits the surgeons to work on a still heart as opposed to a moving one. The various arteries and veins leading in and out of the heart are clamped off while the heart-lung machine operates. With an experienced team, amazingly little blood is lost, and transfusions can be avoided.

The surgeon then sews the grafts to the aorta and over the affected arteries to a point where the artery is not blocked or narrowed. Once all the grafts are in place, the patient is disconnected from the heart-lung machine and his organs take over breathing and circulation once again.

Finally the surgeons close the chest, wiring closed the rib cage, and the patient is sent to recover. After a day or so in intensive care, the patient returns to a regular hospital room to continue recuperation. Hospital stays vary, but average seven to ten days, and it may be up to six weeks before return to the full spectrum of normal activities and work. Of course, some patients do particularly well, and are up and about in no time at all.

Enormous progress has been made since CABG was first performed at the Cleveland Clinic in 1967 on a regular basis. My first surgery in 1978 was highly traumatic. I lost 14 units of blood and was kept unconscious in recovery with tubes down my throat for over 24 hours. It was a full year before I felt fully recovered, at least physically. For 12 months I was easily tired, cried frequently, and was extremely irritable. And, of course, I remained in a state of virtual limbo until the time I had the second surgery.

My second surgery was, in comparison, a resort vacation. Even though it was a "re-do" I lost absolutely no blood; in these days of fear of infection, that, indeed, was a blessing. Recovery was short and my lungs did not fill with mucus from disuse as was the case the first time around. My stay in the hospital was brief, and nurses had me walking the halls early on. Two weeks after I walked into the hospital, I was back at the typewriter. Within a month I was back to normal, doing my rehabilitation program, and well on my way to total recovery.

While there has been some controversy as to whether bypass surgery is performed too often, without sufficient justification, long-term studies at Duke University sponsored by the National Center for Health Services Research and Health Care Technology Assessment have shown that CABG does indeed give one a better chance at a longer life than if heart disease is treated medically. It's also important to recognize one major difference between the time CABG was begun and the situation today.

In the old days, CABG was viewed as a cure. One had the surgery and went back to the same lifestyle that had helped precipitate the disease in the first place. Moreover, the number of arteries that closed down early after the surgery was much greater than it is today, thanks to drugs and techniques used to keep bypass vessels *patent*, that is, open and flowing. And your lifestyle modifications, following the eight steps in this book, can keep those vessels open for years to come.

When I had the opportunity to observe Dr. Jack Sternlieb perform two of the procedures at the Heart Institute of the Desert in Rancho Mirage, California, I was amazed and impressed as to how smoothly the surgery can be done. There was none of the Hollywood-style chaos and yelling and sweating. Instead I watched a practiced team expertly orchestrate their movements. Hours later I spoke to the patients as they lay in their beds. That was in 1990, and progress continues.

But while CABG has become routine throughout the United States, one cannot assume that every cardiac surgeon and every hospital will have equal success. If you face the prospect of having bypass surgery, you owe it to yourself to do some careful research in advance. Every hospital must make its records available to you. You have a right to know how many bypass surgeries are done weekly and what the success rates are at the hospital you might enter and for the surgeon who might do the procedure. Shockingly, mortality rates for CABG vary from as low as one percent or so up to an inexcusably high 15 percent. You deserve the best! Don't settle for less.

The material I've shared with you on testing and treatment has been necessarily brief. Doctors and hospitals have detailed information on every procedure. Ask for it, read it, and become a fully participating member of *your* health team.

CHEST PAIN DOES NOT ALWAYS MEAN HEART ATTACK

Virtually everyone who has had a heart attack or bypass surgery or has been told that he or she has heart disease fears another attack. That fear can take the joy out of life and sometimes can be actually debilitating. All of us know what it's like to have one or more of the symptoms—chest pain, discomfort in the shoulder and arm, gastric disturbance, sweatiness, tightening of the jaw, rapid heartbeat, anxiety—and think that the next one is on its way.

But those symptoms do *not* necessarily signal heart problems at all. A number of quite different conditions can closely imitate the pains of angina and heart attack.

In fact, depending on varying estimates, anywhere between 20 and 33 percent of all patients having an angiogram are diagnosed as being free of heart disease. Yet even then, many continue to fear their symptoms.

It's very important for you to realize that these other conditions exist, and to discuss with your physician the possibility that you might be suffering from them. Indeed, as many as half of all coronary heart disease patients have a non-cardiac condition that also causes chest pain. If that's the situation for you, you need to clear the air and dispel unnecessary fears.

Gastrointestinal Pretenders. Often it's not your heart but your esophagus that's at the root of your pains. That's the muscular tube that conveys food from the mouth down to the stomach. When working properly, the contractions that convey the food are nicely coordinated and no one thinks much about it. However, stress, smoking, alcohol, diabetes, and other disturbances can lead to painful spasms or cramps in the esophagus. One form of the disorder causes contractions so strong and painful that it's known as *nutcracker esophagus*.

Another related condition, which some experts are beginning to think is the most common cause of non-cardiac chest pain, is called *reflux esophagitis* or *acid reflux*. In essence this is an extreme case of heartburn. Muscles across the top of the stomach act like the lid of a pan and keep food and stomach acid from spilling out. As we age, these muscles weaken and allow acid to flow back up into the esophagus. The result can be painful heartburn.

The symptoms often are similar, if not identical, to a heart attack. Patients wake up in the middle of the night sweating, with pain in the middle of the chest, a rapidly beating heart, and tremendous anxiety. The more they think about it, the worse it becomes.

First, one can distinguish this from angina since it tends to last a lot longer. Angina will pass within two minutes, while reflux pain continues, sometimes for hours. Second, there are differences between esophageal pain and a heart attack. The former tends to dissipate when you sit up and when you take an antacid, while those measures will give no relief from the symptoms of a heart attack.

There are diagnostic tests for these and other esophageal problems. You may require the care of a specialist, a gastroenterologist. Talk with your family practitioner or internist first.

Interestingly, esophageal problems can often be eliminated by the very same steps needed to recover from heart disease: quit smoking cigarettes, control stress and work on effective methods of relaxation, and cut way back on fat intake in your diet. I can't begin to tell you how many nights I lay awake in the past with those pains and symptoms, wondering whether I should immediately check into the emergency ward. Now that I've dramatically altered my lifestyle, I have no such scares. A very nice additional benefit.

Vaso-Vagal Response. A condition known as the vaso-vagal response can mimic many of the symptoms of angina or heart attack, including gastric upset, tightening of the jaw, and anxiety. This phenomenon may occur during times of particular stress. The best treatment is to relax as fully as possible with deep breathing exercises at the very onset of the vaso-vagal episode.

Costochondritis. You've been exerting yourself a bit more than usual, and you wonder whether you've really overdone it. Suddenly you have a wrenching pain in the chest, actually in the rib cage. As you breathe in, the pain gets worse. A heart attack? Probably just an inflammation of a rib or the cartilage or muscle between the ribs. Remember that angina and heart attack pain is continuous: changes in position or breathing will not affect it. With musculoskeletal pains, on the other hand, such positional or breathing changes have an immediate influence.

Panic Attack. It's now been estimated that one of every three outpatients who consult cardiologists for chest pain probably suffers from another great pretender known as panic disorder. People suffering from such panic attacks are defined as having discrete periods of discomfort or fear accompanied by at least four of the following symptoms: shortness of breath, choking or smothering sensations, faintness, dizziness, feeling of unreality, numbness or tingling, flushes or chills, trembling or shaking, fear of dying, and fear of loss of mental control. Studies have shown that 100 percent of panic disorder patients report severe palpitations and a rapid heartbeat. Two-thirds report chest pain or discomfort. Most such patients believe they have a physical, not a psychological, condition. Women very often are afflicted.

What really is happening to bring on those symptoms? Panic disorder appears to be a malfunctioning of the sympathetic nervous system, the part of the involuntary nervous system that controls heartbeat and blood pressure. Combine this with the symptoms brought on, as we've just discussed, by esophagitis, and you have a terrified man or woman who's absolutely certain that his or her time has come.

But what can one do? First, remember that nothing you do will have an influence on a heart attack. Then find out whether you can make some of those symptoms go away. Try doing some relaxed deep breathing; realize that this won't bring relief in mere seconds, you'll have to concentrate and really work at it. Do some of your gastric symptoms go away with an antacid?

The first panic attack will be the hardest to deal with and might very well send you to the emergency room for an ECG to be on the safe side. If the doctor can detect no cardiac basis for your symptoms, you might start thinking about these great pretenders. The next time it happens, and it most likely will, you might be better prepared. Better still, in the meantime you will want to work harder on lifestyle modifications that can make such panic attacks a thing of the past.

The mere fact that there are non-cardiac reasons for chest pain points out the need for a good relationship with a family practitioner, general practitioner, or internist in addition to your cardiologist. If you don't already have such a doctor, you'll be interested in the discussion of how to establish a good medical support base on page 177. Talk with your primary-care physician. Discuss your symptoms. It's one more part of your total recovery program.

CHAPTER 6

Women Fighting Heart Disease Too

When most of us think of Betty Ford, we remember the often-outspoken former first lady as the courageous survivor of both substance abuse and breast cancer. It's far less known that her most life-threatening fight was with heart disease. I had an opportunity to chat with her, and I'm happy to report that it's a fight she's winning in her own characteristically upbeat and positive way.

When Mrs. Ford first felt chest pains and shortness of breath, she had no idea the discomfort originated from cardiovascular disease. Climbing the steps of the family's Colorado home and walking up and down the hilly trails would put a strain on anyone, she felt. But an examination revealed serious problems.

Both arteries supplying blood to the brain were clogged. Surgical procedures called endarterectomies were performed to clear the blockage.

Later treadmill testing indicated oxygen insufficiency to the heart as well, owing to obstruction of the coronary arteries.

As luck would have it, the Fords were in Rancho Mirage, California, where they spend most of their time. That put her into the hands of Dr. Jack Sternlieb of the Heart Institute of the Desert. Mrs. Ford needed a quadruple bypass.

Recovery following that traumatic year was difficult. Simply walking from the study to the living room was an ordeal. She found it hard to remember words to complete a sentence, and feared she would never be able to speak publicly again. But recover she did.

"Once you get beyond the physical recovery following surgery, how do you put together all those individual steps toward a full recovery and return to life? They come in small bits and pieces. A very supportive family and cardiac care system was important."

Mrs. Ford took it one day at a time. "When I'd get discouraged, my husband would say 'Look how much better you are today than you were even two days ago.' "

At first the short walk from the study to the living room was a challenge. Then it was the study to the living room to the dining room. Next she began walking to the pool outside. Afraid she wouldn't make it all the way around the tennis court, Mrs. Ford had three chairs set out so she could have places to rest. And soon the progress was coming in leaps and bounds. "I got to the point I was walking a mile. I was so proud of myself."

But that recovery demonstrates the importance of taking it slowly, not expecting too much too soon. "I never set any goals I thought would be too difficult," she says. That way her efforts were paid off with success rather than failure.

Mrs. Ford was 69 years old when she had the surgeries in 1987 and 1988. Today she leads an active life crammed with appointments, commitments, and travel that would tire a person years younger. And she looks wonderful!

The former first lady never has played the role of victim. On the one hand, she's a take-charge person who's very much in control of herself and her surroundings. And on the other hand she takes the philosophy that ultimately she has no control whatsoever, that God has determined her destiny, and that she has to live and enjoy every day since none of us really knows which day will be our last.

Rather than being angry or hostile when cardiovascular disease struck, Mrs. Ford took it in stride. It's not so much that she has the patience of Job or that she plays the martyr role. Rather, there's an acceptance of life, the good and bad.

Today, her efforts at living a heart-healthy lifestyle aren't really focused so much on her former cardiovascular problems. Instead, both she and former president Gerald Ford live a life of moderation that benefits the entire body and would suit anyone striving to fully enjoy the senior years.

At first she apologizes for not being as structured "as I should be, as my husband is" about her exercise. But when she starts describing her day, it's apparent that she's doing things right. While President Ford swims laps twice a day religiously and does formal calisthenics and stretching exercises, his wife keeps moving throughout the day. "I walk a lot."

For her 70th birthday, shortly after her surgeries, the Ford children presented their mother with a cocker spaniel that needs a brisk walk four times a day. She takes that responsibility very personally, knowing the walks are good for both her pet and herself.

The dog goes with the Fords to Colorado, where they enjoy mountain hikes, and Mrs. Ford experiences no chest pains or discomfort at all. She revels in the fact that she can walk the stairs of the four-story home and can do all the preparations and tree-trimming when her four children and five grandchildren come for the Christmas holidays.

Taking great pride in her appearance, the still-photogenic former first lady watches what she eats as much to maintain her figure as to keep her cholesterol count down. The Fords use margarine, never butter. They eat very little red meat, relying on salads, fresh fruit, chicken, and seafood. Both enjoy cereal for breakfast, with skim milk.

Each day begins with 10 to 15 minutes of meditation. While not a regular church-goer, Mrs. Ford professes a strong belief in God, in a higher force or being. Her daily meditations help put life into proper perspective and get the day off to a good start.

"I believe in God's will. I believe I'm powerless, but I have to take the steps to make things happen. That relieves me of a lot of responsibility.

"My spiritual strength has carried me through all my recoveries. Trust in God is very important. Whatever higher power. You have to have trust. Sometimes it's hard to feel that way.

"If you get to a point when you start feeling sorry for yourself—'Why me?' and so forth—usually you can look around and see someone who has things much worse.

"The way I have been able to handle depression—though that doesn't happen too often—is to get busy and find someone I can help. That takes me out of myself, and I get well again."

Her cardiovascular ordeal has happily strengthened the Fords' relationship. "When I had my heart surgery, my husband was so frightened that I had a life-threatening thing that he realized he wanted to spend more time together. He's a very supportive person. We've both tried to cut back and spend more time together."

While many couples make such promises during the times of crisis, the Fords have carried theirs out. Each year they spend a week alone in New York City where they take in a few plays, do some shopping for the upcoming Christmas holidays, and see some old friends. Vacations are shared time in the sun, perhaps in Hawaii or on a cruise.

And although not everyone has the wherewithal to enjoy the lifestyle of a former president of the United States, each of us could benefit from the real heart of the Fords' pleasure: spending time together, nurturing each other, and appreciating one another. I've had the pleasure of being with the Fords at fund-raising events for the Heart Institute of the Desert Foundation. One can't help notice how they care for each other, exchanging a glance here and a touch there.

Love is terrific medicine. Maybe that's why Mrs. Ford takes only a mild anti-hypertensive drug, with no other medications. Today she gives very little thought at all to heart disease. Actually, her only complaint is about her arthritis, which wakes her once or twice every night.

During our interview in the offices of the Heart Institute of the Desert, we discussed the problems many women have with the inevitable scarring that follows surgery. She was surprised when I told her that many women go into depression about this, and hide their bodies from their husbands, undressing in the bathroom or under the covers.

Yes, Mrs. Ford wears dresses that fully cover the front. But she explains that that's more because of her breast surgery in 1974; she never had the breast reconstructed. And she passed on a wonderful anecdote about how she dealt with the issue.

After the breast surgery, Mr. Ford told her "Well, honey, if you can't wear dresses cut low in front anymore, wear dresses cut low in the back." She started to do just that, and with a twinkle in her eyes she says that "Sometimes I think that's sexier than gowns cut low in front!"

And this isn't just a solution to the issue of scarring. It's a marvelous example of the kind of communications and positive attitudes that can strengthen rather than weaken a relationship and speed along one's recovery.

Mrs. Ford provides a living testimony to the potential for a full recovery from heart disease. She has incorporated all the vital steps into a vibrant, productive, and enjoyable life. Annual physical examinations find her in excellent health, and each year her cardiac evaluation is a bit better than the year before. Women *can* beat heart disease and become *former* patients!

But Betty Ford's successful recovery from cardiovascular illness and surgery belies the grim statistics faced by women. The main problem stems from the surprise that Mrs. Ford showed when she was told she had cardiovascular disease. She had dismissed those chest pains and shortness of breath. After all, she was a woman, and women don't get heart disease. Right? Wrong.

Asked what they fear most, the majority of women would quickly cite cancer. We hear a lot about breast cancer and ovarian cancer as diseases that threaten women. But the little-recognized fact is that heart disease, not cancer, is women's number-one killer.

A woman's risk of developing breast cancer is one in nine. The chances of dying of heart disease are 50-50. While our society normally pictures the heart attack victim as a middle-aged man, just about 50 percent of the yearly 520,000 fatal heart attacks strike women.

Statistics from the American Heart Association put the matter into proper perspective.

- Between the ages of 45 and 64, one in nine women has some form of cardiovascular disease. After 65, the numbers jump to one in three.
- Each year heart attacks kill 247,000 women.
- Women who have heart attacks are twice as likely as men to die within the first few weeks.
- During the first year after a heart attack, more women die than men.
- Blacks are at even greater risk. Black women have 22 percent more heart attacks and 75 percent more strokes than do whites.

If you're a woman who's had a heart attack or cardiac surgery, you are far from alone. If you're the wife of a man with heart disease, take this information personally. It could save your own life.

Women aren't the only ones who live in blissful ignorance of the risks of heart disease. Their doctors very often don't take it into account either. A doctor presented with a man complaining of chest pains will immediately investigate the possibility of heart disease. A woman with the same symptoms might be checked for indigestion or dismissed with a prescription for a tranquilizer to ease family or career stress.

Then again, it's not entirely the doctor's fault. It's true that women do have protection against heart disease prior to menopause. Heart attacks in younger women are much rarer than those in young men. Doctors are trained to look for things they're likely to find. They don't think they're going to find heart disease in their young female patients.

The fact is that women's heart disease poses an increasingly massive problem. After menopause, especially, women begin to catch up with men in occurrence. After years of protection, seemingly through their unique hormonal balances, women pour fuel on the fire through their lifestyle risk factors.

Many, like Mrs. Ford, have a family history of cardiovascular disease. Her mother died of a cerebral hemorrhage, her brother died of a heart attack, and another brother also had to have bypass surgery. Yet despite that history, she never gave her symptoms a thought. And her doctors didn't catch the disease until it had progressed to life-threatening stages. Remember: this wasn't 20 or 30 years ago; she had heart surgery in 1988. And this wasn't just an ordinary citizen; we're talking about the wife of the President of the United States.

Up until very recently, research dollars in heart disease were spent almost exclusively on men. The Multiple Risk Factor and Intervention Trial was aptly nicknamed Mr Fit. It involved about 350,000 men in a massive, long-term research study. No women. The information we have about the use of aspirin to prevent heart attacks was gleaned from a study of thousands of male physicians. No women. Today, however, studies getting underway include both men and women, and one major study that we'll look at in detail focuses on women exclusively.

While the information will take time to trickle into every medical office, doctors are becoming more aware of the problem. In the meantime, women face far greater risks than men when heart disease does strike.

A study published in the February 1991, issue of *Circulation*, the official publication of the American Heart Association, shows that female heart attack patients have a significantly higher chance of dying before leaving the hospital than males. The report scrutinized data on nearly six thousand heart attack patients. After adjusting for age, the death rate one year after hospitalization was 12 percent for women, compared with nine percent for men. During hospitalization, 23 percent of women and 16 percent of men died.

Women fare more poorly on the surgical table as well. The risk of death during or immediately after bypass surgery for men is two percent or less, while that for women is at least double.

And coronary angioplasty, the procedure by which the blockage in the heart's arteries is reduced by a balloon at the end of a catheter, produces poorer long-term results in premenopausal women than in either postmenopausal women or men. A study at Duke Medical Center showed that arteries closed up again after angioplasty in 46 percent of premenopausal women, compared with 38 percent of postmenopausal women and 35 percent of men. The researchers feel that premenopausal women may have a more aggressive form of heart disease which calls for stricter attention and more stringent control measures.

Amid such negative statistics, however, you should know that, in the long run, women do as well as men in the years following their initial recovery from either angioplasty or bypass surgery. The problem is getting through the crisis.

But why do women face greater odds of survival and recovery than men? A number of factors enter the equation.

Ignorance is not bliss. Women who don't pay heed to warning signals such as chest pains and shortness of breath allow their condition to degenerate. Thinking that they aren't as prone as men to heart disease, women largely aren't as cautious as men might be regarding the factors that accelerate the process, such as cigarette smoking and cholesterol levels.

Yes, women do have greater protection against heart disease, in most individuals, prior to menopause. But that means that female victims of heart attack tend to be older than their male counterparts. Age itself puts women at greater risk of death and weighs against success in intervention efforts including bypass surgery.

Very often the disease has progressed much further in women who finally get medical attention than in men. More severe disease is more difficult to treat, with poorer results.

Obesity and diabetes are frequently complicating factors, more often seen in women than in men. Both are discussed in detail later in this book.

To make matters even worse, it's far more difficult to diagnose heart disease in women than in men. Treadmill exercise tests, used very successfully in men to determine the heart's ability to get enough oxygen through the arteries, results in a disturbingly high rate of false positives in women.

Fortunately, another form of testing, which utilizes a radioactive drug called thallium injected into the bloodstream to measure the heart's oxygen uptake is quite accurate for women. Unfortunately, the test often is not administered until quite late in the progress of the disease.

And when heart disease is finally diagnosed in women, the tendency is to treat conservatively with medication rather than angioplasty or coronary bypass surgery. The reason doctors give is that women don't do as well in those interventions. We'll look at that rationale in just a moment. But because doctors don't plan to do either procedure for their female patients, they don't do the definitive test, the angiogram. Only an angiogram can provide a direct look at the interior of the coronary arteries in order to determine the exact percentage of blockage. Everything else gives only an estimation of the severity of the problem.

Why do doctors feel that women don't do as well at bypass surgery? They point to female patients being older and sicker, thus poorer candidates for any surgery. They say that women have smaller arteries and smaller hearts that are harder to work on than men's. But they seldom talk about surgical skill.

Bypass surgery has become so commonplace, performed in hospitals in virtually every town and city, that we tend to take it for granted. But not every surgeon has equal success rates. Mortality and complication rates vary widely from surgeon to surgeon. And to make matters worse, with fewer female patients doctors have less opportunity to hone their skills on these more difficult cases.

Most hospitals show double the mortality rate for women when compared with that for men. But that's not always the case. Both Dr. Michael DeBakey at Baylor University's Methodist Hospital in Houston and Dr. Jack Sternlieb at the Heart Institute of the Desert report no differences in mortality rates based on sex. And I'm sure there are other surgeons and institutions with excellent case histories.

If you have been diagnosed as having heart disease, perhaps having suffered a heart attack, you may be a future candidate for bypass surgery. You owe it to yourself to check out the surgeon and the hospital prior to subjecting yourself to this potentially risky procedure. This is even more important for women than for men, although neither should blithely accept a surgeon without investigating his or her skills first.

Ask about their numbers, how many women have been operated on and what the success rate has been. Ask how that compares to the numbers for men. Don't settle for less than the best.

WALKING THE ROAD TO RECOVERY

Now here's the good news. Women can, indeed, expect to make a full and successful recovery. In fact, as one of the most respected heart researchers has pointed out, one of the first examples of the potential for actually reversing heart disease was a woman. Dr. William Castelli, director of the famed Framingham Heart Study which first put together a clear picture of the risk factors for heart disease, described the case during a conference in 1989.

The woman lowered her cholesterol level and got into a program of exercise. The first result was, in Dr. Castelli's own words, to "cure" her hypertension. The second was to reverse the blockages which had developed in her arteries.

In another, more recent, study by Dr. Dean Ornish in San Francisco, women responded to lifestyle modifications far more favorably than did men. The women, in fact, did less than men in terms of restricting their diets, exercising, and reducing stress by way of meditation techniques. Yet the blockage in their arteries lessened. Dr. Ornish concluded that "It looks like women may not have to do as much as men to reverse the disease."

Women appear to be more susceptible to influences both good and bad, according to Dr. Mary Malloy of the University of California at San Francisco, basing her remarks on yet another research project involving women. Those who continue adverse dietary patterns, don't exercise, smoke cigarettes, and don't control their hypertension, obesity, and diabetes do even worse than men. But those who do make those lifestyle changes do better than men.

Ultimately, then, you hold your destiny in your own hands. The first step is to become optimistic about your recovery. Before you can begin to affect your heart and cardiovascular system, you have to be in the proper frame of mind. Read the chapters in this book dealing with attitude adjustment, stress control, and relaxation techniques. Put them into practice immediately.

Perhaps it's owing to a more submissive role enforced on women by society at large, but women suffering from heart disease tend to take a more pessimistic view than men. They don't think they're going to do well, and that attitude becomes a self-fulfilling prophecy.

Women, too, can exhibit the Type-A behavior patterns which make them more prone to heart disease. Type-A women react with more stress to both marital and career conditions. They have more self-reported stress, tension, and physical health problems. Moreover, Type-A women tend to have lower levels of self-esteem and greater fear of failure.

A study of the employees at the Volvo automobile plant in Sweden showed that women managers experience the same kind of blood pressure increases and surges in stress-related hormones into the bloodstream as males. But when the men left work and returned to their homes, blood pressures and hormone levels fell. Women's stress levels continued unabated. The researchers suggest that this might be because men are allowed to unwind, while women carrying multiple roles in life must attend to another set of problems at home.

Dr. Margaret Chesney of the University of California at San Francisco believes that women deal with stress in more unhealthful ways than do men. She says that women under stress sleep less, exercise less, weigh more, feel more anger, and smoke more. It could be, then, that the resulting behaviors, rather than the stress itself, may be directly contributing to women's heart disease.

We do know that the same risk factors that place men in increased danger of heart disease, and that lessen the likelihood of successful recovery after a cardiac event, also apply to women. But in each case, there seems to be a special female twist to the picture. I've discussed each of those risk factors in greater detail in separate chapters throughout this book, and have kept the emphasis on their importance to women in the following sections.

CHOLESTEROL AND WOMEN: THE SAME BUT DIFFERENT

Women with elevated cholesterol levels generally are as much at risk of heart disease as are men. Both men and women should have a total cholesterol of less than 200 mg/dl, an LDL or "bad" cholesterol count of no more than 139, and an HDL or "good" cholesterol count of at least 40 to 45. For those recovering from a cardiac event, the goals should be even better. To stop the progress of the disease, or even reverse it, the total cholesterol should be in the 150–180 range, with an LDL of about 100.

But when it comes to HDL levels, most women have a decided advantage. Their counts are naturally higher than those in men, and respond more favorably to measures to increase those numbers. The factors that can raise HDL levels include exercise, quitting cigarettes, and certain medications.

But before getting too excited about cholesterol levels and making dietary modifications to lower them, it's important to realize that a woman cannot base her cholesterol risk on total counts alone. That's because women so frequently have a much higher HDL count. The result is a much different ratio of total cholesterol to HDL, which is a more accurate predictor of risk than total cholesterol alone.

A man with a total cholesterol (TC) of 260 and an HDL of 40 has a ratio of 260/40 or 6.0. A ratio of more than 4.5 places a man at risk. But a woman with an identical TC of 260 who is found to have an HDL level at 70 has a ratio of 260/70 or 3.7. A ratio of more than 4.0 puts a woman at risk. Thus the woman in this example would be at no increased risk, even though both the man and woman have exactly the same TC.

There have been instances of women being placed on prescription drugs to lower cholesterol levels when a closer look would have revealed a picture similar to the one described above. Moreover, stringent dietary restrictions may actually have an adverse effect for women, lowering the level of HDL more precipitously than that of the TC. The result would be a deterioration of the risk ratio.

However, elevated cholesterol levels which are not counterbalanced by increases in HDL must be contended with. This is especially important for older women. Dr. Castelli has noted that high cholesterol has far more negative impact on females over 65 than those under 65.

And not every woman is blessed with a high HDL. The only way to know for sure is to have a complete blood study done after at least 12 to 14 hours of fasting. Don't trust just one test. Get an average of two or three before making dietary modifications based on any given result. Remember, too, that cholesterol counts are lower for both men and women for the first weeks, perhaps as long as two months, after a cardiac event.

That complete cholesterol analysis, which can be done at your doctor's office or at a clinical laboratory, will also reveal the level of your triglycerides. While the entire picture has not yet been painted, it appears that an elevated triglyceride count has far greater negative impact on women than on men. A normal triglyceride level is between 70 and 150.

If you find that your triglycerides are up, even though your cholesterol count is normal, you should take steps to get them down. You can do that by increasing your activity level, by increasing the amount of omega-3 fatty acids you consume by way of fish, and by decreasing your intake of alcohol, sugars, and saturated fat.

STOP SMOKING THOSE CIGARETTES!

You'll recall that women may respond to stresses in life by smoking more. Both women and men adversely affect their potentially successful recovery from heart disease by continuing to smoke. The statistics on this are clear, as seen in chapter 12. Unfortunately, women appear to have a more difficult time in quitting than do men.

Some studies go so far as to say that cigarette smoking accounts for as much as half of all cardiovascular deaths in women. And younger women are picking up the habit more than men.

The picture is complicated even further for women who both smoke and take oral contraceptives. The combination of the two places women at particularly high risk of both heart attack and stroke.

THE BEST REASON TO LOSE WEIGHT

I know, I know, you've heard it all before, and you've tried a number of times over many years to lose those extra pounds. It's tough, even tougher for women than for men. But now you have the best reason in the world: to save your life.

Most statistics show that women who are more than 30 percent over their ideal weight have a greatly increased risk of heart disease. But data published in the *Journal of the American Medical Association* in 1990 show that there's no magic number. Literally *any* excessive weight, even just a few pounds, raises the risk of death from heart disease.

And, let's face it, we're no longer really talking about risk of developing heart disease for you. You have the disease. Now it's a matter of stopping the progress or even reversing it.

Weight loss provides one of the most obvious demonstrations that you're getting better. You can see the results in the mirror. And as you start looking better, you start feeling better about yourself, and that leads you to further commitment to lifestyle modification in a wonderful cascade effect.

But it's not just the pounds that count. Measure those inches as well.

As you replace fatty tissue with lean muscle, your weight may not drop as dramatically as the inches. And as you increase that muscle tissue you'll be able to burn more calories and thus lose even more weight. That's why men have the edge over women, since they're naturally blessed with a higher percentage of lean-to-fat tissue.

The best way to increase your muscle tissue is through resistance exercise, otherwise known as weight training. Don't roll your eyes up until you've read the data I share in chapter 11 on exercise. Even the most elderly men and women show tremendous improvements in just a short period of time.

You'll also improve your muscle tone by getting regular aerobic exercise, which you'll be doing as part of your cardiac recovery program anyway. Happily, as you'll be reading later on, it doesn't take a great deal of effort. You don't have to run marathons or jump up and down with skinny girls in their twenties. Remember Betty Ford's story. Do some walking.

And, of course, you need to cut back on the calories. The average woman requires 10 calories to maintain each pound of body weight. What's your realistic, if not ideal, weight? Perhaps you weighed 120 when you were in high school. But that was a long time ago, and maybe 135 would be a realistic goal, at least to start with. So, at 10 calories per pound, you'll need 1,350 calories a day.

That's not a starvation diet by any means. You'll be able to get all the nutrients you need from a wide variety of foods. And when you cut back on the fat content as suggested in chapter 13, you'll find that 1,350 calories represents a lot of food. You'll lose weight on a gradual but certain schedule, since you're feeding only the pounds you want, in effect starving away those extra pounds of fat.

Many people need help getting started. Women, in particular, profit from support groups. Weight Watchers offers a very successful, medically sound program that you can stay with for the rest of your life. Many YMCAs and YWCAs provide excellent community services as well. Or talk with your doctor or nurse about a hospital-based approach.

DEFEATING DIABETES

Twice as many women as men have what used to be called "maturity onset" diabetes, now known as type II, non-insulin-dependent diabetes. And here's a frightening figure from the National Institutes of Health: 80 percent of all diabetics die of coronary heart disease. If you have diabetes, there's no doubt that it contributed significantly to your cardiac event. And there's no question that you must bring your diabetes under control in order to prevent future risk and possible if not probable death.

Now that I've gotten that nastiness out of the way, I'd like you to know that you can not only control diabetes, you can actually cause the symptoms to completely disappear. It's entirely up to you, and there are only two things you have to do.

If you have type II diabetes, I can tell without even meeting you that you're overweight and sedentary. While this form of diabetes has a genetic basis, and you were predisposed to develop the disease, you developed diabetes because you gained weight and stopped getting enough physical exercise. Now you can literally reverse the process by losing the weight and increasing your exercise.

That may sound like empty promises to you, snake oil as it were. But talk with your doctor about it. It's true. You can partially or completely turn diabetes around, depending on just how much you're willing to lose that weight and get that exercise in.

You'll get some additional benefits as well. Diabetes, left uncontrolled, can lead to kidney failure, nerve damage, vision loss, and gangrene requiring amputation of the feet. Not a pretty picture.

The flip side is that by simply putting into practice the steps outlined in this book, you'll automatically come to control your diabetes. On a very positive note, you'll flat-out feel better than you have in many years. That's a promise.

BRINGING DOWN THE BLOOD PRESSURE

Elevated blood pressure looms as one of the "Big Three" risk factors for heart disease, along with cigarette smoking and high cholesterol levels. Here, too, there are special considerations for women.

Of the 58 million Americans with hypertension, half are female. Black women are at particular hazard, as are those over age 40 and those taking oral contraceptives. It's been said that blood pressure is second only to cigarette smoking as the precipitating factor for heart attacks in women under 60.

Recommendations from the National Institutes of Health call for treating women whose diastolic pressure (that's the one on the bottom) goes over 95.

A woman's hormones are much different from a man's, and may influence the way medications are used to treat blood pressure elevations. Fortunately, a great deal of data exist to guide doctors, and you and your physician will have to work closely together to determine which medications and at what dosages work best for you. There are many choices, and with diligence and patience you'll find the drug therapy that's just right for you.

But drug treatment is just part of the equation for controlling blood pressure. Once again we come back to diet and exercise. Weight loss can help bring hypertension down significantly, with or without medications. And exercise has both a direct and an indirect effect in getting the numbers down.

Although not everyone responds favorably to sodium restriction (see page 353), women, in particular, can benefit by limiting the use of the salt shaker. Even if this doesn't directly lower blood pressure, sodium restriction can limit the amount of fluid retained by the tissues. This, in turn, can help control weight. No, you probably won't need to go on a strict sodium-restricted diet, but cutting back will do no harm and almost certainly some good.

GETTING ON THE ACTIVE TRACK

It's no surprise that women have a very difficult time following their doctor's advice to do regular physical exercise following a cardiovascular event. For most older women, exercise is as foreign a concept as becoming a circus performer.

Boys get praised for their physical prowess at sports while girls receive attention for more "ladylike" behaviors. Sure, that picture's changing today, but if it's what you grew up with, it won't help too much now.

It's quite possible that you've not done anything very active in years, if not decades. You've become comfortable with your lifestyle, and now you resent the need for change.

To make things worse, cardiac rehabilitation classes are made up principally of men, not women. You may feel uncomfortable about exercising in front of men.

Yes, those problems all exist. They are recognized and acknowledged. But they do not justify refusal to take part in one of the most important aspects of the recovery process. It's just as important for women as it is for men to regularly exercise.

Here are a few tips I've learned over the years that can help you make the transition from "couch potato" to fitness enthusiast:

- Take a positive mental attitude that this is something that's really good for you and that, given a chance, will become actually enjoyable. Almost no one who exercises regularly for six months or more wants to abandon it. You'll feel too good to give it up!
- Treat yourself to a few spirit-lifting exercise clothes. Pick out a nice, comfortable pair of all-purpose exercise shoes that you can wear at rehab, in a gym, or walking in your own neighborhood. Find some perky outfits that reflect your positive outlook and commitment.
- Recognize that it's never too late to start. Just look around you and you'll see other women your age and older doing a variety of active pursuits. Visiting my mother's retirement village, I'm always delighted to see elderly men and women out walking briskly, riding bicycles, playing golf, and swimming.
- Find something you actually enjoy doing. For most, a daily program of brisk walking fits the bill. But you might like something else instead.

Experiment with a number of activities until you decide that one or two are best for you.

- Involve a spouse or friend. It's a lot more fun, and you're much more likely to participate, if you don't do it on your own. Many communities have walking clubs. Maybe you'd like to join a YMCA/YWCA or a health club. A number offer private facilities just for women.
- Keep a record of your daily activities in your daily diary. You'll see how fast you'll progress, and how much better you feel in a short period of time. Reading your own accounts of how you fared just a few weeks earlier will act as a more potent testimonial than any case history I could ever provide for you.
- Realize that you're part of an entire societal change that's gotten millions of men and women active. You're riding the crest of the latest trend, just like getting away from smoking cigarettes. View your exercise as a way to start feeling and looking better, rather than as just a part of a forced medical regimen.

HORMONES AND HEART DISEASE

While we certainly don't have all the answers about how a woman's hormonal balance offers protection against heart disease prior to menopause, there's no question that a clear link exists. And it appears that replacing those hormones later in life can extend that protection. This is particularly important for you, having already experienced one cardiac event.

Estrogen seems to affect the way the body deals with fats and cholesterol in the bloodstream. Numbers of research efforts have demonstrated that with estrogen in the blood, levels of LDL, the "bad" cholesterol, remain down while those of HDL, the "good" cholesterol, are up. We don't know just how that works. Nor do we know how the use of other hormones in oral contraceptives influence the picture.

Taking "the Pill" tends to increase LDL counts, especially when those pills contain a large proportion of progesterone to estrogen. Oral contraceptives also intensify the rate of blood clotting; young women taking them have double the rate of heart attacks, especially those who also smoke cigarettes. Women who once took oral contraceptives, but have stopped, have no continued risk.

Owing to the apparent protection provided by natural estrogen, doctors have long pondered the effects of giving the hormone artificially. For men, the results were disastrous. Those receiving estrogens actually had a higher rate of heart attacks than those not taking it. But that's not the case for women who have stopped producing estrogen owing either to menopause or removal of the ovaries.

As is the case with natural estrogen, supplements given to postmenopausal women appear to lower LDL and raise HDL. This suggests that women would receive protection against coronary heart disease. That might be particularly true for those who have both ovaries removed and thus experience a sudden loss of estrogen production. Such women are at double the normal risk of heart disease unless they get estrogen replacement.

The benefits may not be as clear for those who gradually produce less and less estrogen as they enter menopause. Some studies indicate that risk of heart disease, and the potential benefits of hormone replacement therapy (HRT), would be less for such women. Other studies offer promise that HRT benefits all women who are at risk of heart disease, especially those who have already developed the disease or those who have had a cardiac event.

Of course there are other advantages to HRT, involving a lessening of the ill-effects following menopause including reduction of hot flashes and balancing of masculinizing tendencies. Hormone replacement can also reduce the loss of calcium from the bones.

But there has been a major complication. Estrogen replacement has been associated with increased risk of cancer of the endometrium, the lining of the uterus, when that hormone is used alone. But when it's given in combination with progesterone, HDL levels tend to fall, thus potentially minimizing the protective benefits.

Women should also be aware that estrogen replacement may place them at greater risk of breast cancer. This is particularly true for those who have already developed that disease or who have a family history of it. This has long been a consideration when trying to reduce the hazard of osteoporosis, which is greatly increased after menopause. Give estrogen and the rate of osteoporosis goes down, but the rate of breast cancer goes up.

If this all sounds terribly confusing and frustrating to you, you're not alone. Doctors across the country are concerned. In an effort to answer some of these perplexing questions, the National Heart, Lung and Blood

Institute has begun a detailed three-year study. The Postmenopausal Estrogen Progesterone Intervention (PEPI) should shed some light on this complex issue.

But if you've already experienced a cardiac event, you probably don't want to wait for definitive evidence of the benefits of HRT. You should know that very encouraging data do exist, showing the benefits of an estrogen/progesterone treatment. In a study of more than 1,000 women aged 50–79, those getting HRT showed improvements in blood pressure, cholesterol, and blood sugar.

In two studies presented at the American College of Cardiology, women with known heart disease lived longer when getting HRT. Ninety-seven percent of those receiving estrogen survived for five years, while only 81 percent of those not taking the hormone were alive after that period of time. After 10 years, the number of survivors taking estrogen remained at 97 percent, while those without it had fallen to 60 percent survivorship.

To summarize, HRT offers the benefits of reduced risk of heart disease and future heart attacks, protection against osteoporosis, and alleviation of many of the symptoms of menopause. The disadvantages are potential increases in the risk of endometrial and breast cancer, depending on whether the estrogen is given alone or with progesterone.

HRT can be a difficult decision. Discuss it fully with your physician. A woman who has had a hysterectomy and thus faces no possible risk of endometrial cancer, has no family history of breast cancer, but has a medical history of heart disease might certainly be seen as a logical candidate for HRT. Another woman, having an intact uterus and perhaps a medical history of breast lumps, might not be as clear a candidate.

VISUALIZE A BRIGHT FUTURE

Happily, the long-term chances of having a complete recovery from heart attack and bypass surgery are as good for women as they are for men, once the critical first year goes by. You, too, can become a *former* heart patient.

But, just like men, you'll have to do your share of work to achieve that potentially elusive goal. You'll have to make your own commitment, based upon your own motivation. No one can do it for you.

Like Betty Ford, you can enjoy your life to its fullest, reveling in family and friends, holidays and travel, career and hobbies, and caring for others. Mrs. Ford is far from alone in her achievements. Many other women have proved that you can beat heart disease rather than surrendering to it.

Whether you've just been diagnosed as having heart disease, had a heart attack or cardiovascular surgery recently or some time in the past, or simply want to prevent the disease from taking its toll in your own life, start today by visualizing yourself as a winner rather than as a victim. Quite literally, close your eyes and paint a mental portrait of the vibrant, healthy person you can be. See yourself laughing, playing, working, making love, enjoying all the things that make life worth living. Then follow the steps in this book to make that picture a reality.

THE THIRD STEP:

Getting Back into the Swing of Life

CHAPTER 7

Sex After Heart Attack: This Chapter Rated XXX

I must admit that I'm more than a little biased as I begin writing this chapter. I absolutely and unequivocally like sex. No, make that *love* sex. I like everything about sex, the fondling, the hugging, the closeness, and the act of intercourse itself in all its wonderful variations. Sex is one of life's blessings, something to celebrate, and should be free of any embarrassment or shame.

Having said that, let me now say that there's no reason why having had a heart attack or bypass surgery should change anything in your sex life. If you were active before, you'll be active again. In fact, if you were inactive before, you just might become active again. And, especially if you follow the advice for recovery in this book, your sex life very likely will be better than ever before. That's true whether you're male or female, young or old, married or single.

Yet it's a sad fact that sexual dysfunction is common during cardiac recovery. Problems may be physical or psychological. Virtually any of them, however, can be resolved. There's no reason why your enjoyment of and participation in sex need be diminished at all.

Ultimately, many of the heart patient's difficulties with sex come down to misunderstandings. First and foremost, many fear that sex can be dangerous to their health, that it might even be fatal. That's just not true. Then there's the concern that sexual capacities will be diminished. That's not true either.

If one were to have an injury or a type of illness that would take, let's say, three to four weeks to recover from, and which would preclude sexual activity during that period, one would simply have to accept it and wait to heal. One would realize that the period of sexual inactivity is only temporary. But when it comes to heart disease, too many patients believe that they will never again be able to have sex, or at least to enjoy it as they did before. That's simply not true.

Yes, you might have to take some time off, as it were. That's between you and your doctor. Some doctors suggest that patients remain sexually inactive for anywhere between four and eight weeks following a heart attack. Those who have undergone bypass surgery usually needn't wait as long. Yet there are other doctors who see no reason not to engage in sex almost immediately upon return from the hospital.

Dr. Paul Thompson, medical director of cardiac rehabilitation at Brown University's Miriam Hospital, tells patients that if they want to have sex on the day they get home from the hospital they can. "In 11 years of practice," he says, "I've not lost one patient yet on that first day home. And I think by telling them that it is all right for them to have sex, it's a sign to them that things are going to be okay."

On the other hand, certain patients react very negatively. Dr. Herb Budnick, a Southern California psychologist who specializes in treating heart attack patients, says that following a heart attack sexual desire often disappears, and that it doesn't come back until patients address underlying issues.

Sex is very important to the vast majority of us. This is not a trivial matter. Some patients actually feel embarrassed, not so much because of a reluctance to talk about such a private subject, but rather because they're ashamed that they're concerned about what the doctor or nurse might view as a not very important issue. After all, isn't it enough to be alive? How dare one be concerned about such a mundane item as sex? Combine this attitude with an anger about the heart attack or surgery and a veritable time bomb begins to tick away. Sex becomes buried in a shell of denial and anger, tension begins to build between spouses, additional emotions foment, and soon sex is out of the question completely.

But why is sex so important? First of all, for both men or women, sex is a powerful indicator of self-esteem and self-assurance. And for both men and women, sex is also an important aspect of preserving their relationship. Dr. Chris Papadopoulos at the University of Maryland, observed a deterioration of the emotional relationship of half the couples who did not resume sexual activity. He also noted that a smaller percentage of couples who developed a more distant relationship, although they resumed sexual activity, reported a decline in the quality of sex. Now, more than ever before, the relationship between man and woman needs to be protected and strengthened. Sex, in all its aspects, not just coitus, can be a vital part of cementing that relationship.

Then, too, one should not lose sight of the pure pleasure sex can provide. Life is to be enjoyed, and sex is and should be a significant part of life's enjoyment. And what better time to savor the intimacies of sexual union than after a heart attack or surgery? Possibly for the first time in years, you have time on your hands. I can't think of many more pleasant ways to spend that time than in bed with someone you love.

When was the last time you made love in the afternoon? Or in the morning in the middle of the week? It's always been, "sorry, no time for that now," and off to work you go. Well, now there's plenty of time. Actually, mornings are an excellent time to make love, since you're both rested and relaxed. And, perhaps after a bit of a nap, why not relish an "afternoon delight"?

What about the risk of sex following a cardiac event? The old notion that one is going to "die in the saddle" is simply not founded in reality. As we'll see, sexual activity puts far less strain on the heart than the average patient imagines. All those tales of "going out in a spurt of glory" are greatly exaggerated.

The only exception seems to be sex in an extramarital situation. There are many theories about this one. Most references in the medical literature point to a scenario in which the man has had quite a bit to drink, has eaten a large meal, and is with a much younger woman. The liquor and heavy food have already made the heart beat faster than normal. There may be guilt involving the illicit nature of the affair. The man may attempt to prove his virility in an athletic performance. Perhaps he experiences chest pains but chooses to ignore them lest this younger woman think less of him. On the other hand, there's no proof to any of this. Simply enough, there are very few data because there are so few cases of individuals dying in a compromising position. The one study that's cited over and over in the medical journals is a Japanese reference in which 14 of 18 sudden deaths related to coitus were reported to occur with extramarital sexual activity.

In a marriage, both men and women fear for their spouses. Neither the husband nor wife wants to be responsible for the death of his or her spouse. As a result they may become overprotective. One woman's story is a sad example of just how far that fear can carry.

Every time they made love, the woman tenderly held the man's hand. Actually she was holding his wrist. In fact she was taking his pulse! Can you imagine trying to enjoy sex and to be spontaneous while taking your partner's pulse?

The reality is that the physical effort involved in sexual intercourse between man and wife, especially middle-aged men and women who have been married for quite a long while, is rather minimal. That might come as a surprise if not a bit of a disappointment to learn. The stress placed on the heart has been likened again and again to climbing two flights of stairs. The details of the physiology of sex are fascinating and enlightening, and we'll explore them in depth in the coming pages.

But there are other factors which undermine the enjoyment of sex. A major one is physical symptoms. Needless to say, it's impossible to enjoy sex while experiencing the pain of angina pectoris. Yet even that need not get in the way of a satisfactory sex life. Your doctor can prescribe drugs including nitroglycerin and beta-blockers that you can take prior to having sex which can, in many cases, completely eliminate the symptoms. Certainly this need not destroy the spontaneity of love-making, any more than the use of contraceptive measures would.

On the other hand, certain drugs can have a disastrous effect on sexual activity. The best source of advice, as always, is your personal physician. Ask whether any of the prescription drugs you're taking could have an effect on sexual appetite or performance. While it's not meant to be a replacement for discussion with your doctor, the accompanying table lists the drugs that could potentially affect your sexual activity. Bear in mind, however, that these drugs do not always adversely affect sexual performance. Moreover, certain drugs not listed in the table may affect you.

Prescription drugs are not the only substances that can have a negative impact on your sexual activity. Alcohol is one of the major offenders. This is ironic, since a glass of wine or a cocktail may be seen as a prelude to romance. Yet alcohol is actually a depressant, and a bit too much can ruin the moment. At least during the first weeks and months following heart attack and bypass surgery it's best to strictly limit alcohol consumption.

If you need one more reason to quit smoking cigarettes, your sex life is a good one. Each puff of smoke sends a wave of carbon monoxide into your blood stream, lessening the available oxygen to your heart and

TABLE 1

Drugs That May Adversely Affect Sexual Performance

Drug	Decreased Libido	Impotence	Ejaculation Problems
Heart Drugs:			
beta-blockers	X	X	
clonidine		X	X
methyldopa	X	X	X
guanethidine		X	X
reserpine	X	X	X
hydralazine		X	
digitalis	X		
verapamil		X (rare)	
Diuretics:			
thiazides		X	
spironolactone		X	
Lipid-lowering Drugs:			
clofibrate	X	X	
Drugs affecting the central nervous system:			
tricyclic antidepressants	X	X	X
monoamine oxidase inhibitors	X	X	X
neuroleptics	X	X	X
benzodiazepines	X (high doses)		
Anticholinergic Agents		X	
Miscellaneous:			
cimetidine		X	
ranitidine	X	X	
disopyramide		X	

Adapted from *The Medical Letter* 29 (July 17, 1987).

increasing the potential for angina pains during sex. Do something really sexy: quit today.

Some men have sexual problems prior to their heart attack or bypass surgery. In fact, many believe that the coronary bypass operation will cure their impotence and they're terribly disappointed when that doesn't happen. While there are many reasons for impotence, both physical and psychological, one cause may be a clogging of the arteries which supply blood to the penis to achieve an erection. If blood can't flow properly and abundantly to the penis, impotence can result.

In some cases, penile bypass surgery has been performed on men to overcome this problem. You might want to talk with your physician about this, and he might refer you to a surgeon to discuss the possibilities. On the other hand, we do know that arterial blockage can be reversed. One could certainly expect at least as much improvement in arteries supplying the penis as in those vessels providing blood to the heart and the legs. This should be even more inducement to practice the heart-healthy dietary and exercise lifestyle which will lower cholesterol levels and control blood pressure.

Whether you're having sexual difficulties or not, a good exercise program will, without doubt, improve your sex life enormously. I know it has mine.

Thus far we've been discussing some very real and solvable problems which can have an adverse impact on sex. But there's one that remains entirely between the man and woman involved. Simply enough, some patients use their heart attack or bypass surgery as a convenient excuse not to have sex with their spouses. If this is the case in your relationship, honesty is the best policy. It's cruel to your spouse and unfair to your physician to pretend that some other factors must be involved.

For some couples, the decision not to have sex can be mutual and will not affect the relationship. Friendship and companionship are enough for certain individuals. If this is the case for you, that's fine. If a lack of sexual activity is driving a wedge between you, however, perhaps a few sessions with a marriage counselor would be worthwhile. You might just find that, on a subconscious level, you've been getting away from sex in the past because of symptoms of angina. Perhaps by dealing with the disease directly by way of your surgery and the guidelines in this book, you'll find that you can once again enjoy a full sexual relationship in a way that's eluded you for years.

Although sex is so important, it's absolutely amazing that so little attention is paid to it in counseling for patients. Numerous articles in the medical literature bemoan the fact that patients are not given vital information, that they have so many misconceptions, and that their lives are being damaged because of this lack of attention. Most patients want counseling, but they just don't get it.

You may have specific questions that pertain to that most important patient in the world: you or your spouse. By all means, don't be shy about getting your questions answered.

Do you feel confident in talking with your cardiologist? Your family physician? Is the cardiac nurse who has been assigned to your case someone you can place trust in? Do you feel more at ease talking with a man or with a woman? Whatever the case, talk with someone.

Perhaps sex is so private a topic for you that you have a difficult time talking face to face with either a doctor or nurse. Have you thought about using the telephone? That might diminish the personal confrontation you fear, and allow you to talk more openly. You might even take this a step further and ask for the phone number of someone you haven't personally met so you can speak with him or her in complete anonymity.

For most individuals, sufficient information matched with a sound program of cardiac rehabilitation will quickly restore sexual normalcy. For others, additional assistance may be in order. By all means seek that assistance. You might want and need to spend some time with a psychologist or a marriage counselor. In some areas you'll have access to sex therapists, professionals who specialize in this field.

You may be unfamiliar with such therapists. They are not sex surrogates, individuals with whom a patient actually has sexual activity. Rather, these are professionals who provide counseling and who try to find the solutions for specific difficulties you may be experiencing.

On the other hand, you may have a very specific problem. You may be having angina pains or cardiac arrhythmias when you have sex. You've talked with the doctor about this, but you're still concerned. "If only he could see my EKG when I'm having sex," you may have said to yourself. Well, you can accomplish just exactly that. You doctor can equip you with a Holter monitor which gives a 24-hour electrocardiogram. You'll have a few electrodes attached to your chest which lead to a portable ECG machine the size of a Walkman on a belt you fasten around your waist. You'll be given a diary in which you'll record your daily activities, including sex and any other events which may affect your heart. The physician can then review your ECG for the day, comparing it to your diary. You'll benefit from the Holter experience in either of two ways. One, the doctor may give you the all-clear signal that even though you might have thought those blips you were feeling were significant, you have no irregularities to worry about. Then you'll be able to enjoy sex to its fullest, without worry or concern. Two, he might spot something for which he can prescribe a specific therapy. Perhaps that might be a low dose of a beta-blocker or a nitroglycerin tablet.

THE PHYSIOLOGY OF SEX

As you might imagine in this high-tech era, just about every function of the human body has been scientifically analyzed, and sexual activity is no exception. You've probably never given it any thought, but there are four major stages or phases your body goes through during sex.

Arousal: Your skin gets warm and flushed, your breathing and pulse rate start to increase, and your blood pressure goes up just a bit.

Plateau: You experience an increase in all the aspects of the arousal phase, with skin getting warmer, breathing and pulse faster, and blood pressure going up a little more.

Orgasm: This is when your heart works the hardest. Your pulse rate may go as high as 150 beats per minute while blood pressure rises. *But* this phase lasts only 10 to 15 seconds, perhaps up to 20 seconds.

Resolution: Your body returns to its resting heart rate and blood pressure within just a few seconds.

For most men and women who have been married more than a few years and who are in their middle years, the actual time expended on all four phases of sexual activity is relatively short. On average, total time elapsed is only 10 to 16 minutes. Of that amount of time, only four to six minutes involve elevations in heart rate and blood pressure.

The first, and still definitive, study measuring the intensity of effort and body changes during sexual activity in normal and postcoronary individuals was done by Drs. Herman Hellerstein and Ernest Friedman at Case Western Reserve University in Cleveland in 1970. Others have replicated those efforts and come up with similar figures.

Physiologically, young volunteers showed that during sexual activity, maximum heart rates vary from 114 to 180 beats per minute. Systolic blood pressure increased by 40 to 100 percent. Most of these changes happen in the minute preceding orgasm and return close to baseline within two minutes into the resolution phase. Of the different positions studied, the traditional "missionary" man-on-top position was the most physically demanding.

Dr. Gordon Walbroehl wrote in the *American Family Physician* that during sexual intercourse, a group of individuals who had had a heart attack achieved a maximal heart rate of 107 beats per minute. In a group which had had heart surgery, the maximal rate was 117 beats.

While there aren't a lot of studies with elderly men and women, figures most often recorded show an average maximal heart rate of 120 beats per minute for less than one minute and an average systolic blood pressure of 146. In one study that directly compared reactions, there were no differences between physiological changes in men and women.

What do those numbers really mean? Simply enough they indicate that sexual activity places no more stress on the heart than normal daily activities such as walking or climbing stairs or typical work duties.

Many men experience an erection while they're still in the hospital. I know I did, and more than just once. A good number of patients actually masturbate while still in their hospital bed. And they tend to start flirting with the nurses. Yes, I did that, too. All this is quite healthy, showing that the body is recovering.

So, since the sex drive is pushing you forward, yet fear may be holding you back, you want to know, right off the bat, how soon can you engage in sex once you get home? As I noted at the beginning of this chapter, the final decision is going to be in the hands of your doctor. Most will probably suggest a "rest" of a few weeks at least, with many still opting for the traditional four- to eight-week period of abstinence. On the other hand, a good number of well-informed physicians realize that sex will put their patients at no greater risk than the physical activities they're prescribing for them. Such doctors will give you the green flag much sooner.

Don't let your doctor off the hook. Get specific information. Sex is important to you. You've already gone without it for a while in the hospital. You want to express affection for your spouse or some special person. You want to experience that special feeling that comes with being alive and well. Ask him point blank: just exactly when can I have sex?

If you're having severe angina, if your tests have shown problems, or if you're having significant arrhythmias, the doctor very likely will ask you to refrain from sex until you have those problems stabilized. Even so, don't think that you will never have sex again. You *shall* return!

While you're talking with your doctor or nurse, ask how often you can enjoy sex. Probably the answer will be as often as you wish. That doesn't mean you have to prove anything to yourself or to your partner. No one is keeping score. Relax and enjoy it.

How do you you get started? The rule of thumb is to take it easy and not rush. Spend some time getting reacquainted with your sex partner. Do some hugging and kissing. Touch one another with no demands implied or intended. A simple caress is a sexual act, or at least it can be. A massage is always nice to give and to get.

If you're not quite ready to have sexual intercourse, consider the alternatives. Maybe you'd like to see how you experience orgasm. Will there be any discomfort? Pain? If it doesn't offend your moral standards, you might want to try masturbating. That's perfectly fine. Or you might take that opportunity to hug and pet a bit and have your partner provide manual stimulation leading to orgasm.

Another possibility is oral sex. Once again this will depend on your background and sense of morals. If you've never given nor gotten oral sex, certainly this is not the time to start. But if this is a normal part of your sexual repertory, oral sex can be a great way to enjoy your first orgasms. This is particularly true for bypass surgery patients who have to be careful because of their chest incisions.

Once you're comfortable with having sex and want to indulge in intercourse with your partner, you can select a position that suits you. There's a bit of controversy in the medical literature about this. Some say it doesn't make much difference which position you choose, others say to choose one that demands the least effort. The traditional man-on-top position is generally felt to be the most demanding. You might want to try a side-to-side approach, woman-on-top, or rear entry, otherwise known as doggy-style. Needless to say, surgery patients must avoid the man-on-top position for the first month or so until the chest incision heals and the chest bone mends.

More than a few couples enjoy anal sex, and so that particular variation should be considered. There seems to be a bit of controversy in the literature on this topic. Some say that anal sex stimulates the vagus nerve which, in turn, affects heart rate. As such they say to avoid anal sex during cardiac recovery. Others are less concerned. If this is something you and your partner mutually enjoy, do discuss it with your physician before engaging in anal sex. If you find it a topic a bit too taboo to discuss openly, perhaps it would be best to avoid anal sex until you're completely recovered.

In general, the guidelines for good, healthy sex during cardiac recovery are the same for good, enjoyable sex at any time. It's best to have gotten a good night's rest. Choose a comfortable place in a warm room. This is not the time to start experimenting with positions from the *Kama Sutra*. Nor is it a good idea to try it on the beach or under a bush in the park. If nothing else, placing additional burdens upon yourself or your partner is likely to make your sex experiences during recovery less than totally enjoyable.

You'll find yourself getting tired more easily after your heart attack or bypass. That's a perfectly natural part of the recovery process. Your body is working very hard to heal itself. Don't be disappointed in that. And don't try to prove your virility in the evening when what you'd really like to do is go to sleep. Give each other a hug and kiss, and a wink and a promise that something very special will be awaiting you in the morning.

By all means don't push yourself after having a big meal or alcoholic beverages. As it is, you very well may find that your heart is beating a bit faster than usual after indulging in heavy food or alcohol. Wait for a while, perhaps up to a few hours, before having sex.

It would be wonderful to say that there are never any problems with sex after a heart attack or surgery. Certainly such sex is safe, as we've discussed. Yet the reality must be faced that you're dealing with a very real illness, and you should be aware of some warning signals. If you experience any of the following danger signs, be certain to report them to your doctor, even if they happen just once. It's always best to be on the safe side.

The warning signs associated with sex include:

1. Shortness of breath or increased heart rate for more than a quarter hour after intercourse. Remember that heart rate should return to its resting level within two to five minutes after orgasm.
2. Extreme fatigue the day after having had sex, especially if you can't attribute the tiredness to anything else.
3. Any feeling of pain, pressure, or other discomfort in the chest during intercourse. Associated with this might be other symptoms of angina such as radiating pains down the arm or tightening in the jaw.
4. Irregularities in heartbeat during or immediately following intercourse.

5. Sleeplessness after intercourse that can't be explained by any other cause. Obviously this doesn't mean that you should fall asleep every time after sex in the morning or afternoon.

Your doctor may assure you that all's well and that there's nothing to worry about. Or he may ask you to note whether any of the above warning signals happen again. Or he may decide to try a medication to prevent such discomfort. Regardless of his decision, let him be the judge.

SPECIAL CONSIDERATIONS FOR WOMEN

The reality, unfair though it might be, is that most research in cardiac recovery, including sexual activity, has been done with men. Very few studies have concentrated on women. Yet women certainly have heart attacks and bypass surgery, and the numbers are growing every year. And women want to return to a healthy sex life just as much as men do.

Dr. Chris Papadopoulos at the South Baltimore General Hospital and University of Maryland interviewed 130 female patients who had had heart attacks. Of those women, 30 percent of those who had been sexually active before the cardiac event were concerned about resuming sexual activity. Primarily owing to fears, 27 percent of the women did not go back to sex, 27 percent were unaffected in their sex lives, and 44 percent reported that sexual activity had been decreased. Only 45 percent of all those women said they had received sexual instructions before leaving the hospital, and in only 18 percent of the cases was the discussion started by the physician. Fully 57 percent of the women told of symptoms during intercourse. Dr. Papadopoulos concluded that heart attack has a negative impact on female sexuality, yet the women were not getting the attention and information they needed to include sex in their full cardiac recovery.

Women are concerned not only whether they will be in danger during intercourse. They're worried that they won't be attractive to their husbands, that their spouses won't desire them any longer. Moreover, they fear that they won't be able to satisfy their husband's sexual needs.

This is all the more tragic when one considers that, for the vast majority of female patients, none of those fears is founded in reality. As we've seen, there is no more reason to discontinue sexual activity than to become physically inactive in any other sense. As we now know, quite the opposite is true. Doctors want their patients to be physically active, and that includes sexual activity as well.

Husbands need to be reassured just as much as wives that sex will not harm their spouses after heart attack or bypass. If anything, this is a time when even more caring, touching, caressing, and hugging are called for. And sex is a natural, healthy, wonderful extension of such loving.

While it's true that there has been very little formal study of women following heart attack, some observations have been made. Women may have a decreased ability to lubricate and to achieve orgasm. On the other hand this may be more the result of the stresses and fears associated with sexual activity than of the underlying cardiac illness. Unfortunately, problems women experience have a domino effect on their husbands, who may have problems with premature ejaculation, impotence, and a generalized fear of having sex lest it harm their wives.

The best advice for women must be identical to that for men. Sexual activity should no more be limited than any other physical pursuit. As cardiac recovery progresses, sexual activity is likely to increase in both quantity and quality. And all efforts directed at improving general health are certain to have a positive impact on a woman's sex life.

Women face problems whether they are patients or partners. As wives of patients, they share their husbands' fears, and in some cases they exceed them. That can be emasculating for their men. It's a fine line any spouse must walk, to care rather than to cripple.

What about the woman who has had a very lusty enjoyment of sex, and who has frequent if not regular orgasms. Her husband takes pride in her satisfaction. But immediately after heart attack or surgery her husband may not be able to perform at the physical level previously achieved. Now she may not have that expected orgasm. Should she fake it?

Honesty and openness are necessary now more than ever before. It would be a mistake to fake orgasm in order to protect the husband's sense of manhood. A more appropriate response would be to reassure the man that the sex was fully enjoyable and that it won't be long before the couple will be back to a full level of sexual intensity.

That doesn't mean that a woman should resign herself to frustration for the duration. While some may be quite content with hugging and touching and rather mild-mannered sex for the coming weeks, others may have a more difficult time in coping with the situation. Again, openness in the relationship is the key. You might want to ask your husband to help you achieve your orgasm manually, even after he has experienced his own orgasm.

By all means, talk about sex. It's been part of your lives for years, and we certainly expect that it'll be there for years to come. Talk about it now. Talk together. Talk with your doctor and nurse. If necessary get some counseling. But don't, please don't, let sexual frustration for either of you develop into marital discord. There's just no reason for it.

But what about single people or gays? They have special needs and considerations in their sexual lives which cannot be ignored. For virtually everyone, sex is an integral part of life.

SEX AND THE SINGLE HEART PATIENT

When I had my heart attack and first coronary bypass surgery I was 35 years old and single. One of my first reactions was anger that somehow my newly diagnosed disease was going to undermine my sex life. Not that I was a swinger by any means, but I had a normal, healthy sex drive.

Even in the hospital bed I began to have erections, and the nurses seemed particularly attractive. I managed to get the phone numbers of three of them, who subsequently came to my apartment to cook some meals for me during my recovery.

But what about sex? Was I going to die in action? There's no doubt that fear affects us all in this area, and age makes little or no difference.

Soon, however, I learned that the anxiety provoked by asking a girl out for a date was far greater in intensity than that generated by sexual activity, as measured by the rapid heartbeat I experienced in both situations. It became apparent that if other events which caused my heart rate to increase didn't bring on another heart attack, certainly sex wouldn't either.

In this discussion of sex and singles, I'm making a definite assumption that most if not all readers in this category are male, since heart attacks are relatively rare in younger females. Let's talk, guys . . .

We all know that women are different in many ways. They actually revel in their greater sensitivity. This is the time for you to put this to your advantage. Talk with your sexual partners. Explain your needs and your limitations.

You'll find that virtually all women will respond in the most wonderful way. Do some hugging, caressing, and snuggling rather than passionate, bouncing-off-the-ceiling sex. Women love it. Spend some time holding hands in front of the fireplace? Wonderful idea. Wait until the morning? Great, we can fall asleep curled up together.

Remember, too, that the same healthy practices you'll want to follow—low-fat diet, moderation in alcohol intake, and so forth—are just what the ladies want and need to keep their figures under control. Let them prepare some meals for you. It's a great way to spend some evenings.

But of course you also want to keep your sexual partners fully satisfied. First recognize that you'll be slowing down only temporarilly. Soon you'll be enjoying a state of health and vitality better than you knew before the heart attack or surgery. The time will pass quickly, and you'll be doing your Olympic-level sexual athletics.

In the meantime, you can provide full sexual satisfaction for your partners in a variety of ways. Oral and manual stimulation are, quite often, more effective in bringing a woman to orgasm than penile penetration anyway. You can perform in these ways without much sapping of your strength and without greatly increasing your heart rate.

Again, the operative word here is talk. Communicate with your lover. Find out how to please each other, both in bed and out.

But what if you aren't currently seeing someone? This is not the very best time to cruise the singles bars. Keep the true time frame in mind here. Many men have gone months without sex while in the military service, out at sea, or on foreign assignments. The time of your slight disability will pass quickly. And this will give you even more incentive to get back into shape as soon as possible.

In the meantime, call a few friends and spend some time catching up with old acquaintances. Maybe someone will know a girl you might like to meet.

Just don't allow yourself to get caught in a cycle of depression. View your cardiac event as you would an injury. Unfortunate, but just one of those things.

In talking with singles who'd had a heart attack or bypass, I was amazed that they and I had very similar mental attitudes at the beginning. Would women think less of us because we were "heart patients"? Most if not all of us go through a kind of emasculated phase for a while. Well, you should know right now that you have nothing to fear. Women don't react negatively at all. Many, in fact, welcome the notion of finding someone they might be able to take care of. In the years that have passed since I had my heart attack in 1978, I've never known anyone who's said that he had a woman turn him down because of having had a heart problem.

The reality is that, because you're now going to get into terrific physical condition, you'll certainly be actually better at sex than ever before. You'll be more confident in meeting women because of your glowing health.

Heart disease doesn't mean an end to your sex life. Play your cards right and it can be just the beginning.

SEX AND THE GAY HEART PATIENT

Problems for gays simply are more intensified. But the same principles apply for all of us. And whether you're gay or straight, you can learn something from this section.

Simply put, the threat of AIDS and other sexually transmitted diseases poses far more danger than that of sex itself. Fortunately, most members of the gay community have responded to the AIDS epidemic with intelligence and restraint, and the incidence of the disease in that community appears to be declining. That same intelligence can be put to use in assuring the safety of sex following a heart attack or bypass surgery.

As with heterosexual sex, sexual positions and practices vary in their appropriateness for early activity. Those requiring less strain are preferred. At the beginning, oral and manual sex are best. Anal sex may be overly strenuous. Moreover, anal sex has been thought to stimulate the vagus nerve which, in turn, affects heart rate. For both gay and straight patients, it's best to put off anal sex until the patient is fully recovered.

The other dangerous practice more often seen in the gay community than in straights is the use of various types of drugs. Amyl nitrite and numerous over-the-counter "poppers" adversely affect heart rate and can provoke cardiac irregularities. Cocaine, in all its forms, can be disastrous for the heart patient. Regardless of sexual preference, cocaine has been increasingly implicated in heart attacks in otherwise healthy young adults. Don't just cut down cocaine use, cut it out entirely.

The same applies to cigarette smoking. Cigarette smoking kills. To help you kick the habit permanently, read chapter 12.

Communication remains an essential part of good relationships and good sex after heart attack. If you're lucky enough to have a monogamous lover, talk about the situation and work on personal caring and tenderness rather than worrying about the temporary stops on more active sexual athletics. This is the time for touching, hugging, and loving.

If your sexual activity in the past has been largely impermanent, with meetings at bars and resultant sexual encounters, it's best to curtail such behavior temporarily. It's not the sex that might negatively affect your recovery, but rather the associated hazards of drugs, smoking, and excessive alcohol intake.

What to do during the weeks following heart attack for those without a companion? Immediately following the AIDS outbreak and its association with promiscuous sexual behavior, many gays turned to autoerotic stimuli including X-rated videotapes. This is probably best during the recovery period as well.

All things pass, and this period of recovery and sexual inactivity will as well. Your mental state is crucial here. Never lose track of the fact that you are now at the beginning of a new high in physical fitness. That same physical fitness which will confer protection against heart disease will also make you more sexually attractive and a better lover. It's well worth the work and the wait.

GOING FOR THE SEXUAL GUSTO

Most sexual activity places little strain on the heart. But what if you want more? What if you really want to get athletic? What if you want the judges to be holding up score cards of 9.5, 9.7, 9.6, and 10.0? Well, just because you've had a heart attack or bypass surgery, there's no reason not to go for the sexual gusto. You've just got to get into physical shape for those more exciting bedroom antics.

Here we can make a direct comparison. If regular, ordinary, rather run-of-the-mill sex takes the energy of climbing two flights of stairs, how many flights does it take to seek a new endurance record between the sheets? If this sounds just a bit exaggerated, let me assure you, it's not.

If you want to participate with full fervor, you certainly don't want to be wondering if that little twinge in your left arm means The Big One. You don't want your lover to be taking your pulse to see if you're

OK. You just don't want to let anything get in the way of this extra-special pleasure in life.

But how can you fully enjoy sex if you fear that overly enthusiastic love-making just might precipitate a cardiac event? The answer is to view sex as one more of the many physical activities of life. As you get into better and better physical condition, you'll be able to perform at higher and higher levels.

The man just out of the hospital is not ready to run a marathon or ski down an expert trail in Colorado. But all such things are possible, right along with dynamic sexual performance. Fitness comes gradually.

Today you can walk a few blocks. Tomorrow a bit longer. Soon it will be miles. And on and on. You'll feel better. You'll look better. You'll do better at all sorts of activities. Once you're regularly pushing your heart rate up to the training zone in your aerobic fitness regimen, whether in the gym or on the jogging trail or in the swimming pool, and keeping it there for 20 minutes, 30 minutes, or more, you sure won't be concerned with a rising heart rate in bed. As your sexual partner sees your increasing fitness, she won't be concerned either. The result: probably better sex than you've had in years!

CHAPTER 8

Returning to Work Without Hassles or Fears

Call it the Protestant work ethic or just the need to be productive, but most of us enjoy some sort of work in our lives. The notion of sitting around and doing nothing isn't at all attractive to the majority of men and women. As the old joke goes, the problem with doing nothing is that you can never stop and take a rest.

We've all known friends and relatives who died or deteriorated physically and mentally soon after retirement. Keeping active and alert seems to be essential to both health and happiness.

For those of us recovering from heart disease, return to work assumes an even greater importance than before. It signals a return to normalcy. Getting back to work really means we're OK again, back in the swing of things.

Certainly the money involved remains important to most heart patients. Sure, some are in retirement or close to it, but most of us are still in the prime of our lives, at the peak of our productivity between 40 and 65. The bills need to be paid, and even if disability is picking up some or all of the tab, we'd rather be writing those checks ourselves. That's a natural part of feeling independent.

But the sad truth is that a large number of men and women who have had a heart attack or bypass surgery simply never go back to work, despite the fact that they're perfectly capable of doing so from a medical standpoint. This has baffled and disturbed not only the medical community but also the insurance industry for many years.

Of course some patients are simply too ill to work again. Their disease is severe, and the cardiac event has left permanent, irreparable damage. But those patients are in the minority!

If you haven't already done so, it's time to have a frank discussion with your physician. The bottom line: are you one of the majority of heart patients whose event was uncomplicated and for whom the future looks perfectly rosy, assuming that you take the steps necessary to prevent another occurrence? Assuming you are, there's no reason not to go back to work as soon as possible.

If you happen to be at an age when that return to your job or career is optional, owing either to your personal financial security or your proximity to a normal retirement date, make your decision carefully. Don't burn any bridges. Your first impulse might be to "really start living" and spend lots of time with the grandchildren, do some fishing and traveling, and catch up with those things you've been meaning to do for years but just haven't gotten around to doing. Ah, that sounds great at first, but it might wear off faster than you'd think. And after you accept that gold watch, you probably won't be able to return to the desk or office you were so hasty to leave.

Talk it over with your spouse and friends as well, maybe even with a clergyman or other counselor. You and your spouse may be marvelously in love, married for many years, and each other's best friend. But being together day after day, every hour of every day, may prove to be a bit much.

Why not give yourself a bit of a transition? Make that return to work and spend some time really thinking about whether you want to give it up just yet.

If the time comes when you retire to more leisurely pursuits, be certain to factor in some productive activity as well as leisure time. Could you become involved with some charitable organizations? Are there some opportunities for consulting? Do you have an interest in the arts? Or education? Or health care in your community? Remember, like the television ad says, a mind is a terrible thing to waste.

Having something to do outside the house, rather than getting in your spouse's way, might also keep your marriage happy.

RATE OF RETURN TO WORK POOR

Discounting those who decide to retire or whose disease precludes further work, a disturbing number of heart attack and surgery patients never go back to the job. In reviewing the issue in an article in the *Journal of the American Medical Association,* the authors point out that in the past 30 years there have been major advances in reducing the mortality associated with heart disease. But the percentage of patients disabled by this disease has not been substantially reduced.

What seems to be the main reason for this loss of productivity and man power? It's not the severity of disease by any means; that accounts for just a small percentage. Rather, it's the patient's own perception of his or her health status. Simply enough, these people think they're a lot sicker than they really are.

Here are some of the reasons patients don't go back to the job. Some are valid, some not.

- They suffer from anxiety and depression.
- They exhibit symptoms of marked hopelessness and excessive worrying.
- They embrace the role of being a "sick person."
- They stayed away from work for quite a while, and then decided never to return.
- They have insufficient knowledge of heart disease in general, and their own condition in particular.
- They have a poor body image and are ashamed to have suffered a heart attack or to have had surgery.
- Their friends and relatives tell them not to work or exert themselves in any way.
- They misinterpret their physicians' analysis.
- Their physicians are too conservative and facilitate the patient's role as a sick person.
- They view their jobs as stressful, contributing to their heart disease in the first place.
- They perceive their workplace as detrimental to health in terms of noise, hazardous materials, or dangerous activities or assignments.

There are also certain categories of patients who are less likely to return to work. Women return far less often than do men. The older the individual, the less likely he or she will be to go back. White-collar workers return more often than blue-collar workers. Those who have had previous heart attacks return less frequently than those having their first cardiac event. And if disability payments are generous, there's less motivation to work.

Some believe that having had a heart attack or surgery will keep them from promotions and the assignments that could lead to promotions. There's a nugget of truth in that fear. Society still views heart disease as some sort of final disqualification from the game of life. Not as bad as cancer, perhaps, but the attitude is there.

When I left my job in Chicago to come to California to pursue a freelance medical writing career, I never told any prospective employer about my past medical history. The irony is that I frequently landed assignments writing about advances in cardiac surgery and instrumentation. I never let on that I had special insight, but I must say that it often gave me an edge. It was only when I needed my second bypass that the cat got out of the bag.

The surprise was that by that time no one cared. The only question was when I'd be able to get back to the typewriter to take on more assignments.

Many patients have done just as I did, never saying anything about their heart disease when applying for a job. Most of the time no one asks, so why bother to volunteer the information?

Ultimately the return to work comes down to a personal attitude about oneself. Anxiety and depression get in the way of recovery in all aspects. And the ability to deal with stress becomes a valuable tool in a successful recovery in general and return to work in particular. More about that in the pages to come.

MEDICAL AUTHORITIES DRAW RETURN-TO-WORK GUIDELINES

In 1989 a 70-member blue-ribbon panel of cardiologists, other health professionals, psychologists, and sociologists, along with representatives from industry and insurance companies, drew up a set of guidelines regarding patients' return to work following a cardiac event. The panel, headed by Dr. Robert DeBusk, director of the cardiac rehabilitation program at Stanford University, published their recommendations in the *Journal of the American College of Cardiology.*

- Most occupations don't increase the risk of heart disease.
- A clinical examination and testing to evaluate left ventricular function, heart muscle at risk, and oxygen deficit to the heart muscle can be easily performed in most cases to provide an accurate prognosis. Cardiac catheterization is not usually necessary.
- Those whose occupations call for sudden or sustained high levels of physical effort, or exposure to temperature extremes, should be thoroughly evaluated.
- Based on such evaluations, most patients can be advised to go straight to full-time work. But some may need a gradual comeback or a trial period.
- Those whose work involves or potentially endangers the lives of others (such as air traffic controllers) should be carefully evaluated.
- The patient's functional capacity should be evaluated as soon as he or she becomes stable. That generally means five weeks after an uncomplicated heart attack, seven weeks following bypass, and one week after angioplasty. This will determine any abnormal responses to exercise. A full treadmill stress test at six months will be more definitive. Assuming that cardiac rehabilitation efforts have been faithfully followed, one can assume that the six-month stress test will show significant improvement and work capacity.
- If routine testing procedures don't give clear-cut information, more definitive measurements should be performed, including, perhaps, angiography.
- Psychological profiles, including reactions to stress and Type-A behavior patterns, should be taken.
- If necessary, appropriate tranquilizing medications can be prescribed. Others may respond well to psychological counseling.

Dr. DeBusk, who is considered to be one of the world's authorities on this aspect of cardiac rehabilitation, stressed the importance of the doctor–patient relationship. The doctor should spend significant and adequate time with the patient to discuss return to work, providing guidelines which should instill confidence and allay fears.

We're going to talk more about the importance of that doctor–patient relationship, and how to make sure you get the best possible treatment and counseling, in the next chapter.

Not only should most heart patients return to work, but also they can and perhaps should do so sooner rather than later. For openers, surveys have shown that putting off a return to work lessens the odds that the patient will return at all. The quicker you get back to a routine lifestyle—and that includes work—the better your chances for complete recovery.

Dr. DeBusk and his associates at Stanford studied the benefits of an occupational work evaluation in terms of shortening the time to return to work. About 200 patients recovering from an uncomplicated heart attack were assigned to one of two groups. In the first, they were given occupational work evaluation consisting of a symptom-limited treadmill test performed about 23 days after the heart attack and a formal recommendation to the patient and primary physician that the patient could return to work within the next two weeks. The other group received usual care, without the emphasis on work. There was no difference in age, medical status, or occupation between the groups.

By the end of six months, 92 percent of those getting the testing and encouragement had returned to work, while 88 percent of those who did not get the additional attention also were back on the job. That's not a big difference. *But:* return to full-time work occurred at an average of 51 days in those receiving special intervention, and 75 days in patients getting usual care. This 32 percent cut in recovery time meant an average of $2,102 in additional income! There were no more complications in the group that went back to work earlier. Couldn't you use an extra two grand?

You have a right to know about your health status. There's no point in being a cardiac cripple, performing at less than your full potential. That's essential to enjoying your life whether at work or at play.

The American Heart Association has come up with a very complete way of making recommendations for both recreational and occupational activity. The following breakdown for patient recommendations was published in the November 5, 1986 issue of *Circulation,* the AHA's official publication.

Take a copy of it (or take the whole book along) to your doctor and ask that he or she fill in the appropriate blanks. Then you'll "have it in writing" as to what your limitations and restrictions, if any, are, and you can proceed to live your life to its fullest.

FIGURE 3

Recommendations for Recreational Activity

Name _____

Diagnosis _____

Date _____

[ ] Category I   No Restrictions
                       Activities may include endurance training, interscholastic
                          athletic competition, contact sports.

[ ] Category II   Moderate Exercise
                       Activities include regular physical education classes, tennis,
                          baseball.

[ ] Category III   Light Exercise
                       Activities include nonstrenuous team games, recreational
                          swimming, jogging, cycling, golf.

[ ] Category IV   Moderate Limitation
                       Activities include attending school, but no participation in
                          physical education classes.

[ ] Category V   Extreme Limitation
                       Activities include homebound or wheelchair activities only.

Addtional Comments _____

_____

_____

Physician _____

Address _____

_____

_____

Phone _____

Recommendations for Occupational Activity

Name _____

Diagnosis _____

Date _____

[ ] Category I   Very Heavy Work
Peak load of 7.6 cal/min and above. Involves lifting objects in excess of 100 lb, with frequent lifting and/or carrying of objects weighing 50 lb or more.

[ ] Category II   Heavy Work
Peak load of 7.6 cal/min and above. Involves lifting 100 lb maximum, with frequent lifting and/or carrying of objects weighing up to 50 lb.

[ ] Category III   Medium Work
Peak load of 5.0 top 7.5 cal/min. Involves lifting 50 lb maximum, with frequent lifting and/or carrying of objects weighing up to 25 lb.

[ ] Category IV   Light Work
Peak load of 2.6 to 4.9 cal/min. Involves lifting 20 lb maximum, with frequent lifting and/or carrying of objects weighing up to 10 lb. Even though the weight may be negligible, a job is also in this category if it requires considerable walking or standing, or if it involves sitting most of the time with some pushing and pulling of arm and/or leg controls.

[ ] Category V   Sedentary Work
Peak load of 2.5 cal/min and below. Involves lifting 10 lb maximum and occasionally lifting and/or carrying such articles as dockets, ledgers, and small tools. Although a sedentary job is defined as one that involves sitting, a certain amount of walking and standing is often necessary. Jobs are sedentary if walking and standing are required only occasionally and other sedentary criteria are met.

Additional Comments _____

_____

_____

Physician _____

Address _____

_____

_____

Phone _____

YOU CAN AFFECT YOUR OWN ATTITUDE

We know that the best predictor of whether a patient will successfully return to work is the patient's own opinion, regardless of what his or her physicians have to say about the current state of medical affairs. Those who come up with comments such as "Oh well, I guess I'm unlucky; fate has struck me down," "I had a friend who had a heart attack, and she was dead within a few months," and "It's completely out of my hands, I have no control over this," are unlikely to have a good recovery. It's a case of self-fulfilling prophecy.

But you can change your own attitude. You don't have to steep and stew in your own misery, waiting for the pitiable outcome. How important is optimism? Researchers at the University of Pennsylvania checked it out. Here's what they found.

- Optimistic patients recover more quickly from bypass surgery and resume a normal life much faster than the pessimists.
- During surgery, optimists had significantly less physiological damage to the heart. Those happy-thinkers had fewer Q-waves (a sign of heart attack) than those who think the worst.
- Optimists released less of the enzymes following a heart attack than pessimists.

An article in the *Journal of Psychosomatic Research* revealed that patients who anticipated few problems regarding their future work had a threefold higher rate of return to work when compared to those who expected the greatest reduction in work capacity. Remember *The Little Engine that Could:* "I think I can, I think I can . . ."

Sometimes, in fact, patients seem to know better about their recovery prospects than even their own doctors. Israeli psychologist Dan Bar-On interviewed 89 first-time heart attack patients and their physicians. He found that patients knew more about how fully they would recover, and did a better job at predicting their recovery, than did their doctors. Those patients who made the best recoveries were likely to blame a combination of controllable and uncontrollable factors. They admitted that they were often hostile and angry and were under a lot of pressure at work. To aid in their recovery they intended to draw on their own strengths as well as on the advice and support of others.

On the other hand, Dr. Bar-On found, those least likely to return to work and other activities cited "fate" as the cause of their attack and the determining factor as to whether or not they would recover. They believed that being "unlucky" had led to the attack, and hoped that they would be "lucky" in recovering.

The realists, who were also the optimists, took matters in their own hands. Yes, they took the advice of their doctors and others and made some important lifestyle changes regarding diet, smoking, and exercise. And they made some changes in the ways they dealt with the stresses they knew were part and parcel of their lives and their work.

Here's another one of those adages that are laden with truth: "The Lord helps those who help themselves." Yes, ask for help. But don't forget your own responsibilities.

STRESS AT THE WORKPLACE

Ask a doctor why you had the heart attack and he or she probably will list the litany of high cholesterol, high blood pressure, cigarette smoking, and family history. Ask the patient, and you'll probably hear that the number-one reason was stress, either in his personal life or, more often, at work.

Now, it's not that those doctors are wrong. Those risk factors definitely come into play, and without them one isn't likely to develop heart disease. But the role of stress, notably in the workplace, is coming more and more into focus. For many patients it may, indeed, have been the precipitating factor.

Note that I say "precipitating" factor. I mean that literally. It's what may have caused the heart attack at that particular time in your life. I know that it played an integral role in my own heart attack, and I've listened to dozens of others recall how they were under a particularly difficult time just before the heart attack struck. It's the last straw.

Dr. Alan Rozanski at St. Lukes/Roosevelt Medical Center in New York, has shown that non-exercise-induced stress can show up as depressed ST segments on the ECG as well as or better than it can be shown on the traditional treadmill workout. He induces that stress by asking the patient to solve a series of mathematical problems or by discussing aspects of the patient's life. Can stress influence the heart? It's right there on the ECG tracing.

One way many men and women deal with stress, especially when that stress shows up as anger and hostility, is to try to console themselves with food. At those times when you'd like to kill the boss, you might turn instead to devouring brownies. And the weight starts to go up. What's one of the risk factors for heart disease? Obesity.

Of course, when you take your anger out on the refrigerator, you don't head for the carrot sticks and a glass of skim milk. High-fat goodies seem to have the greatest soothing properties at such moments. And up goes the cholesterol level, bringing in yet another risk factor.

Anxiety and depression are known to be associated with the kinds of patients most likely to have a heart attack. And according to a Gallup poll of 201 corporations in the United States, work-related stress and its resulting anxiety and depression are more prevalent than ever. At least one in every four workers is directly affected.

Today's stress-stoking situations include the threat of layoffs, mergers, takeovers, or labor disputes. Such incidents affected 84 percent of all the companies questioned in the Gallup poll reported in January 1990.

Workers are responding by filing more job stress claims than ever before. In California alone, stress-related complaints now are the fastest-rising type of job disability claim and may be costing hundreds of millions of dollars each year, according to the California Workers' Compensation Institute.

But You CAN Control Stress on the Job. By now you're probably thinking that on the one hand I'm telling you to hurry right back to work, and on the other hand I'm letting you know that the job's going to kill you. The fact is that you can, in this instance, have your cake and eat it too. You can control, at least to some extent, the stress in your job that could be detrimental to your recovery.

The first step to take is going to be the hardest, because you're going to have to admit to a flaw within yourself. You *allow* the factors or individuals at work to get to you. Only you can change this in yourself. You have more control over your world than you realize. No, you may not be able to control the physical world in which you live and work, but you can control the psychological world you create for yourself. Who really makes you angry? You do. You see something or hear something and you let it eat at your insides.

As Dr. Arna Munford, the psychologist at Cedars-Sinai Hospital in

Los Angeles, points out, people often say they have no control over things at work. Yet they really do. Take her example of an insurance executive who had experienced an MI and was afraid to go back to the office. Yet he was on a high-level career track, and not too far from retirement.

Dr. Munford talked to him about the things that made him really hot. He said that people demanded impossible things of him. Like what, she asked? Like the secretary always sticking a pile of notes and messages at him as soon as he'd walk into the office. He never had a moment to organize the day before the deluge she delivered. Asked what he was doing about it, he shrugged and indicated that there was nothing he could do. That was the way the day always started. The psychologist gently suggested that he refuse to take the secretary's stack, and ask her to hold them until he'd had time to organize his day. He'd never thought of that. He took the suggestion, and that was enough to turn his life around. Soon he found that he could say "No" to any number of people and obligations.

One of the first rules a recruit learns in the Army is: Never volunteer. Yet so many of us seem unable to keep ourselves from doing just that and bringing on more and more work even though we're already bogged down.

Is your boss unreasonable, asking too much or doing things the wrong way? Are you out of control? Now's the time to do something about that. It doesn't need to be a confrontation, just a private discussion. Listen to his side of the story as well. See if you can't come up with a compromise.

Can't do it directly? How about speaking with someone who has the boss's confidence and ear? Ask that person to intercede for you. You might just be surprised at the receptivity.

No such personal contact? Try an anonymous letter.

Some people aren't able to express their anger for fear that it will precipitate another heart attack. So instead of having an argument with the boss (or coworker, or spouse, or whomever), the patients stews.

Mark Twain advised writing a letter venting one's spleen, signing it, putting it into an envelope, and then filing it away in a drawer for a few days. By that time the anger, and often the offending incident, would pass, the writer's steam would be released without repercussions, and all would be well. Just another way of saying "count to ten."

The fact is, there's no evidence that hard work is a predictor of death. Many people like a busy schedule of work, and those at the top, including company executives, physicians, and engineers, have a significantly lower rate of death from heart disease than others who work at lower levels, even though they put in much longer hours and seem to be battling all the time.

You have a number of ways of coping with stress at your disposal. But it's up to you to use them.

- Take advantage of labor arbitration if its available. Talk to the union steward. File a grievance.
- Delegate responsibility to others. Even if they don't do as terrific a job as you know you could do, that's just fine.
- Learn to expect less of yourself. That doesn't mean that you've got to become a goldbrick, but just don't come down so hard on yourself.
- Stand up to the boss if you have a just complaint. Do it directly or indirectly. Maintain a "paper trail" of letters and messages with dates to fall back on; in most states, you can't be fired without just cause.
- Don't take it all that seriously. Your job or career is important, but it's not worth dying for, is it?
- Stop taking work home with you. That way you won't be tempted to keep at it to all hours, and you won't feel guilty when you see that briefcase in the corner.
- Give yourself a margin of time and space between home and work. How about taking a walk around the block between parking the car and entering the house? Or stop off to browse through a bookstore. Do something to "come down" before walking through the door.
- Try not to take it out on your family, especially your spouse. Instead, enlist them as allies, sources of refuge in this tough, cruel world.
- Do something nice for yourself now and then. Mark something like an appointment for a massage on your office calendar, and make a point of looking forward to it.
- Keep your car nice and clean, with some good tapes to listen to during the commute back and forth.
- Maintain a sense of humor. Learn a new joke now and again and share it with someone at the office. Rent a comedy video to view that evening. Life may not be a laughing matter, but laughing can make it easier.
- Keep a diary of the things that upset you. Then at a calm, collected moment, sit down and figure out some ways to cope with those situations. Maybe seek the input of others.

- Join a health club to go to after work. Do a bit of exercise and relax in the bubbling waters of the spa.
- Take a walk instead of going to the coffee break where you'll wind up eating the wrong foods while griping about work with your coworkers.
- Take a course in something you always wanted to learn more about. Maybe at the art museum. Or at the zoo. Every community offers some program of non-credit classes.
- Get into yoga. That may seem far-fetched to a level-headed person like you, but forget about those Eastern Zen origins. This is a great way to relax and unwind.
- Be diligent about your exercise program. There's probably no greater stress-buster on earth.
- Eat sensibly, avoiding those high-fat foods and trying not to eat late in the evening when the digestion process could interfere with sleep.
- Make certain to get enough sleep. Watching another late-night movie or talk show won't give you the rest that only a solid night's sleep can provide.
- Read a novel rather than watching a lot of TV. Reading is soothing and relaxing, while TV tends to be agitating, especially when you first come home from work and just before you go to sleep. If you have favorite shows, schedule them, watch them, and then turn off the set.
- Limit the amount of caffeine and alcohol you drink. Caffeine can keep you jittery all day and into the night, and can make you more likely to become easily agitated at work. Alcohol may seem the answer to a tough day, and the first effects are, indeed, relaxing. But alcohol interferes with a good night's sleep.
- Admit that you're not an island unto yourself and seek comfort from others. That might be a clergyman, an old friend, or a professional counselor.
- View life as more compartmentalized. There's time for work, time for sleep, time to eat, time to play, time for yourself. Work is just one part of life.
- Express your love more freely. Hug your spouse and kids and grandkids and others you care about.
- Spend some time at work as well as at home doing some meditation. That might be a formal kind of biofeedback, a few minutes of prayer, or a short period of deep-breathing exercises in a darkened office with the door closed. Review some of the relaxation techniques discussed in Chapter 4.

- Take a break from the day's stresses and distresses by doing some stretching exercises. Here's a technique developed by the Pentagon's John W. Woodmansee Jr.

Hand Rubs. Lean forward in your chair, rub the palms of your hands together as fast and hard as you can for two minutes. Relax.

Here are some additional ideas you can use in the office, in your car, at the airport, or while waiting for an appointment—all times when stress levels can rise.

Big Mouth. Lean your head back, open your mouth as wide as you can, and hold it like that for about five to ten seconds. Repeat two or three times.

Arm Reaches. Slowly stretch your arms out to your sides, then up toward the ceiling, reaching as high as you can, and finally grasping your hands together. Hold that for 10 to 15 seconds. Repeat.

Elbow Pull. Put your right hand on your right shoulder, lift the elbow toward the ceiling until you feel the pull. Repeat with the other arm.

Shoulder Shrugs. Let your chin drop to your chest, and simply shrug your shoulders for a few seconds. Relax and repeat.

Back Pulls. Grasp your hands behind your back and lift upward, causing your torso and head to lean forward. Hold for a few seconds. Then lift your head back, with the nose now pointing to the ceiling. Hold and relax.

Mark your calendar, put little notes for yourself around your desk and office and in your attaché case, and otherwise remind yourself to do those simple stretches frequently during the day. You'll be absolutely amazed at how much good they can do for you. In fact, to prove it to yourself, try each one of the stretches right now so you don't just pass over this extremely valuable pointer.

- Avoid eating candy for those quick little pick-ups you might feel you need during the afternoon. A better energy boost is to take a walk. Want proof? It comes from researchers at California State University at Long Beach. They found that a brisk, 12-minute walk provided more energy and less tension than eating a candy bar.

The researchers worked with 18 volunteers, 15 women and three men. For all of them, both the candy and the walk provided an energy lift. But one hour after eating the candy, participants reported feeling more tense. Two hours later they felt increasingly tired and had less energy. But those who took the walk felt energetic and reported less tension two hours after walking.

Now, that's 27 different ideas to reduce stress on the job. They all work, but only if you do them. I'm certain you'll find some of them are particularly suited for you.

Take This Job and Shove It! OK, you've tried it all. You've done stress-busting techniques. You've tried talking with the boss. You've done it all. After all these years, you realize that the job is killing you, and that the heart attack was a warning that you shouldn't ignore.

There comes a time when you have to ask yourself, is this worth dying for? The answer of course is no, no job in the world is worth your life. They'll get along very well without you, one way or the other.

If you're ready for early retirement, you might want to consider taking it. Even if the money might be tight, you can probably come up with a way to make a few extra dollars with a part-time job of some sort. For a cut in salary you just might get a few years more of life.

If it's a matter of quitting the job in order to find another one, perhaps you'd be well served to check out the job market first. Talk about this with your spouse and family to get their support. They love you, and they want what's best for you, not just a meal ticket.

You might want to take some of the vacation time you have coming to look for another job. Or start sending out your résumé and making some phone calls. Talk with employment agencies and recruiting firms. Just don't make the mistake of quitting in your mind before being ready to make the big step; consider yourself in transition.

Don't limit yourself to the same sort of work you've been doing. It's very likely that the kinds of stresses and problems and politics that played havoc with your cardiovascular system in one place will be repeated in another. Maybe it's time for a complete make-over of your job options and choices.

Are there some things you do as hobbies, as avocations, that just might expand into money-making opportunities? Many a man has retired and taken up a special interest, only to find that he could then make a lot more money by doing what he had always wanted to do.

Consider spending some time with an employment counselor to discuss your options. He or she just might come up with something you'd never have thought of doing.

Beating the Monday Blues. OK, let's face it: not everyone loves his or her job and can't wait for the weekend to be over. When Howard University researchers studied 185,000 workers, they found that the majority go through some level of depression come Monday morning. But there are some ways to beat those first-day blues.

- Arrange your day so that you'll have meetings, work sessions, breaks, and lunches with people whose company you actually enjoy.
- Set your alarm clock a bit earlier than usual to give yourself a bit more flexibility in time. Feelings of being rushed bring on stress and aggravate negative attitudes you may already have about going to work.
- Start off the week with something you don't mind doing, especially something that can give you satisfaction in completing. One of the ways to get a flying start is to get back to a job that wasn't quite finished when you left it. That way you know just where to start, and you'll get a sense of fulfillment when it's finished.

TAKING THE FIRST STEP BACK

The first step back to work is really the first step you take when you take your first walk in the hospital corridor. Next it's the steps during your walks at home. Then it's the steps on the treadmill during a structured program of cardiac rehabilitation. Simply enough, those who "graduate" from those rehab programs feel more confident about themselves. They feel stronger, more energetic, more capable of taking on their weight in wildcats.

Recognizing that the workplace today is what the battlegrounds and hunting fields of yesterday were to our ancestors, you'll need all the strength and capability you can get! To succeed in your return to work, you need to succeed in your total program of cardiac recovery.

CHAPTER 9

Building a Dynamic Support Base for Healthy, Happy Living

No man, no woman, is an island. Never is that adage more filled with truth than following a cardiac event. We need all the help we can get. In fact, a number of studies have shown that those with plenty of support from spouses, families, and friends do the best job of recovery.

Patients with a strong support base demonstrate better compliance in doing the things that will help them recover both for the short- and long-term return to normal life. We've discussed the role of optimism in the recovery process, and once again this comes into play. Except this time it's the spouse's and family's optimism that's important.

If the spouse and family treat the patient like a sick person, the patient will act like one. Again, studies have demonstrated that "playing the sick role" can have disastrous consequences. An upbeat patient, living with an upbeat family, is most likely to have a spectacular recovery.

The properly functioning support base is effective in cutting through a major stumbling block for virtually all heart patients. After a heart attack or cardiac surgery, we feel tremendous loss of control over practically everything in our lives, including our own health. This lack of control leads to depression. And depression keeps us from doing the very things needed to ensure recovery. The support base can provide that control and lessen depression. Not, as we'll see, by dictating the patient's life, but by facilitating it.

When it comes to the support base, the more the merrier. Spouse, children, friends and relatives, doctors and other health professionals, and various support groups are all important. But for the heart patient, the spouse is the person best positioned to help the loved one through this emotional crisis.

Ironically, it's the spouse who is typically left out of the rehabilitation process. And his or her own problems are very much underestimated if not completely ignored.

In many cases spouses receive minimal information about their roles and responsibilities during their loved one's recovery. This puts both the patient and the spouse under stress due to a perceived lack of control. One study found that stress was higher for spouses than for the patients.

What are spouses concerned about? During the second and third weeks of convalescence, worries center on the amount, type, and level of appropriate activity. They have questions about returning to work, dietary restrictions, medications, and other aspects of rehabilitation and treatment. To top things off, tension mounts when the spouse becomes uncommunicative and is subject to wild mood swings.

Especially for older couples, there are problems with role reversals. For years the man took care of the "little woman" who now has to write the checks, pay the bills, direct the household, drive the car, and, in general, care for the man. All this while worrying about a second heart attack.

Conversely, for younger couples the woman has her own career concerns. How can she take care of her husband while maintaining that career? And is this the way it's going to be for the rest of their lives together?

Finally, although most heart patients are male, we have an increasing number of women recovering from heart attack and bypass surgery. In many cases, the husband has already died and isn't available to provide convalescent care. And when he is around, he's typically not equipped as a nurturing care-giver in our society.

In the coming pages I'll discuss some options and strategies for various households. Unless specifically addressing the female patient, I'll assume that the spouse is the wife. However, the concepts remain valid for either sex.

Let's cut to the chase: how long is this whole recovery process going to take? Asked another way, how long is the household going to be in emotional upheaval? Certainly every case is special and there will be wide variances. But on average, complete recovery takes about a year.

The recovery process gets easier and easier as the weeks and months pass. Certainly those first few weeks will be the worst. As the patient enters the formal, structured rehabilitation program he or she will rapidly return to the person you knew and loved. Yes, there will still be mood swings, easy fatigue, grumpiness, and concerns. But it will get easier.

I've suggested that all cardiac patients should keep a daily diary to keep track of progress in diet, exercise, stress management, general feelings, and so forth. All the same benefits would accrue to the spouse who keeps a daily log. In fact, there's something very therapeutic about putting one's thoughts to paper. Don't hold back, let it all come out, all the anger, all the anxiety, all the emotions.

Yes, this will be an emotionally fraught year. But haven't you gone through some tough times in the past? Try to put this into a proper perspective of taking the good with the bad. Remember the problems that the two of you faced through the years: worrying about buying a house and paying the mortgage; times when you thought you were going to go bankrupt; troubles with the children; automobile accidents. You made it through those and other times together, and you'll make it through this one too. Because heart disease does *not* mean that life as you have known it is over. You can beat heart disease and make it, like other problems, a thing of the past.

The cardiac event does place an additional stress on any marriage, whether rocky or idyllic. But there's some really good news from a British study that found many couples actually reported an improvement in their marriage. About one out of four said their lives together became better and richer. Couples stopped taking each other for granted and several made deliberate efforts to show more tolerance and consideration for each other. (Of course, that all took time; those first few weeks are tough for everyone.)

The experience in America seems to be about the same. About 20 percent of spouses rate their marriages as worse while 25 percent note an improvement; the other 55 percent indicate no changes one way or the other.

Needless to say, if the marriage wasn't good to begin with, a cardiac event may be just the straw to break the camel's back. While most couples in such circumstances remain together during the initial recovery, divorce may be forthcoming. In some instances, the heart attack or surgery may lead to a rethinking of the rest of one's life. Some decide that they'd be happier alone, or with someone else.

No matter what the state of your marriage before the event, this is the time to improve communications rather than clamming up. Often spouses keep their anger within, fearing that an argument might trigger an attack. That leads to even more resentment. Keeping all channels of communication open is essential. You might even consider some family counseling at this time if communication seems impossible.

Los Angeles psychologist Herb Budnick specializes in helping individuals and couples in their emotional recovery from heart disease. The advice he give heart attack survivors is to "increase your quality of life by communicating more, by addressing your emotions, by reaching out to your spouse, and by allowing her (or him) to reach out to you."

SURVIVAL STRATEGIES FOR SPOUSES

You can't love someone else unless you love yourself first. And you can't help someone else unless you have the physical and emotional capacity to do so. Therefore, before dealing with how a spouse can help a patient with his or her recovery, we have to deal with the problems of the spouse.

"What?!" you might say in amazement. "No one has ever asked how *I'm* doing." "No one cares about me." "It's always him." "I love him, but . . ." Don't feel ashamed or embarrassed if those statements could be your very own quotes. It's natural to feel that way.

In fact, it's even natural to be angry and resentful that your spouse had the heart attack in the first place. It's "ruined" your life. All those plans you had. You were just about ready to start really enjoying yourselves. Maybe the kids have finally gone and now there was going to be some time for yourself. Now it's all ruined.

Well, let's not say ruined, OK? Let's say that your plans have been postponed for a while.

Next, don't feel guilty about the heart attack itself. Some patients can be truly vicious at this time in their lives, lashing out at those around them, making them feel as though it was their fault that they had the heart attack to begin with.

Let's put that argument away right off the bat. Heart disease, culminating in heart attack or surgery, is the result of years of deterioration beginning in childhood. There is the family history of the disease. There are the contributing factors outside of our control including diabetes and thyroid dysfunction. And there are the controllable risk factors including high blood pressure, elevated cholesterol levels, cigarette smoking, overweight, and sedentary lifestyle. Those are the things responsible for your spouse's heart disease, not you! Never forget that!

Just as you didn't cause your spouse's heart disease in the first place, you're not going to make it go away. Only the patient can do that. Yes, with considerable effort and lifestyle modifications as discussed in this book, heart disease can be stopped and even reversed. For most patients, heart disease can become a thing of the past, with a life free of fear of another occurrence. But you can't do that for your spouse. You can help. You can facilitate. You can encourage. But you can't do it for him or her. And you can't force the patient to do to it for himself or herself.

Don't lay guilt on yourself. Don't believe you are capable of more than is truly possible. Moreover, don't become a nag. Making the patient's life miserable by never-ending comments on diet, exercise, medications, and so forth will just lead to marital strife. Neither of you needs that.

Certain patients seem bound and determined to let heart disease "finish them off." They refuse to change their lives one iota. They eat high-fat foods, never exercise, lead stressful lives without ever relaxing, smoke cigarettes, and refuse to take medications. If you happen to be married to or involved with such a person, you must start planning for a future alone.

It may be morbid to say, but estate planning should be one of your priorities. Make sure the life insurance bills are paid up. Make sure you understand the household finances. Start living a life of your own, so it won't be as traumatic when being alone becomes a reality.

But regardless of your spouse's attitudes and willingness to make a full cardiac recovery, and even though you're willing to help every step of the way, you still have your own life and health to consider, even during the earliest stages of the patient's convalescence. You can't sacrifice yourself entirely. In fact, that can be self-defeating and ultimately you'll come to resent your spouse for it.

Here are some strategies for coping with the inevitable stresses in the coming weeks and months.

Maintain your own health. You've got to stay healthy and strong for your spouse's sake and for your own sake. Letting stress cause you to begin smoking again would be a huge mistake. Food can sometimes be used as consolation; be careful not to allow yourself to gain weight in the process. Maintain your own exercise schedule, both for physical fitness and as a way to deal with stress.

Pay attention to grooming. This is not some movie tragedy in which you're playing the suffering victim, looking haggard and worn, with no makeup, hair in disarray, and clothes crumpled and soiled. Give yourself the gift of good grooming. Keep your hair styled and your makeup well done. Dress stylishly as always. Don't ignore the little details. Maintaining pride in your appearance will help you to keep things in perspective, and will help keep you from feeling insignificant or unimportant.

Make time for yourself. Despite the added demands on your time, schedule a little space for yourself. Your spouse can survive an hour or two without you very easily. Go out for a facial and a manicure. See a movie. Take a long walk through the park. Even if there are things you could just as easily do at home, such as reading a book, leave the house for a while. Go to the library to read that book, for example.

You need to have some time on your own, time when the phone can't ring and your spouse can't make a request of some sort. Do so regularly, perhaps even every day.

Believe this or not, your spouse will appreciate the time alone as well! Many patients start to feel like their every move is being monitored, and they resent it. Being left alone can be a breath of fresh air for them as well. Maybe there's a video your spouse has been wanting to watch, but hasn't because you don't share his tastes. Rent the video for him, and then go out to see a movie you'd enjoy.

Keep in touch with your friends. This one comes under the category of self-sacrifice and how to avoid it. Many spouses feel guilty about having friends visit, or going to visit them, during the recovery period. Having a good friend or friends can be a wonderful aspect of your own therapy. Yes, give them a progress report, but then talk about the things you'd normally discuss.

Continue your own job or career. Sure, you'll probably want to take some time off to take care of your spouse during the first few weeks of recovery. But you have your own life to lead as well, and sacrificing a job or jeopardizing your career isn't the thing to do. Now, you may ask who's going to do all those things you've been doing for your spouse? Get someone else to do some of the tasks that you can't handle once you've returned to work.

If you stay home, you'll lose income. So why not take that income and pay someone to come into the house while you're gone? Every community has services available for just such circumstances. Often the person is a nurse, or has some training in caring for post-heart attack or post-surgery patients, and will also do some shopping and cooking.

In many cases, it's financially expedient to pay such a person, resulting in a positive balance. But even if it's a negative balance, consider the benefits to your own well-being as well as the future of your job or career.

Keep a sense of humor. Laughter is the best medicine both for the spouse and the patient. Tell a joke. Rent a funny video. Tape a comedy rerun on late-night television. Keep laughing; it can keep you from crying.

Manage your own stress levels. Remember that recovery is just as stressful for the spouse as for the patient, and maybe even more so. The same techniques that can help the patient can help you. Read and practice some of the suggestions in chapter 4.

Don't deny your own needs. Consider yourself a full partner in the recovery process. As such you're entitled to all the privileges of your relationship as well as the obligations. If you have an itch on your back, it's perfectly all right to ask your spouse to scratch it. If you have an opinion, voice it. If you have sexual yearnings, let them be known and express yourself. Sex is not taboo. Read chapter 7.

Many women resent the fact that they're expected to change their own lives and habits and tastes just because the spouse happens to have heart disease. Diet can be a big problem for some. Certainly, there are a lot of advantages in making the lifestyle modifications a family affair. And the low-fat, low-cholesterol diet that's best for the heart patient is really a healthful diet that's advised for all men and women. But you may not have to be as stringent.

In my own case, I haven't eaten a single egg yolk since the second bypass in 1984. But my wife's cholesterol level is perfectly normal. So when we're in a restaurant, she has the poached egg and I have the egg substitute.

I don't personally resent her eating those eggs, although now and then I wish I could have one. But if your spouse makes a big fuss about it, then just make a point of going out for breakfast or brunch once or twice a week and indulge your tastes. And don't feel guilty about it.

Seek your own counseling. Sometimes having a good friend serves to get things off your chest and to put things into perspective. But sometimes it takes a professional to help you cope. Get the help you need. Perhaps you can talk with a clergyman. Maybe the hospital has a counselor you could schedule some time with. There may be support groups for cardiac spouses, with people who have gone through the same things and are willing to share their experiences and insights. Or perhaps your doctor can suggest a good professional counselor with training in family matters.

PROVIDING THE BEST SPOUSAL SUPPORT

When it comes to caring for your loved one, there's a fine line between facilitating and incapacitating. While proper social support improves patient compliance and speeds the recovery process, overprotectiveness undermines and impedes that recovery.

The question was put to 201 patients: "How were you treated by your family and friends after the heart attack?" Eighty percent said they were protected "much more than before" from physical exertion. Almost half said "My responsibility is taken away." And 10 percent said they were "treated like an invalid."

The spouse plays an incredibly important role here. A study in the *British Journal of Medicine* concluded that "the role of the wife is a major determinant of the patient's readjustment during convalescence."

Unfortunately, in their eagerness to help, some spouses actually cause more problems. After their spouse has had a heart attack, some people just shut up and don't say anything for fear of making the situation worse. Wrong. Spouses may also fall into the trap of being overly supportive and protective. Equally wrong. This coddling and babying only contribute to a sense of dependence. This increases emotional distance and the recovering spouse may even begin to resent the partner. Eventually, the wife will also come to resent the husband for forcing her to handle things. It's easy to see how a household can quickly become a hotbed of anger and suppressed emotion.

GETTING INVOLVED IN THE ENTIRE PROCESS

An ability to view the recovery period and process through the eyes of the patient helps the spouse provide adequate support. Conversely, an inability to comprehend the experience results in anxiety. What are the patient's limitations, and what are the capabilities? Not many spouses really know.

A Stanford University study compared 10 wives who did not observe their husbands' treadmill exercise test with 10 who watched and another 10 who not only watched but also participated in the test themselves. Wives who rated their husbands before testing tended to rate them substantially lower than the patients rated themselves, reflecting the spouses' serious doubts about their loved ones' capacity for physical effort. In fact, husbands tended to judge themselves moderately robust while wives termed their husband's cardiac capacity as "severely diminished and incapable of withstanding physical and emotional strain."

Of course, the patients' own perception of their physical and cardiac abilities improved considerably after the treadmill test. Even watching the husband undergo the stress test did not change the wives' impressions. Why? Because women focused on symptoms and signs of their husbands' high workloads. But the wives who literally followed in their husbands' footsteps and walked the treadmill themselves showed a sharp increase in their perceptions of their husbands' cardiac and physical capabilities. Subsequent counseling was also more effective with the women who participated in the treadmill testing.

The bottom line of the spouses' thinking: If my husband can do that much work, sweating and straining, and be perfectly fine, then he'll be fine at home and I won't have to worry about him; let's get on with the recovery!

Getting involved in the process does *not* mean becoming a warden or watchdog. If the spouse is asked to make certain that the patient complies with the medical and rehab program, he or she assumes a great deal of the responsibility. The mate thus becomes accountable for the patient and any transgressions that may occur. Needless to say, this induces stress and resentment.

The flip side of the coin is that patients whose spouses become watchdogs feel like they are invalids, children, or a combination of both. The nagging can be deafening.

Instead, try to live your lives as normally as possible. That means both of you. The patient will still be able to do many if not most of the normal chores in the household. Perhaps there will be limitations at first, but those will rather remarkably diminish in the weeks and months to come. There's no reason why a patient can't take his or her own plates to the sink after dinner! Being a patient doesn't equate with privilege!

For the spouse, helping out doesn't mean taking over. How about working on the bills together? Maybe one person can sort out the bills and the other can write the checks. How about planning and preparing a low-fat dinner for the two of you, or for the entire family? Here the patient will have to be honest about saying when enough is enough and it's time to stop and rest.

I must admit that one of the toughest things for me after the surgery was dealing with the fatigue. I was so used to my previous level of activity, that it was difficult to admit when it was time to quit. So many times I'd push myself beyond my limits, and this would result in my feeling lousy for the rest of the day. Finally I came to the realization that pushing myself was ultimately self-defeating since I could do more work by not exceeding my limits and requiring a period of recovery.

Sharing the rehabilitation process makes it much easier for the patient and can have significant benefits for the spouse, but it may become a source of conflict. Some spouses may balk at making changes just because the patient's life depends on it.

Every family is different. My wife Dawn had worked out in a health club when we lived in Chicago. So when I joined the club here in Los Angeles, she was eager to share a membership. Now we both do our workouts regularly, and it gives us one more thing in common.

On the other hand, I've mentioned that she doesn't need to avoid the saturated fat and cholesterol as much as I do, and I've mentioned the egg compromise. Another is that when we're in a restaurant, I don't make a big to-do about her putting butter on her bread, even though butter is forbidden in our home. Ironically, as time has passed since 1984,

Dawn has leaned more and more toward vegetarian foods as a matter of personal taste, while I still enjoy my fish, poultry, and meat. We've worked it out for ourselves, and you'll have to do the same.

Dawn gave me a T-shirt that expresses a very basic need for every cardiac patient. It's red and white, with some little hearts here and there. The inscription reads: "Daily Prescription: 4 Hugs for Survival; 8 Hugs for Maintenance; 12 Hugs for Growth." I love that T-shirt, and I believe its message implicitly. Which brings me to another crucial aspect of cardiac recovery . . .

If hugs and kisses could be bottled, we'd have a magic elixir. Affection is so effective, it's almost like snake oil: Cures what ails you.

This is the time to come closer together as a couple and as a family. Make it a point to give and get lots of hugs and kisses. Promise yourselves that you'll never go to bed without a good-night kiss. Wake up in the morning with a hug. Punctuate the day with affection.

When's the last time you held hands while watching a movie? How about a little nuzzle behind the ear? A pat on the backside can recall a younger, friskier time in your relationship. Yes, sex is important and a terrific source of physical pleasure and a feeling of togetherness. But those little expressions of affection throughout the day can mean even more. And you can do them much more often!

IT'S A FAMILY AFFAIR: CONSIDER THE CHILDREN

If Dad broke a bone skiing down a challenging run on the slopes, the kids would probably be proud of him, although they might kid him about "acting his age." An automobile accident might bring weeks in the hospital and lots of sympathy. But a heart attack somehow reminds children that Dad (or Mom) is mortal indeed and that they won't have him or her around forever.

Every child, whether 8, or 18, or 28, has some strong fears and anxieties when they hear the term HEART ATTACK. It's right up there with the word DIVORCE as a basic dread of the real world.

The dream of every child whose parents get divorced is that they'll get back together. Almost never does this happen, and some real psychological damage can result. But when it comes to heart attack and bypass surgery, you can honestly explain that the outcome is going to be positive.

The explanations should be at the child's level of understanding, but should cover the basics of the anatomy of the heart, the process of the disease, the factors that led to the heart attack and/or bypass, and the lifestyle modifications that will ensure a speedy recovery and a likelihood that this isn't going to happen again. This would be the time to start encouraging the kids to take an active role in making this a family affair in terms of everyone adopting a healthier lifestyle. Whether the children are in elementary school, college, or on their own, they know the basic truths of what you're saying and have heard them stated time and again in the media. Now the reality has struck close to home, and it's time to take this all to heart for everyone's sake.

Realize, however, that there can be some backlash. The kids, if they're living at home, may resent dietary changes. It's a long way from the standard teenage diet of pizzas, burgers, and tacos to a low-fat diet. Creativity and effort can make all the difference. My books *The 8-Week Cholesterol Cure* and *Cholesterol & Children* contain recipes that are more in tune with real American tastes than most heart-health cookbooks. I talk about ways to make those pizzas, burgers, and tacos, and a lot of other foods, with all the fun and flavor but without the fat. Give it a try. While you're at it, it would be a good idea for the kids to read *Cholesterol & Children* themselves.

Get the children involved in the recovery process all the way. Divide up some of the chores that need to be done. Then balance that off by planning some involvement together. No matter how jaded today's kids tend to get, they still yearn for expressions of parental love. Spending an hour or so playing a board game such as Parcheesi together can be a boost for everyone's spirits.

But don't put too much of the burden on the children. Imagine the horrors and potential damage of the following true stories. In one case, the mother told her eight-year-old son that he'd have to be the man of the house now that Daddy was sick. In the other instance, a boy came out of the parent's bedroom wearing Dad's wedding ring with the announcement that he was now the man Mom could depend on. Placing such heavy burdens on young shoulders will almost certainly result in psychological scars that will carry into adulthood.

Don't leave Dad (or Mom) out of the picture. Continue to seek his advice. Let him maintain his sense of authority. To do otherwise will be harmful to all parties.

No matter why a person is "under the weather" he or she will tire more easily and will tend to be a bit more grumpy or more easily irritated than usual. The entire family will have to learn, and accept, new limits.

Finally another comparison with the modern blight of divorce in the family. Children of divorced parents very often feel somehow guilty for having caused the divorce. Little boys and girls frequently promise "to be good" if Mom and Dad will get back together. Even older children wonder whether they were somehow responsible for fomenting family discord that led to the break-up.

So it is with heart disease. Quickly defuse any idea that the children are responsible, even in the smallest way, for the parent's heart attack.

The best rule for dealing with cardiac recovery for the family is to keep life as close to normal as possible. The patient must also realize that his or her temperament might, in fact probably will, change for the worse. But the change will be temporary. So try to be a little more understanding. All of you.

WITH A LITTLE HELP FROM MY FRIENDS

If ever you had need for some good friends, this is the time. And that works both for spouse and patient. Friends give us an opportunity to say what's on our minds, sometimes in ways we won't even share with our mates. And maintaining friendships during the convalescent and full recovery period is a wonderful way of actively demonstrating that life goes on.

In fact, it's good to continue normal activities that would include friends as soon as possible and as much as possible. If you normally have a game of bridge every Wednesday evening, return to it as soon as you're able. If on Fridays you meet a couple for dinner, resume doing so.

But your friends should become a part of the total recovery team, along with your family. As such they should understand as much about the recovery process as you do. A really good friend will want to read this book. That way they will understand your diet, your exercise, and your other lifestyle modification efforts. In fact, you might enlist one or two to go along with you. It would do them a world of good as well.

But when you're together, try not to dwell on the aspects of heart disease. That can get really boring after a while. After a few minutes of the normal social amenities of asking about each other's health, get on with what you'd normally talk about.

Explain your limitations right up front. Yes, you can do a lot of things, but you're likely to get tired a bit easily for the next few months as you get your strength back. Set a definite time limit as to when you'll call it an evening.

Make sure your friendship isn't a one-way street. If there's something you can do, now that you have some time on your hands, offer to do it. That will help reciprocate for the times you might need a little assistance.

As with virtually all things relative to the recovery process, your friendships will go on as usual, and they should. Recognize your own limits and those friendships will speed the process along.

GETTING GOOD MEDICAL CARE

When the cardiac event occurred, you came under the care of a cardiologist and possibly a cardiac surgeon. In an ideal situation, those specialists will keep in close contact with your family physician, general practitioner, internist, or whomever you rely upon for usual care, if, indeed, you have a regular doctor. If you're from a small town, and you received cardiac care away from home, reports will be sent back so that your doctor will know what's happened, what to expect, and how treatment should be continued.

During the first weeks, you'll rely a lot on your cardiologist. He'll be the one, most likely, to do your exercise treadmill tests and to set the course for your rehabilitation program. He'll also be the one to prescribe special medications that you may take for a short period of time or possibly for the rest of your life. For details on cardiac medications see chapter 16.

But there'll come a time when your care will and should be transferred back over to your regular doctor if you have one. Indeed, you're better off with a family practitioner or an internist rather than relying on a cardiologist for too long a time.

First, the cardiologist is highly specialized and may not be up to date on other physical and medical conditions that you're dealing with. Second, the general practitioner or internist has a great deal of knowledge about cardiology and can make a smooth transition.

In fact, it's the general practitioner or internist who is more likely to provide expert advice for your specific, individual situation. Cardiologists don't normally give dietary counseling, stress management input, hypertension management, and so forth on a daily basis. It's the family practitioner who does those things routinely and is best suited to do so.

Of course you probably will go back to your cardiologist periodically for reevaluation, including an annual treadmill test and perhaps other testing as called for. But when it comes to normal aches and pains and ongoing cardiac recovery, your family practitioner, GP, or internist will have principal responsibility for your health.

Some patients become overly dependent upon their cardiologist, feeling that he and only he has the expertise needed. Think of this another way. If your doctor referred you to a urologist for a specific problem, would you continue to rely on the urologist for all your medical attention?

Because your family doctor will be such a vital member of your health team from now on, it's really important for you to have confidence in him or her and to feel comfortable with his or her care. (Yes, there are many female physicians, but for the sake of brevity for the balance of this discussion, I'll refer to the doctor as he. No sexism intended.)

This is the time to ask yourself quite candidly, do you really like your doctor? Do you think he has the medical horsepower you need to feel confident? Is he the kind of person you can sit and talk with, expecting to get the answers you need for the questions that are so important to you? If so, count yourself as quite lucky. Not everyone has such positive feelings about his doctor. If you're not completely happy with your current doctor–patient relationship, this is the time to do some shopping.

Unless you live in a very remote area where you're lucky to have any medical care at all, you have your choice of quite a few doctors. In fact, in many if not most major population centers doctors are in abundance and actually are anxious to get new patients. You're in a buyer's market.

We all have warm, fuzzy feelings about having a doctor like Marcus Welby, M.D. He always had time to talk with his patients, to take a walk with them through the palms, and to get to know their entire family intimately. Although that situation was obviously exaggerated for the purposes of television drama, there are many caring physicians who feel deeply about their patients. I've personally known dozens of them.

As a side note, I've been asked a number of times whether I feel doctors are jaded and uncaring, and whether working on my books has given me a negative impression of the medical community. I'm very happy to say that the result of my work has been exactly the opposite. Sure, there's a doctor here and there who cares more about his real estate holdings and stock portfolio than his patients, but those are in the minority. Both the doctors who are in practice and those doing research in medical centers and universities are highly dedicated, compassionate people. I've been proud to be associated with them, both directly and indirectly.

So how do you find a good doctor? First consider the characteristics that are important to you. Would you feel comfortable with a very young person, or do you need more maturity? Bear in mind that age does not always equate with knowledge, however, and many "youngsters" have state-of-the-art information and training that their seniors lack. Should the doctor have privileges in a certain medical center or hospital that you've come to like? Do you need a doctor with a marvelous bedside manner, or would you prefer a practitioner who has tremendous medical credentials?

Many studies have shown that some women feel much more comfortable with a female rather than a male physician. This is particularly true for older women. There are certain subjects that are just too personal to be discussed with a man, even though he's a doctor. If that's the case for you, by all means make an effort to find a good female physician. There are plenty of them.

I personally think that a very important characteristic for any physician is his or her own optimism. I've mentioned this trait as a predictor of success in recovery for the patient. It's no less vital for the physician, who can convey that sense of optimism, that you're going to be fine. Optimism is highly contagious. You want to catch it from your doctor!

For years, many have recognized the physical as well as psychological benefits of the so-called "laying on of hands." Just a doctor's warm and caring touch seems to be a conduit for reassurance, just as a Mommy's kiss seemed to make that scraped knee "all better." It turns out that there's actually a scientific basis for this phenomenon. The University of South Carolina has been gathering data under a National Institutes of Health grant to learn just why tender loving care works. Apparently there is an electromagnetic field that transfers energy from the hands of an accomplished and caring healer to the patient. Is it all in the mind? Researchers at McGill University in Montreal have shown that the principles even apply to animals, as shown in terms of wound-healing in mice.

But a word of warning. Beware of quacks and charlatans who are expert in bedside manner and providing reassurance, but have no scientific basis for their treatments. Those who practice chelation therapy fall into that category. Chelation is an unproven treatment which purports to remove arterial blockage through a series of injections. Sure, they can tell you about "thousands" of patients who "feel 100% better" after their treatments. But they have no proof to show that it was their ministrations that made the difference. If a patient is willing to shell out thousands of dollars on chelation therapy, it's likely that he'll also make dietary changes and get additional exercise. Here's the bottom line: if chelation therapy really worked, virtually every doctor in the country would be happy to add it to his medical repertory, not only to aid his patients but also to be able to collect additional fees. If you'd like to have additional information on chelation therapy and other aspects of medical quackery, write to the American Heart Association, 7320 Greenville Avenue, Dallas, TX 75231. They have a good booklet called "Questions and Answers about Chelation Therapy." Another good source of information is the National Council Against Health Fraud, Inc., P. O. Box 1276, Loma Linda, CA 92354. Or you can call them at (714) 824-4690.

You need help. You don't need hindrance. Not only will quacks and charlatans take your money, they could wind up taking your life by standing in the way of sound medical care that could help you beat heart disease.

So how do you find this doctor who's just right for you? Talk with your friends. Are they happy with their physicians? Ask your cardiologist for a referral, telling him what you're looking for in a family physician. Call the local medical society for a listing of doctors with the qualifications you seek in your area.

Then go talk with them. There's absolutely nothing wrong with doing a bit of "shopping" for a person who will be providing services that are, quite literally, a matter of life and death. If a doctor refuses to spend a few minutes with you just to get to know you, you know right off the bat that he or she won't have time for you later on when you really need it. But remember, of course, that time is precious to all doctors. Keep the meeting short and to the point, having your list of questions in hand. Some questions might include:

- How long have you practiced?
- How many patients do you see per day?
- What hospital(s) have given you privileges?
- Are you board certified in your area of practice?
- What is your availability on weekends and holidays?
- How often do you attend continuing education programs?
- How many medical journals do you read weekly?
- Have you been sued for malpractice? More than once?
- Can you provide a list of references?

Before your meeting, while waiting in the reception area, chat a bit with the nurse or receptionist. You'll quickly pick up on how they feel about the doctor. Good doctors have staff members who practically worship them.

If your doctor suggests a certain treatment, and you're not certain about whether it's right for you, by all means seek a second opinion, even a third opinion. No good doctor would be insulted by that, and he should be willing to provide whatever X rays and lab results necessary.

And if your doctor or cardiologist has suggested that you need angioplasty or bypass surgery, you'll certainly want to interview the potential practitioner. Cardiologists normally do angioplasties, although some radiologists do them as well. And bypass surgery is strictly the domain of the cardiovascular surgeon. Again, have your list of questions in hand.

- Where did you receive your training?
- How long have you done this type of surgery?
- How many surgeries do you perform weekly?
- How many surgeries are done at your hospital weekly?
- What is your morbidity (medical complications) and mortality (death) rate?

If you're not completely comfortable in interpreting the answers to those questions yourself, consider discussing the matter with an objective third party such as your family practitioner.

We've come to take bypass surgery for granted in this day and age in our society, and we sometimes believe that it's as easy as having a decayed tooth filled. (Even at that, don't you want a *good* dentist to fill your tooth?) The fact remains that the mortality rate differs enormously from one doctor to another and from one hospital to another. It's your heart and your life. You deserve the best. Don't settle for less.

Happily, excellent cardiac surgeons are available in virtually every area of the country. If you have to travel a few miles, or even more than a few miles, to get to the best one, it's worth the trip.

MAKING THE BEST USE OF A DOCTOR'S APPOINTMENT

You walk into the office, wait for your turn to see the doctor, read an old magazine, and before you know it you're back in the elevator on your way out of the building. What happened in the appointment? What about those questions that you had? Why didn't you mention the pains you were having?

Most patients leave the doctor's office with a vague feeling of disappointment and frustration. That's because they weren't really prepared and the doctor, whose time is always limited, didn't probe for questions. You can assure a successful and satisfying appointment by literally writing an agenda for the meeting, listing all your questions in advance. Keep a running tab through the days prior to the appointment, and then organize it all on a piece of paper you bring in with you and literally read to the doctor. You'll be happier, and so will your doctor. Besides, you'll get better care that way. Here are some sample questions.

- What do those red pills do?
- If I miss my morning dose, should I take two at lunch?
- Is it OK if I take an extra walk in the evening?
- Does this pain in my upper back have any significance?
- Is it OK to take an extra aspirin when I get a headache since I already take one a day?
- My neighbor says a special bracelet wards off angina. What do you think about that?

Remember that no question is "dumb" and you need the answers to all the questions you come up with.

OTHER PROFESSIONALS TO RELY ON

The term "medical team" is frequently used, and with good reason. It takes a close-working, well-coordinated effort to achieve the best results. You, of course, are an integral member of that team, not just the recipient of care. Those who passively sit by and nod during meetings, then assume that everything will be done for them with little or no effort of their own, typically do not do well. Those who actively participate, ask lots of questions, seek the best professional input, go for second opinions, utilize all the collateral services available, and then put good advice to practice are likely to come out as real winners. As I call them, *former* heart patients.

Many medical and surgical groups have nurses specifically assigned to cardiac patients. If the service is not offered to you, ask your doctor if you couldn't be introduced to someone who could act as that kind of contact. It'll make your life, your spouse's life, and your doctor's life, a lot easier and less stressful.

Next there is your cardiac rehabilitation team. If you follow my advice and take advantage of a structured, hospital-based cardiac rehabilitation program, your recovery will be easier, faster, and more successful in all ways. Your job is to do exactly what they tell you to do, to the letter, and never miss a single session. Their job will be to provide the training and education you'll need for a marvelous—and, yes, even enjoyable—recovery. They'll also be there to answer questions that come up. This in itself makes the hospital-based program invaluable; imagine being able to ask any questions you have three times a week, every week, and have nurses, exercise physiologists, psychologists, nutritionists, occupational therapists, and doctors to ask. It's truly the ideal situation.

Similarly, I hope that the suggestions and coping strategies I've given you in this book will help you deal with the psychological aspects of cardiac recovery. But you may have individual questions that pertain to you and only you. Again, it's time to rely on an outside expert. Your doctor or hospital can refer you to a psychologist, marriage counselor, family counselor, or occupational therapist who can help you come to grips with the problems that currently burden you.

The next group of professionals may not be in the health field, but they can exert a profound influence on your well-being and recovery.

These are the people who can make you feel good for at least a little while, and who can make you feel better about yourself. They include those who provide such marvelous services as massages, facials, manicures, and pedicures. Just having an appointment to look forward to can make the week a bit brighter. And allowing someone to totally pamper you for just a little while can have positive effects that can last for the entire day. Be nice to yourself now and then. It doesn't have to be expensive, you don't have to go to the most exclusive club or salon in town. But taking advantage of those little things that can mean so much can help your recovery by putting you into a better frame of mind.

SUPPORT GROUPS AT YOUR SERVICE

You're not alone. You know the statistics well enough to realize that heart attacks, surgeries, and angioplasties happen millions of times to millions of men and women each and every year. While you may not derive a great deal of comfort by simply knowing that, you may very well get a lot of benefit from talking with and getting to know some of the men and women in your "cardiac club."

Many hospitals and medical centers have established regular group sessions for patients to get together and chat about this and that. They share ideas about things to do, low-fat recipes to prepare, wonderful restaurants that serve delicious food while catering to special heart-healthy requests, and just plain old-fashioned camaraderie. Some groups even offer special meetings for cardiac spouses. Ask your hospital whether they have such programs, and, if not, where you might find a group.

One cardiac spouse took this to the limit. Rhoda Levin began by writing a book called *HeartMates*, recalling her experiences following her husband's heart attack and offering suggestions as to how to cope with the reality. The book is in paperback, and you might want to read it. My only criticism is that the emphasis is on living with heart disease rather than beating heart disease.

Marion Laboratories, a pharmaceutical manufacturing company, has sponsored a series of videotapes under the *HeartMates* name, offering tips for working things out in the family. The advantage of seeing the tapes is watching other, very real men, women, boys, and girls and hearing them portray their own situations. Ask your hospital whether these tapes are available for your viewing. If not, the hospital can call for information from Marion Laboratories in Minneapolis at (612) 929-3331.

I'm a member of Mended Hearts, a group I think you should learn more about and get involved with right from the start. Originally the group was formed by patients who had had heart surgery and who visited other patients in hospitals to give them moral support and encouragement and to answer questions on a patient-to-patient basis. Started several years ago, there are now more than 200 chapters of Mended Hearts in the United States and one in Ontario, Canada.

In addition to hospital visits, Mended Hearts members conduct educational and social programs in their communities, assist in community health care programs, and can work with the American Heart Association in a number of ways including fund-raising efforts. Membership includes a subscription to *Heartbeat*, a quarterly magazine featuring educational material and articles of interest for heart patients and their families. Some local chapters also publish newsletters.

As you're first recovering, Mended Hearts can help you in your own rehabilitation efforts. And as you get better, you'll be able to return the favor by visiting others. I've done my part by speaking at chapter meetings, sharing my own experiences and especially my knowledge of diet and cholesterol.

Ask your hospital if they know of the local Mended Hearts chapter in your area. If they can't help you, write to them at 7320 Greenville Avenue, Dallas, TX 75231.

The cost of Mended Hearts membership is nominal. But there is no cost at all if you simply would like some of their members to visit you personally or would like to attend one of their meetings. I've never attended a meeting that I didn't benefit from in some way, mostly in terms of meeting a bunch of really nice, caring people who share my enthusiasm for the potential of beating heart disease, not just living with it.

Many of us who've had bypass surgery refer to ourselves as members of the zipper club owing to the scar on our chests. But there really is a formal Zipper Club on the East Coast. They give talks and visit hospitalized surgery patients in New York, Philadelphia, and New Jersey. For more information you can write to the Zipper Club through its president, Walt Chacker, 1161 Easton Road, Roslyn, PA 19001.

THE ONGOING VALUE OF ALL SUPPORT

No matter who you are, rich or poor, weak or powerful, young or old, man or woman, you need others. Accept their caring and their loving and give back as much as you can. You'll not only recover faster, you'll be a better person for it.

THE FOURTH STEP:

Building a Strong Heart and Body

CHAPTER 10

Taking Advantage of Cardiac Rehabilitation

Cardiac rehabilitation should be just as much a part of the recovery process in the case of heart attack, bypass surgery, or other heart surgery as physical therapy would be after a body injury. The very definition of purpose of cardiac rehabilitation is very upbeat: to prevent future heart attacks, to prolong life, and to improve its quality. The medical community in this country is ambitiously optimistic in this regard. Compare even the term with that used in France: *Cardiac readaptation* implies a far more cautious approach, a certain degree of surrender to the disease.

It's our typical American "cowboy" attitude that comes through in cardiac rehabilitation. We just make the assumption that every uncomplicated case of heart attack or surgery will have a successful outcome and that every patient can and should be a winner.

This is one time that you can and should close the barn door after the horse has run away. It's almost never too late. We now have the programs at our disposal to facilitate an almost miraculous recovery from heart disease, to get that horse right back into the barn, as it were.

That was not the case back in 1978 when I had my heart attack and first bypass surgery. As I've said earlier, I was released with the flimsiest kind of advice and counsel: walk more and take it easy. I had no idea how much was enough or too much exercise. How much exertion would be dangerous? Which activities could pose problems? Those questions formed only the tip of the iceberg of my concern. The result was a level of depression, anxiety, and virtually neurotic attitude that today is termed the "cardiac cripple."

Compare that with my experience in 1984. Following my second bypass procedure I entered the cardiac rehabilitation program at Santa Monica Hospital Medical Center. My progress was dramatic. This time I had the guidance I needed. My confidence grew daily. And I was learning about the lifestyle modifications I'd need to make a spectacular recovery. That's just what I wanted: a *spectacular* recovery. And I got it.

BRIEF HISTORY OF CARDIAC REHABILITATION

The first record we have linking exercise with successful cardiac recovery came in 1772. An English physician noted that a patient who had had a heart attack was "nearly cured" after six months of sawing wood for a half hour a day. In 1799 another doctor wrote that physical activity benefited his patients who had chest pain. Those reports came long before the medical community knew what a heart attack was or what caused heart disease.

The original clinical description of a heart attack was written in 1912. The author of that paper stated his concern over physical exertion and the risk of aggravating the condition. He urged a conservative treatment of bed rest for six to eight weeks after the heart attack, medically termed a myocardial infarction (MI).

Needless to say, long periods of inactivity drained a person's energy enormously. In the 1940s, Dr. S. A. Levine stated that "long continued bed rest saps morale, provokes desperation, unleashes anxiety and ushers in hopelessness of the capacity of resuming a normal life." In a move which seemed wildly progressive for the time, he recommended that patients be allowed to sit in a chair for one to two hours, beginning the first day after the MI.

There were no complications to Dr. Levine's approach, and his "chair treatment" rapidly caught on. This method, which improves circulation and lessens the risk of thrombosis, remains in use today. Remember how you were told to sit in the chair next to your bed in the hospital?

By 1950, medical authorities began to seriously question lengthy bed rest, pointing to the lack of evidence that it did any good and suggesting that it might do far more harm than good. Yet for many years more, well into the 1970s in various parts of the country, doctors continued to prescribe immobilization of heart patients.

Inactivity is detrimental even for the healthiest individuals, much less for heart patients with compromised circulation. Put a healthy young man or woman in bed for any length of time, much less two to four weeks, and you will deplete energy, lead to easy fatigue, and create dizziness. Of course those are exactly the symptoms that the heart patient finds so troublesome and depressing.

By the 1960s, a number of studies showed that early activity after an MI safely eliminates the adverse effects of prolonged bed rest. An appropriate time of training is needed to restore patients to pre-bed rest condition. One study demonstrated that functional capability of normal, healthy subjects dropped by one-third after three weeks of bed rest. It took the same amount of time to get back to normal. After three months of twice-daily rigorous exercise programs, all exceeded the level of functional capacity prior to bed rest.

TODAY'S MODERN CARDIAC REHABILITATION

Cardiac rehabilitation can be divided into three or four phases of recovery. Phase I includes the five to ten days of hospitalization after the heart attack or bypass surgery. Immediately upon release from the cardiac care unit (CCU) patients begin to be active.

At first it's just dangling the feet over the side of the bed. Then it's sitting in a chair. Next comes a bit of walking with assistance down the halls. More progressive institutions incorporate some gentle stretching exercises to maintain muscle tone and begin to overcome the effects of bed rest.

By the time of your discharge, you're able to walk the halls confidently and to climb a flight of stairs. Often you're given a treadmill test to determine your physical status. Your doctor is assured that you'll be able to function quite well at home, and that you don't need to have round-the-clock medical and nursing attention.

It's important to realize that if your cardiologist thought that you were at risk of having another heart attack by leaving the hospital, he or she would not release you! Many patients feel tremendous anxiety at this time as they are pushed, as it were, out of the nest and urged to fly. A certain amount of anxiety is understandable and natural, but it must not be incapacitating.

Your recovery will continue at home for the next four to six weeks, sometimes as long as eight weeks. During that time you'll walk regularly as prescribed by your doctor. This is a great time to start thinking about the lifestyle changes necessary for making a spectacular comeback.

What should you do during those weeks at home? First of all, don't be surprised if you're really tired a lot of the time. Your body has experienced both the trauma of your cardiac event as well as the debilitating aspects of remaining inactive. You'll be more easily tired than before, and there's no point in getting frustrated about it. Accept the fact that you're recovering from a major occurrence and that this is going to take some time, just as though you were in traction after an auto accident.

Yes, you'll want to take those walks, but you don't want to overdo it. Don't get overtired. Again, don't get frustrated when a little walk tuckers you out. It's all part of the game of recovery.

Your doctor had you take a shower before leaving the hospital. The main reason was to show you that you were able to do so without significant problems and that it would tire you. Yes, taking a shower is a major activity during those first days back home for all of us. We all need to lie down afterward.

We tend to take things, including life, for granted. All of us do it, so don't feel guilty. I remember a time many years ago when I broke a bone in my right foot. I was in eighth grade at the time, and the doctor put my foot in a cast. I could walk only with crutches. For the first time ever, I became fully aware of the phenomenon of walking. I watched other boys and girls daily, noting how they swung one leg forward, balanced, then swung the other rhythmically, the knees bending, the foot flexing, the body swaying. A marvelous piece of engineering! I discovered. When that cast was finally removed six weeks later, I reveled in the idea of walking. But, as might be expected, the process became routine, not to be considered at all. I wonder if those without a leg or, worse, those having lost both legs, give a great deal of thought to the process of walking. I'll bet they do.

Use your heightened emotions positively, to focus on the marvels of life and living. Instead of complaining about taking a walk, think about the blessing of being able to walk. Give some conscious thought to the process. Note the movements of your legs. Observe how your arms swing to and fro.

Feel your heart beating inside your rib cage. Notice how your breath is quickened, in and out, in and out. How far have you walked today? Isn't it more than you did last week? Far more than you did in the hospital? You're making progress. Maybe not as fast as you'd like it to be, but progress nonetheless. See the future in your mind's eye. Picture yourself briskly walking along a mountain trail, or jogging along the beach, or bicycling with a friend, or swimming effortlessly lap after lap. You can make that picture a reality.

Just how fast should your heart beat during those first few weeks of recovery at home? There's no magic formula that works for all patients. Your age, former level of fitness, and severity of disease will all come into play as your doctor writes your personal exercise prescription.

To understand that prescription, you must realize that your heart has both a minimal and maximal rate of beating. When at rest, the average individual's heart will beat about 72 times per minute. More physically fit persons will have lower resting heart rates; their hearts are stronger and capable of pumping out the blood the body needs with fewer strokes. Endurance athletes such as marathon runners may have heart rates all the way down into the 40s. On the other hand, resting heart rates may be higher than average owing to age, poor physical condition, and heart disease as the muscular wall of the heart is weakened.

The resting rate is the minimal rate your heart must beat to provide the body's tissues with oxygenated blood. As you engage in various activities, the heart must beat faster as the demand for blood and its oxygen increases. But there's a limit. And as we get older, our maximal heart rate decreases. We can calculate the absolute maximum by subtracting our age from the number 220.

Thus, a 40-year-old man will have a maximal heart rate of 180. A 60-year-old woman's rate is 160. And so on. But no one exercises at the maximal heart rate for any length of time; that would be likened to a steam engine pushed to full throttle. Neither the heart nor the engine can withstand the strain for long.

As we engage in any physical activity, the heart beats to match demands. Some activities require 50 percent of the individual's maximal capacity. Others call for 60 percent. Still others may need even more.

At the same time, our lungs are pumping air in and out. Again, we have maximal capacities for vigorously breathing. The scientific term for this is VO$_2$ max. There's no practical reason for you to know any more detail than that.

Put the two, heart rate and breathing rate, together and you have a measure of physical performance or level of activity. This is termed the *metabolic equivalent*, commonly referred to as the *MET*. Virtually every human activity can be broken down to the effort required, measured in METs. You probably never heard the term before, even if you were physically active. But for those professionals engaged in physical conditioning and rehabilitation programs of all sorts, the MET is a very useful measurement. Take a look at Table 2 for a listing of daily activities and their MET ratings.

TABLE 2
Energy Requirements of Common Activities in METs

1 MET (Metabolic Equivalent) equals the amount of energy needed when the body is at rest.

  Sleeping
  Lying in bed
  Sitting quietly in a chair

2 METs equal *twice* the amount of energy used when at rest.

Standing	Playing cards
Talking	Light housekeeping (dusting)
Walking (1 mph)	Typing/Word Processor
Reading	Shaving
Writing	Dressing/Brushing hair

2–3 METs

Walking (2 mph)	Moderate housekeeping (light laundry)
Playing piano	Meal preparation
Playing golf w/ electric cart	Bicycling (5 mph)
Bathing/Showering	Bowling
Washing hair	

3–4 METs

Walking (3 mph)	Heavier housekeeping (scrubbing)
Bicycling (5 mph)	Playing golf w/ pull cart
Driving a car	Ballroom dancing (foxtrot)
Climbing stairs	Factory labor

4–5 METs

Walking (4 mph)	Playing badminton/light tennis
Bicycling (8 mph)	Heavy housekeeping (mopping)
Gardening/Raking	House painting
Light carpentry	Driving car in heavy traffic

5–6 METs

Walking (4.5 mph)	Social dancing (tango)
Bicycling (10 mph)	Very heavy housekeeping (hauling)
Rollerskating	Light shoveling/digging

6–7 METs

Walking (5 mph)	Lawn mowing
Bicycling (11 mph)	Square dancing
Playing tennis (singles)	Splitting wood
Waterskiing	Snow shoveling

7–8 METs

Jogging (5 mph)	Playing football
Bicycling (12 mph)	Horse riding at gallop
Downhill skiing	Climbing hills (moderate)
Canoeing	

8–9 METs

Jogging (5.5 mph)	Cross-country skiing
Bicycling (13 mph)	Playing basketball

10+ METs

Handball, racquetball, squash	Jogging (6 mph and more)
Climbing hills with load	

Routine activies such as dressing and undressing, washing your face and hands, doing some light work at the desk, or taking a very slow stroll take only one to two METs. More energetic efforts including taking a shower, working in the kitchen, and bicycling at 5 miles per hour require two to three METs. Activities in the three- to four-MET range include scrubbing floors, slow dancing, and working as a stock clerk. When you start raking leaves, walking at four miles per hour, and doing light carpentry, you've reached the four to five MET level. And on and on.

So why do I go into these details? Certainly you're not going to start calculating your daily METs! But here's the good news. Before your doctor discharged you from the hospital, he or she made certain that you are capable of doing activities requiring an energy output of five METs or less. You should be aware, on a very positive level, that virtually anything you'd really want to do during your first weeks of recovery falls into that range.

But what is a reasonable, convenient way to monitor your own effort levels? How much is enough and how much is too much? For those first few weeks of recovery at home, you'll rely on your heart rate.

As we've seen, the way to determine your maximal heart rate is to subtract your age from the number 220. Those who have not had a recent heart attack or cardiac surgery calculate a proper heartbeat range during vigorous exercise by multiplying their maximal heart rate by 60 percent when they begin a workout program and by up to 85 percent as they increase their fitness levels. You may have seen this kind of equation before, providing a formula to reach the so-called "training rate" whereby the heart is beating fast enough to achieve cardiovascular benefit.

As an example, a 50-year-old person would subtract his or her age from 220, giving 170 as the theoretical maximum the heart can beat. Then multiply the 170 by 60 to 85 percent to provide a range of 102 to 144. (See Table 4 on page 224.)

However, those who have recently had a heart attack or cardiac surgery should follow a more conservative formula. This is determined by calculating 60 to 80 percent of the heart rate reached on your most recent treadmill test.

Let's say that your doctor found that your maximum heart rate was 130 when you began to demonstrate symptoms. For the time being, then, you would multiply that maximum rate of 130 by 60 and 80 percent to give you a range of 78 to 104. Every individual will differ. Discuss this with your physician to get your personal exercise prescription.

Your doctor concluded the test for a number of reasons. Perhaps you were beginning to have symptoms when exercising at that maximal rate. Or you may have begun to tire to a sufficient degree that your doctor saw no reason to continue. Or maybe he or she saw an abnormality on your ECG reading and decided it was not wise to continue past that point.

For the time being, therefore, you would be prudent not to exercise to the same extent as an individual who has not had your recent cardiac history. Again, limit your exercise to a level which brings your heart rate up to a range between 60 and 80 percent of the top rate achieved on your treadmill test. Your doctor probably will give you the exact numbers for your convenience. If he or she does not do so, please ask.

There are two ways to measure your heart beat manually. The first is to place your forefinger and middle finger over the inside of your wrist lightly until you feel the pulse. Then, using your watch, count the beats for ten seconds and multiply that number by six.

The second method is to lightly place your two fingers alongside the Adam's apple just under the jaw in order to find your pulse. Again, count the beats for ten seconds and multiply by six. If you use the throat, be careful to use a light touch. Don't push down too hard limiting the flow of blood through the carotid artery that supplies oxygen to the brain, causing lightheadedness or even fainting. While this is rare, forewarned is forearmed.

A number of pulse-taking devices have been marketed for use at home. Some of the cardiac rehabilitation facilities and some gymnasiums and fitness centers provide very sophisticated (and costly) equipment that digitally provide your heart rate at a finger's touch. While they may seem convenient at first, after a few days of practice of taking your own heart rate manually, you'll probably agree with me that there's no need for the extra expense.

Does the multiplication seem difficult? Practice taking your resting heart rate while sitting in a chair at home. Do it a few times during the day. It's natural to notice some variation at different times of the day. Then do the multiplication. Soon you'll begin to see a cluster. Here are some examples of resting heart rates in a typical cluster:

$$11 \text{ beats per 10 seconds} \times 6 = 66 \text{ beats per minute}$$
$$12 \quad '' \qquad\qquad\qquad = 72$$
$$13 \quad '' \qquad\qquad\qquad = 78$$

As you get into your walking program, you'll similarly see a clustering of rates. Again, here are some examples:

$$18 \text{ beats per 10 seconds} \times 6 = 108 \text{ beats per minute}$$
$$19 \quad '' \qquad\qquad\qquad = 114$$
$$20 \quad '' \qquad\qquad\qquad = 120$$
$$21 \quad '' \qquad\qquad\qquad = 126$$
$$22 \quad '' \qquad\qquad\qquad = 132$$

It's important to reiterate that there's no magical formula for determining the right amount of exercise in terms of intensity or time or the right heart rate for everyone. This becomes a medical prescription that must be written exclusively for you by your own physician.

You may find, for example, that symptoms will limit your walk after just a block or two. Or you may get very tired at first. Other physical conditions may also come into play, forcing an adjustment in your prescription.

But two factors remain the same for everyone. First, do your exercise regularly, probably every day unless told to do otherwise by your doctor. Don't make excuses for not doing your walk or your ride on an exercycle. This is the most important job in your life right now, and it deserves your highest priority. Second, you'll be pleasantly surprised at how much progress you make in a relatively short period of time. Today you can do only one block at a time. Three days from now you're walking two blocks. Then three, and four, and five, and on and on.

Can you overdo it? Here are two simple guidelines. One is to stay within your heart rate prescription as prescribed by your doctor. If you find your heart rate going over the 60 to 80 percent range, it's time to slow down or call it a day. The other rule is to quit whenever you feel yourself physically tiring or when you feel any angina pains or other heart-related distress including, for the time being, the leg pains known as intermittent claudication. We'll discuss that specific problem in the coming pages.

If you abide by those two easy-to-follow guidelines, there is no reason to fear overdoing it. Remember that you were released from the hospital because your doctor was confident that you were able to begin your recovery process without round-the-clock supervision.

Drugs such as beta-blockers slow heart rate. You'll be able to exercise your heart to a sufficient level while taking such medications, even though your rate will not go up as much as you might expect. Talk with your doctor about the ideal range of heart rate for you if he has prescribed those drugs.

By all means keep track of your exercise program in your daily diary. Note the time, duration, and length of every exercise session. This will serve two functions. First you can share the log with your doctor at the next visit so he or she can accurately review your activities. Second you will really find it edifying to look back and read how, just two or three weeks earlier, you were a bit tuckered out after walking only a fraction of what you can comfortably do today.

YOUR HEALING HEART

As you know, your heart attack or myocardial infarction was the result of your heart's muscle not getting sufficient oxygen for a prolonged period of time. Depending upon the severity of the heart attack, a certain amount of heart muscle tissue was damaged. As in other injuries, the body begins to heal itself by forming scar tissue at the site of the damage.

Scar tissue does not form overnight. You know that from other injuries you've sustained over the years. Even a scraped elbow takes time to heal. The same goes for your heart muscle.

The healing process begins eight to twelve days after the heart attack, following a period of acute inflammation. By two weeks, scar tissue begins to form; the damaged area of muscle is slowly replaced by a hard, firm scar in the following weeks. Depending upon the severity of the heart attack, the formation of the scar will be completed in from three to six weeks, sometimes a bit longer.

Your recovery period at home allows the formation of that scar tissue. The extent of exercise and other activities allowed during this time span is calculated to not interfere with the healing process. Once the heart has been sufficiently healed, and the scar tissue has been properly formed, you're ready to go on to the next level of your cardiac rehabilitation program.

FORMAL CARDIAC REHABILITATION PROGRAMS

Following your initial, at-home recovery period of from four to six weeks, your doctor will probably do another treadmill exercise test. This time he'll want to push you a bit further, to see just what you can do. You and your doctor will see how well you've recovered thus far. And the test will provide a blueprint for the next phase of recovery.

In the past, this would be virtually the end of a planned approach to recovery. You'd be pretty much off on your own, armed only with some vague suggestions for diet, smoking, and exercise.

But today you have a marvelous option at your disposal. Hospitals and other medical centers and facilities in virtually every community provide formal programs of cardiac rehabilitation. This is an optional program, and not every doctor feels that it's necessary. I strongly disagree, hundreds of medical authorities disagree, and I vehemently hope that by the time you finish reading the next few pages you'll disagree as well. Most importantly, I hope that you'll opt to get into one of those programs and turn your life around once and for all.

When Dr. Albert Kattus suggested the program at Santa Monica Hospital Medical Center, I grudgingly went along with it. He'd given me excellent care both before and after my second bypass, I reasoned, so why not give the program a try, at least for a little while. Even then, I thought that I'd be better off doing things on my own.

My first day was a disaster. I entered the gym and saw a lot of people I just couldn't relate to. I was only 41 years old at the time, and I preferred to be with those my own age rather than older men and women. Some of them were well into their 70s, walking on the treadmill, cycling on stationary exercycles, working the wall pulleys.

No exercise was planned for me on that first day; rather, I filled out some forms and answered a lot of questions. Boring. Then they asked me if I could come in at 7:45 A.M., or whether 9:00 A.M. would be better. Well, I thought, I don't like either time slot. Why not 8:15 so I could sleep a bit later and then get back to the office? But, OK, OK, I'll come in at 7:45.

My schedule called for Monday, Wednesday, and Friday. That meant my first day of exercise would be the following Monday. Come in comfortable, loose-fitting clothes and sneakers, they told me. And with more than a little bit of resentment, I showed up (a little late) at just before 8:00 A.M. Monday, expecting to do some strenuous exercise.

Well, surprise. I couldn't do as much as I thought. Electrodes affixed to my chest sent signals to the front desk where the nurses and exercise physiologists could continuously monitor my heart's activity and rate. My assignment was to bounce up and down on a mini-trampoline or rebounder with handles attached to it. What kind of Mickey Mouse thing was that? But I soon found that it was more than enough to get my heart up to the prescribed rate. Then it was on to the bicycle, and a little time on the treadmill. Of course there was also time for stretching exercises, something I'd really never done before, rather stupidly putting up with aches and pains instead. Oh, and I had to keep an ongoing, daily record including the date, time, resting heart rate, kind of exercise and rate reached, final resting rate after exercise, and any comments. I did *not* want to do that. But I did.

The amazing thing was that there I was, doing what I considered pretty wimpy things, while those gray and bald-headed men and women were doing a lot more than I could. In fact, the closer I looked, they were doing, in some cases, more than I could have done in the weeks *before* my bypass. Astounding. I learned that those patients had been at it for a long time, and had simply stayed on at the hospital's gym after the formal, monitored program had ended. Hm, I thought, if *they* can do that well, what can I achieve if I really put my mind to it.

That was the turning point. For the next 12 weeks, I faithfully attended every session. Almost miraculously, my progress skyrocketed. In fact, I'd be walking on the treadmill or cycling and one of the nurses would shout, "Hey Bob, step it up a bit more." Here I was, doing as much as I thought I should, and they told me I could do more. So I did, knowing confidently that they knew what they were doing and that if anything happened, they'd know what to do. After all, they were looking at my ECG every step of the way.

Within a very short time, well before completing the full 12 weeks, I knew that I was exercising a *lot* more than I'd normally do on my own. I wouldn't have pushed myself that much. My anxiety would have limited my efforts.

Moreover, I knew that nothing I'd do on the outside was likely to come close to the exertion I was experiencing at the hospital. Bingo! That meant that there was nothing in my life that could cause a problem. During exercise I experienced a number of those "funny feelings" you wonder about: the left arm twinges, the tightness of the jaw, and so forth. Since I was "wired" the nurses saw nothing out of the normal ECG, and I knew that those feelings were not heart related. So when they happened outside the hospital, I no longer feared them at all. What a feeling of freedom!

I also had the opportunity to attend a number of sessions dealing with topics that every heart patient should know more about, including stress management, diet and cholesterol reduction, controlling blood pressure, commonly prescribed heart drugs, and so forth.

Very importantly, I got to know the other patients in rehab, and actually looked forward to working out with them in the mornings. It was nice to have someone to talk with, side by side on treadmills. No one there was trying to compete, or to act "macho" as might be the case in a sports club or gym. Some of those friendships have lasted through the years.

By going through the program I was able to enforce a kind of discipline that I might not have had on my own. I had my appointment at 7:45 each Monday, Wednesday, and Friday morning. If I missed that time slot, I was out of luck, since I couldn't do a "makeup" at other times when other patients were using the equipment. Little by little, it became routine, a routine I actually enjoyed.

When the 12 weeks came to an end, I decided I wanted (and needed) that kind of structure and routine. So rather than exercising on my own, I signed up for an unmonitored program whereby I came in as usual, but without the electrodes on my chest. Again, it was about an hour three times weekly, with some extra walking or cycling on the weekends. I thought I'd do that for just a few extra months.

But then the progress I was making in my increasing level of fitness really kicked in, and I was feeling terrific. Dr. Kattus simply beamed when he did my next treadmill test, calling my recovery phenomenal. I wondered if I could do that much in just a few months, what would be possible in a year? So I stuck with it. And continued for another year after that.

Why did I finally leave the hospital program? I found that I wanted to do even more, and I was being limited by the available time slots and the length of time I could work out on any given piece of equipment. It was time to move on, to graduate to an independent setting. I joined a place called Sports Club L.A. because they had a limited membership, which meant I wouldn't have to wait in line for equipment. My early habits have stuck with me, and I now make physical exercise my first appointment of the day Monday through Friday, five days a week without fail. But I'll get into some specifics on continuing exercise and conditioning in the next chapter.

It turns out that the program of cardiac rehabilitation I went through was pretty typical of those available all over the country. The 12-week length is standard, with three hour-long sessions per week. Some concentrate exclusively on the exercise segment, while a large number include educational segments to focus on other lifestyle modifications necessary to achieve total recovery.

There's a bit of controversy regarding the monitoring aspect. Some programs use the chest electrodes allowing continuous ECG monitoring only for higher-risk patients, while others utilize the system of wireless transmittal known as telemetry for all patients. Personally, having gone through it myself, I'm glad I had the electrodes. They gave me the confidence I needed.

Who's eligible for entering a cardiac recovery program? Anyone who's had a heart attack, bypass or other cardiac surgery, angioplasty, or confirmed existence of heart disease with or without the symptoms of angina and claudication. All programs call for an exercise treadmill test documenting the safety of such an approach. We'll get into the safety aspects shortly, but for now suffice it to say that cardiac rehabilitation is warranted for all heart patients except those with significant damage done to the heart muscle, severe arrhythmias, and extremely high blood pressure. As we'll see, even patients with heart failure have done well. Both men and women benefit, in all age categories.

While doing the research for this book, I visited a number of cardiac rehabilitation programs both large and small. Certainly the size of the hospital, medical center, or outpatient center will have a lot to do with the level of sophistication that the program can attain. But that's not always true. Sometimes a very small hospital can set up a very effective and well-equipped approach.

Everyone I spoke with echoed the same thoughts about their patients. The drop-out rate is very low because the participants quickly see the benefits. According to Dr. Michael Lawlor, exercise physiologist and Director of Cardiac Rehabilitation and Fitness Programs at the Heart Institute of the Desert in Rancho Mirage, California, almost everyone says "I've never felt better, not just OK, but fantastic!" Barbara Else, R.N., director of the rehab program at Cedars-Sinai Hospital in Los Angeles, points out that "the faster we get somebody in, the faster they start to feel good about themselves."

Dr. Lawlor notes that the majority of people just don't know what it's like to feel really terrific. "If at one time you were in good physical condition you know what it's like to be in good shape, to feel great," he says. "But if you've never been physically fit, it's almost impossible to relate to what it can feel like."

Virtually all the rehab directors agree on one thing. Once a person gets beyond the first six weeks, no one wants to quit. Time and again, I've spoken with men and women at the start of their rehab program and told them how they were going to love it once they got past the first few weeks' hump. They'd grunt "Yeah, sure." But then a month later I'd see them again, or they'd call on the phone and say, "Bob, you were right, I never thought I could feel this good this fast!"

But the benefits of cardiac rehabilitation can be objectively measured as well as subjectively felt. Here are some of those benefits:

- *Counteract the effects of inactivity.* There's nothing that can compare with a structured program to bring back your body's vigor.
- *Improve functional capacity.* Both your lungs and heart will work more efficiently, reducing the strain on the cardiovascular system. This can increase the level of day-to-day activities you want to participate in without getting tired and with lessened heart symptoms.
- *Improve cardiovascular efficiency.* As your heart pumps more oxygen-rich blood to tissues with less effort, your heart rate and blood pressure begin to come down. The body appears to be more capable of stripping the oxygen off the blood's hemoglobin, as well.
- *Increase in collateral circulation.* Just as a railroad might lay new tracks around a blockage, your arteries can form new branches around areas of blockage, providing a new supply of oxygen-rich blood to the heart muscle. The more one exercises, the more one begins to see the development of such collateral circulation.
- *Reduce heart disease risk factors.* Sedentary behavior has, itself, been identified as a risk factor in the development and progression of heart disease. But exercise can also help in efforts to maintain or attain ideal weight, to control blood sugar for those with diabetes, and to regulate cholesterol levels. Not only will exercise help reduce the "bad" LDL cholesterol, but it will also raise the levels of the "good" HDL type.

A number of well-controlled studies both in the United States and abroad have demonstrated the advantages of cardiac rehabilitation. The *Journal of the American Medical Association* published a review of 10 trials with cardiac rehabilitation and found a 24 percent reduction in all causes of death and a 25 percent cut in cardiovascular mortality. These studies involved 2,202 patients in comprehensive rehab programs compared with 2,145 who were not in programs.

Thus we have the evidence that enrolling in a formal cardiac rehabilitation can actually save your life. In one way, that should be reason enough. But, as mentioned earlier, we have both physical improvements and psychological well-being as bonuses.

As I said, that evidence comes from around the world. A five-year Swedish program found that the incidence of future heart attacks was cut almost in half, and the number of all cardiac events was reduced by nearly 40 percent.

SAFETY OF CARDIAC REHABILITATION

Unfortunately, not all patients are physically able to participate in cardiac rehabilitation. Among the contraindications are congestive heart failure that is uncontrolled, severe damage to the heart muscle with resultant ventricular incapacitation, unstable angina pectoris, thrombophlebitis, severe arrhythmias, and uncontrolled hypertension.

The most complete review of the safety of cardiac rehabilitation was published in a position paper by the American Association of Cardiovascular and Pulmonary Rehabilitation in 1990. The data were collected from 167 programs throughout the United States and involved more than 51,000 patients who exercised more than two million hours between 1980 and 1984. The rate of complications was one cardiac arrest per 111,996 hours, one heart attack per 293,900 hours, and one fatality per 783,976 hours of prescribed, supervised exercise. The authors attribute this high rate of safety to proper patient evaluations, education, careful exercise prescription, appropriate use of ECG monitoring, well-trained personnel, and rapid handling of emergencies. In other words, the safety of a structured, formal program is, by its very nature, much better than would be expected if the patients were on their own.

THE ELDERLY AND CARDIAC REHABILITATION

In its report on cardiac rehabilitation services, the U.S. Department of Health and Human Services covers the benefits of rehab programs for the elderly. The conclusion is simple and straight to the point: "Although the absolute work capacity of the over 65 group was significantly lower than that reached by the younger groups, *the magnitude of favorable change was equivalent.*" And no additional risk due to greater age was found. The elderly patients benefit from early rehab in the same ways that younger individuals do; they experience enhanced functional capacity and improved psychological outlook.

A number of studies back up those conclusions. The effects of exercise training in 60- to 69-year-old patients with hypertension were studied by researchers at Washington University in St. Louis. They found that both low- and moderate-intensity training lowered blood pressure.

Older patients who exercise have a brighter outlook both literally and figuratively. A Stanford University study demonstrated that older people who exercise have better thinking than those who don't. Those who exercise regularly do the best when tested in the areas of vocabulary, memory, reaction time, and reasoning. Those who exercised the most tended to regard their health as better and showed more satisfaction with their lives.

JOINING A STRUCTURED PROGRAM

Despite all the marvelous things that can be said about a formal cardiac rehabilitation program, the sad fact is that only about 17 percent of patients take advantage of it. In fact, since the participation rate is so low, some critics have suggested getting rid of all such efforts! That's like saying since antibiotics work only for those who take them when prescribed, that all those pills should be tossed out. Ridiculous.

Some have pointed to the high costs of a structured rehab program. Both Medicare and most major insurance programs pay for a 12-week, structured, hospital-based cardiac rehabilitation effort. In documented cases of need, Medicare will also pay for an additional 24 weeks. The irony here is that no one argues against the use of physical therapy for recovery from broken bones and other orthopedic injuries and surgery. Such programs are also expensive. But they work. In the case of cardiac rehabilitation programs, they work too. And they can save your life.

Unfortunately, not all physicians have read the documentation on effectiveness of such programs in the medical literature. Physicians who become involved with cardiac rehab programs will see the results: they'll see their patients get better. When that happens, more doctors will recommend such programs.

Actually, doctors themselves benefit when their patients enter rehab. Such patients tend to ask fewer questions, since they have them answered during their sessions. They're easier to work with since they're better informed and better motivated, with a better attitude. And they have a better long-term prognosis.

The most active physician-advocates of rehab are those who have gone through it themselves. Barbara Else at Cedars-Sinai Hospital has seen a number of doctors go through her program in Los Angeles. While many are skeptical at first, they become zealots, both for themselves and for their patients, she says.

Talk with your doctor about rehab programs at your hospital or in your area. Don't let him tell you that taking a walk now and then is "just as good." Demand your rights to have the best possible care, with the best possible outlook for the future. When you need a fine-tuned sports car to win the race, nothing else will do.

Your doctor or the cardiology department at the hospital will have information on rehab programs in your community. But if you need further information on locations and availability, you can contact the American Association of Cardiovascular and Pulmonary Rehabilitation. Their address is 7611 Elmwood Avenue, Suite 201, Middleton, WI 53562. The phone is (608) 831-5122.

The AACPR can also tell you about YMCA locations and other facilities which may be able to provide rehabilitation assistance. Many of those are remarkably good.

CARDIAC REHABILITATION AT HOME

While I strongly advocate a structured, medically supervised cardiac rehabilitation program, there are admittedly times when this is simply not possible for all patients. You may live in a remote area, too far from the nearest facility. You may lack the insurance or the financial ability to pay for such a program yourself. Whatever the reason you cannot enroll in a formal program, you owe it to yourself to engage in a home-based effort to the very best of your abilities.

Talk with your doctor about this. You'll need to undergo a detailed physical examination including a treadmill exercise test to work out your personal exercise prescription. The physician will need to rule out severe myocardial ischemia (whereby your heart is getting insufficient oxygen) and dysfunction of your left ventricle.

Ask whether you might be able to join an abbreviated supervised program for two to four weeks. This will get you started on the right course and will enable the health professionals to detect any difficulties and to answer your questions on a regular basis as they occur.

If working out at home, you'll need to have your treadmill test updated on a regular basis to allow you to go on to the next level of exertion. There are also programs by which patients can attach their own electrodes to their chests and send the cardiac information over the phone by way of special equipment and a telephone modem.

As in medically supervised programs, keep your home activities to a low level at first. It's far better to gradually increase your work load than to overdo it at the beginning. If at all possible, it's best to work out on a number of different types of equipment. Vary your exercise as much as possible, both to utilize and condition all your body's muscles and to maintain interest. Alternate walking, biking, swimming, and gardening.

You may decide that you do want to buy or lease at least one piece of equipment to use at home. When the snow is flying, the rain is falling, or the temperatures are sinking or soaring, having a treadmill or an exercycle at home can be a real blessing.

The variety at your disposal is formidable, and I'd advise you to check out all your alternatives before making a decision. Many stores offer a lease or a rental with a purchase option. That way you can see if you'll really use the equipment and decide if this is exactly what suits your needs. *Consumer Reports,* a publication of Consumers Union, offers a completely unbiased, straightforward evaluation of exercise equipment. If you want specific information that's been published, you can write to *Consumer Reports* at 256 Washington St., Mount Vernon, NY 10553.

Fortunately, there's another way to follow a regular exercise program in your own home, with a series of videotapes specially designed and developed for those recovering from heart attack and surgery.

The series consists of three videotapes, progressing through the stages of recovery. Level One contains instruction, counseling, and warm-ups for beginning exercises that last 20 minutes and are the equivalent of walking at a level of two to four METs. Level Two continues the program with intermediate exercises equal to 30 minutes of brisk walking at a four- to six-MET level. You finally graduate to Level Three, which brings you to 30 minutes of exercises that are the equivalent energy expenditure of jogging (six to eight METs). All the exercises are low-impact.

The tapes all include pre- and post-exercise checklists to monitor your progress and to provide encouragement and feedback. The program has met the standards of the American Heart Association and the American College of Sports Medicine. It was developed by Dr. Alan Xenakis.

To order the *Cardiac Comeback* videotape series, you can call (800) 345-3371 between 6 A.M. and 6 P.M. Pacific Time. The tapes are very reasonably priced and are fully guaranteed.

In addition to exercise, spend some time doing gentle stretches during any activity session. To derive the greatest advantage of stretching in terms of increasing flexibility and preventing aches and strains, do a bit of warm-up exercise first. The ideal approach would be an easy 10-minute ride on a stationary exercycle, followed by about five to eight minutes of stretches, then on to another 35 minutes of aerobic activity, and finishing up with about five minutes of cool-down until your heart rate returns to its resting range.

By all means keep tabs on your heart rate. Take it before, during, and after your exercise, and make certain that you don't exceed your exercise prescription. This is definitely not the time to believe that if a little is good, then more must be better!

Keep an accurate log of your activities, marking the date, time, type of exercise, heart rates, and comments. Share your diary with your doctor whenever you see him.

There's no question that a structured, hospital-based program is more efficient in getting you started. But you can definitely achieve a successful recovery by way of a home-based approach. You'll need more self discipline and motivation, but it can be done. Good luck!

Whether working in the hospital or at home, remember the story of the man in England way back in 1772 who achieved a remarkable recovery by sawing wood. We've come a long way since those days, and a long way since the time when heart patients were kept in bed. We know today that while doctors, cardiologists, surgeons, and others in the health team can do much to get us off to a good start, in the long run it's still up to us as individual patients to make total recovery a reality.

With every step you take, with every turn of the cycle pedals, with every stroke in the swimming pool, think of yourself as getting closer and closer to becoming a *former* heart patient!

CHAPTER 11

Living a Dynamic, Active Life

THE EXERCISE PRESCRIPTION

Exercise is an essential element in the recovery process. This is your life we're talking about. Get to know more about the exercise prescription and how to make it an integral part of your life.

What we have here is a circular path. We start off with what has to be viewed as a medical prescription; in order to recover, you have to follow the medical prescription of exercise. Yet this same exercise will enable us to live a dynamic, active life, free of the limitations that hindered heart patients in the past.

Rather than viewing your exercise prescription entirely as something you have to do because your doctor told you to, start thinking about it as the way you're going to improve your life. It truly will do that, it will improve your life beyond your wildest expectations.

It's no accident or coincidence that virtually every culture in the world has stressed the importance of fitness and exercise. The link between the body and mind and disease is strong in both Eastern and Western societies. The ancient Greeks paid homage to their athletes and stressed the value of exercise as highly for students as academic pursuits. All Oriental cultures place high value on exercise and fitness; it was the Chinese monks who developed the martial art form of kung fu.

Western religions also place the responsibility for the care of our bodies squarely on our own shoulders. Look up Paul's first letter to the Corinthians in the Bible and you'll read that your body is the temple of the Holy Spirit. We are entrusted with the care of that body. And physical fitness is an important aspect of that care.

You'll begin as a patient dutifully taking your medicine, but I hope you will continue as a fit person who is "hooked" on the benefits of exercise. Like many who have gone before you, you just might wind up singing its praises.

Ironically, when I took the President's Fitness Test back in the '50s when I was in elementary school, I flunked badly. I couldn't run the mile in 10 minutes, I couldn't do the required push-ups and sit-ups, or any of the other physical tests. Quite bluntly, I was a pathetically out-of-shape kid who grew up to be an out-of-shape adult. As I've stated earlier, I didn't welcome the idea of entering the cardiac rehab program. But once I got into it, I never stopped. And today I'm in better physical condition than I've ever been in my life. When I tell people that I feel better than I did when I was in my twenties, I'm not exaggerating.

Here's some very good news for those who might rate a workout in the gym just above having one's stomach pumped and just below watching the paint peel off a wall. It takes very little exercise to achieve a heart-healthy status. We will get into the details of that in the pages to come, but I just wanted to let you know right off the bat that you're not going to be asked to become a marathon runner.

THE BENEFITS OF EXERCISE

Physical activity does so many good things for you that if it were bottled the advertising would make it sound just too good to be true. Here's a list of advantages that puts the situation in a nutshell.

Physical activity decreases:

blood pressure
resting heart rate

vulnerability to cardiac arrhythmias
abnormal blood clotting
effects of stress on the body
depression
cholesterol levels
triglycerides
high blood sugar levels
glucose intolerance
body fat

Physical activity increases:

blood flow to muscles including the heart
blood vessel size
heart muscle efficiency
oxygen usage efficiency
HDL "good" cholesterol
muscle mass
insulin sensitivity
metabolic rate

Now let's take a closer look at the role exercise can play in your life. In its report on cardiac rehabilitation and exercise for the U.S. Department of Health and Human Services, the Public Health Service listed chapter and verse extolling the virtues of physical activity. The authors reviewed the available medical literature and concluded that exercise facilitates the ability of muscle, including the muscle of the heart, to extract oxygen from hemoglobin in blood. Blood flow to the muscle also goes up. The result is that muscle can do greater levels of work with less effort. When the heart muscle needn't work so hard, the episodes of angina go down.

Your heart will also get more blood pumped to it, as the size of vessels increase and the number of tiny arteries increases. The latter is called collateral circulation, which we mentioned in the last chapter. All this means more oxygen getting to your heart.

But it's not just a matter of less pain from angina. On a far more positive note, the level of energy you'll achieve will soar to beyond anything you've probably experienced before. It's amazing how bright and alert you'll feel. You just won't tire as easily. It won't happen overnight. Remember that you've got some healing to do first, then some catching up from the incapacitation of prolonged inactivity, but then your progress will take off like a rocket. You'll see the payoff both at work and at play.

Here's how bypass surgery made me a better skier.

I'd been skiing since I got out of college, but was never really good at it. In fact, I could never get beyond a low-intermediate classification. Then came the bypass surgery and my cardiac rehab program. The next season I couldn't believe myself on the slopes. I was in total control, my body responded like it never had before; all those lessons suddenly kicked in. I took run after run without tiring. What a glorious feeling!

And as much as you'll enjoy your newfound energy, you'll love the way exercise improves your sleep. You'll fall asleep more easily, without tossing and turning and watching the hands move around the clock. And you'll stay asleep longer through the night. It's better than any sleeping pill ever invented.

Exercise is a wonderful way to control stress, and it's one of the best ways to keep tabs on your emotions. Here, too, it's not just the negative idea of diminishing stress; the positive flip side of the coin is a feeling of well-being that often reaches euphoria. That's because exercise causes the body to release chemicals into the bloodstream known as beta-endorphins. Those substances are chemically related to morphine, and produce a very blissful, serene feeling that's hard to match. And it's both legal and healthful!

Bear in mind that this isn't just my personal opinion. Researchers at the University of New Mexico found that sedentary people report more perceived stress and have more stress-related hormones in their bloodstream than a group who did regular exercise. The director of the university's human performance laboratory, Dr. Dennis Lobstein, said that exercise decreases anxiety, hostility, and other stress-related disorders.

In another study, scientists at Purdue University concluded that depression does not automatically or necessarily increase with advancing age, but instead may be associated with controllable variables including fitness. Even the smallest amount of physical activity has positive impact.

A paper presented at the 1988 meeting of the American College of Sports Medicine (ACSM) reviewed 79 published and unpublished studies and concluded that exercise significantly decreases depression. They saw benefits both in apparently healthy individuals and in those with medical and psychological problems.

At the 1990 ACSM meeting, Loma Linda University researchers offered the first randomized, controlled long-term study looking at psychological well-being and exercise. Subjects walked 45 minutes, five times a week. Even after just six weeks, exercising patients scored significantly better than their sedentary counterparts in tests measuring well-being. A similar study from the University of Missouri determined that a 12-week exercise program generally slashed depression scores to less than half, sometimes to less than a third, of the pre-exercise levels.

Next on the list of marvelous things that exercise does for you is weight control. Since obesity is a condition that afflicts an estimated 33 million Americans, and one that has a direct impact on the risk of heart disease, this is a mighty important consideration.

First, of course, exercise of all kinds helps burn extra calories. But it's more than that. Even after you've stopped exercising, your body continues to burn calories at a faster rate because your metabolism gets stepped up a notch or two. So you burn more calories for several hours after your workout.

Second, the more you exercise the more you replace fat with lean muscle tissue. Only muscle can burn calories, not fat, so now your body has more ability to use the energy you supply in the form of food.

Now what happens when you feel better, you deal with stress more effectively, you are less depressed, you sleep better, and you've lost weight and put on a bit more muscle? You look better! No question about it, this has happened to more than one former heart patient.

If all this isn't enough, increasing the amount of physical activity you do will also keep you alive a lot longer. Virtually every study of longevity ever performed has agreed on one conclusion: Those who live the longest are those who are most physically active and fit.

Exercise expert Dr. Ralph Paffenbarger published the first evidence of the exercise–longevity link in 1986 in the *New England Journal of Medicine.* He studied the exercise habits of nearly 17,000 Harvard University alumni. Physical activity was reported as walking, stair climbing, and sports and was inversely related to total mortality, especially due to cardiovascular disease. Death rates declined steadily as the amount of energy expended on any kind of activity increased from less than 500 to 3,500 calories per week.

It's fascinating to note that Dr. Paffenbarger's results were statistically exclusive of hypertension, smoking, family history of death, and overweight. Not that those things aren't important, too, but basically his data indicate that an exercising smoker tends to live longer than a nonexercising smoker. By the age of 80, the amount of additional life attributed to adequate exercise was one year to more than two years.

But do these figures hold up for those who have already had a heart attack or other evidence of heart disease, or is it too late? A study published in the *Journal of Cardiopulmonary Rehabilitation* found that exercise has a positive influence for everyone.

In that study, a group of older persons was surveyed in 1976 and again in 1984. The results showed a direct relationship between mortality and aerobic exercise. The more active the person, the more likely he or she was to live longer. Of those individuals who had reported having had a heart attack in the 1976 survey, more were alive in 1984 if their energy expenditure was high.

Until 1990, we had to rely on small, isolated studies to prove the benefits of exercise in terms of living a longer, healthier life. The ultimate proof was published in the November 3, 1990 issue of the *Journal of the American Medical Association*. Researchers at the Institute for Aerobic Research in Dallas had studied physical fitness and risk of mortality from all causes, not just heart disease, in 10,224 men and 3,120 women. Fitness was actually measured by treadmill testing; in the past, studies often relied on questionnaires. The project ran a full eight years.

After screening out all irrelevant variables, the rate of death was 64.0 per 10,000 person-years in the least fit men to 18.6 in the most fit men. The trend held true for women as well, with mortality rates in the least fit at 39.5 and down to 8.5 in the most fit. Higher levels of physical fitness seem to delay death from all causes, the researchers concluded.

At about the same time, investigators at Rockefeller University in New York looked at why exercise offers protection against heart disease. Their ten-week study linked exercise to reduced serum triglycerides and increased lipoprotein metabolism. The study included six healthy men. During a seven-week exercise period following a three-week baseline determination, the men jogged on a treadmill for an average of 15 miles a week. At the project's completion, triglycerides were down by 16 percent, and total plasma lipoprotein levels dropped an average of 32 percent.

How much exercise is enough? Virtually every study to date has shown that you'll benefit from any amount of aerobic exercise. Whether you walk, jog, or cycle, the trick is to get your heart rate up for a minimum of 30 minutes three to five days every week. The Dallas study indicates, though, that a little exercise does the job, and that after a certain level there's a point of diminishing returns. The equivalent of 15 miles a week seems to be the point to shoot for. That would be a three-mile brisk walk or jog five days a week.

We'll look at specific recommendations for exercise in the coming pages. But first I'd like to dispel a number of myths regarding exercise and to put to rest any concerns you might have about safety.

MYTHS ABOUT EXERCISE

Exercise makes you tired. Actually, the reverse is true. Properly done, you won't even have sore muscles or any aches and pains. In a very short period of time, you will find you have more energy, less fatigue, and a better night's sleep so that you're less tired than before.

Exercise takes too much time. The amount of time you need to devote to exercise is quite small, with a minimum of 30 minutes three to five days a week. Once you get into a routine, you'll never miss the time spent. Moreover, you'll get that time back in terms of increased productivity and energy. And you'll live longer. View exercise as time put in the bank for future, extra years.

Older people don't need exercise. Literally everyone benefits from a program of regular physical activity. In the coming pages we'll see how even the oldest individuals benefit tremendously.

Exercise must be very strenuous to work. The good news here is that you don't have to turn into a "jock" to see real health benefits. As we'll see, recent research has shown that even a brisk walk on a regular basis will get the job done.

Your heart has a limited number of beats. Strange as this one sounds, some people have believed that the heart is somehow "programed" to beat just so many times in one's lifetime. The illogical thinking was that if you "wasted" those beats by speeding up the heart during exercise, you would use up your number of beats. An article in the *New England Journal of Medicine* in 1988 put that old myth to rest. The more the heart is exercised, the more efficient it becomes and the longer it's likely to last.

Former athletes need not exercise. In his study of Harvard alumni, Dr. Ralph Paffenbarger found that those who were college athletes but who no longer exercised were at the same risk as any out-of-shape individual. Athletic performance in the past has no benefit for the future.

Exercise can kill you. Look at Jim Fixx. A small number of individuals die each year while exercising. Far more are protecting their lives and health by physical activity. Exercise is very safe when conducted properly.

Jim Fixx is a sad case that proves a point. The man had a terrible history of heart disease in his family. He had smoked cigarettes most of his life, had been sedentary, and was very overweight. Moreover, he had never had an exercise treadmill test, despite the urging of his physicians. After Fixx died while jogging in Vermont, his autopsy showed very significant blockage in his arteries, a condition which would have been detected during a treadmill test and which could have been successfully treated.

Exercise has no proven benefits. Dr. Henry Solomon attacks the concept of exercise in his 1985 book *The Exercise Myth*. He maintains that there is no proof that exercise will help you live longer or improve health. As we've seen in the research data published since that time, we now have definitive proof. Dr. Solomon's criticisms are simply out of date.

"LITE" EXERCISE

Gone are the days of "no pain, no gain" and going for the "burn." After scaring off most of the adult population by stressing the importance of all-out physical training programs, the scientific and medical communities have now come to the conclusion that it just doesn't take very much at all to achieve cardiac fitness.

The fact of the matter is that for some individuals, just getting up off the couch to change the channel rather than using the remote control may get the heart rate up. No, I'm not exaggerating that one bit. Many men and women have done absolutely no exercise for years. For them, a walk needn't even be brisk to increase the heart rate.

What we're seeing today in the ever-expanding data coming out of research laboratories is that a *performance fitness* training rate isn't the same as a *cardiac fitness* rate. That is to say, a young man or woman who's training to compete in track and field contests will push the heart rate to 80 to 90 percent of maximum for his or her age. But there's no need to do that in order to achieve cardiac conditioning. Bringing your rate up to 60 or 70 percent, in fact 60 to 70 percent of a submaximal heart rate attained on the treadmill, will get you where you need to go for your heart's fitness.

Dr. Henry Miller, medical director of the Bowman Grey School of Medicine in Winston-Salem, North Carolina, goes even further. He conducted a study that found no difference in the recovery of heart attack patients whether they were on a low- or high-intensity exercise regimen. Dr. Miller says "You have to do something to increase the use of your muscles, to make your heart rate come up, but I don't think there's anything really magic about getting your heart rate up to 80 to 90 percent of max." He believes that even activities which will bring your heart rate up to 40 percent will provide a healthful effect.

Dr. Miller's opinion is shared by Dr. Arthur Leon, professor of epidemiology at the University of Minnesota. He reports that working in the garden and on the lawn, making home repairs, and even participating in sports such as golf, hunting, and bowling all appear to reduce coronary risk.

Dr. Leon bases his conclusions on an analysis of nearly 13,000 high-risk men who participated in the coronary prevention study known as the Multiple Risk Factor Intervention Trial, commonly referred to as the Mr Fit study. Individuals were divided into three groups: those whose activity level was termed "light" as defined as 15 minutes of light activity per day; moderate, defined as 47 minutes of light activity daily; and heavy, with 134 minutes of light activity each day.

Men in the moderate group showed a marked reduction in coronary heart disease compared with men whose activity level was defined as light. Interestingly, there was little added advantage in being the most active.

Dr. Leon says that an average increase of about half an hour a day of "predominantly light and moderate physical activity" reduced by one-third the risk of heart disease, sudden death, and heart attacks in this population of middle-aged men at high risk for coronary heart disease.

What kinds of activity was Dr. Leon referring to? In order, the most popular activities in the groups studied were: lawn/garden (84%); walking (70%); home repairs (64%); water sports, mostly swimming (56%); other sports, notably bowling (52%); dancing (40%); biking (25%); and golf (25%). Only 12 percent reported themselves to be joggers.

What level of exertion do you have to reach to get the beneficial effects? In Dr. Leon's group, moderately active people averaged only about 1,500 calories a week of activity. Take a look at Table 3 to see how those calories might get burned.

In Dr. Ralph Paffenbarger's study of Harvard alumni, research subjects who exercised enough to burn 2,000 calories a week were a third less likely to have died over the course of the ongoing study than those who got little or no exercise. In fact, those who did very heavy exercise, burning 3,500 calories or more a week, had a higher death rate than those in the moderate-activity category.

The watchword is to take it easy, to start off slowly and surely. Dr. Peter Raven, head of the department of physiology at Texas College of Osteopathic Medicine and the 1990 president of the American College of Sports Medicine (ACSM), says it should take 12 weeks to develop a

TABLE 3
Calorie Expenditure of Common Activities*

Walking (2 mph)	240 calories per hour
Bicycling (6 mph)	240
Swimming (25 yds/min)	275
Walking (3 mph)	320
Tennis (singles)	400
Bicycling (12 mph)	410
Walking (4.5 mph)	440
Swimming (50 yds/min)	500
Running in place	650
Cross-country skiing	700
Jogging (5.5 mph)	740
Jumping rope	750
Jogging (7 mph)	920

*For adult men and women of 150 pounds. For every 15 pounds over 150, one burns 10 percent more calories. For every 15 pounds less than 150, one burns 10 percent fewer calories.

good exercise program. "If you take that kind of time you'll stop the injuries and the muscle soreness that often accompanies the beginning of any activity program."

You'll recall the study done in Dallas at the Institute for Aerobics Research in which both men and women benefited from an increase in physical activity. Subjects fell into one of five categories of fitness, from level one (virtually inactive, literally the couch potatoes), to level five (serious joggers and runners who put on 40 miles or so each week).

Not surprisingly, couch potatoes fared worst, with the highest rates of death from heart disease and other causes. As one left that group and entered the next level or two of light to moderate activity, death rates dropped precipitously. But, much to the surprise of the researchers and others who had long advocated a "the more the better" approach, those at the highest levels of fitness didn't do much better than those moderately active individuals.

Dr. Steven Blair was the principal investigator of the study, which was published in the *Journal of the American Medical Association*. He attended the 1990 meeting of the ACSM and put his feelings quite bluntly: "The public health message needs to swing a bit and we need to get people off their butts and up and moving, even if that just means getting them out for a 15- to 20-minute walk once or twice a day. I don't care what their heart rate is! There is certainly evidence that that kind of light to moderate activity produces health benefits."

But how does one define that level of activity? Dr. Blair thinks that if one exercises hard enough to increase the breathing rate noticeably and—assuming that you're not in a cold climate—you sweat a little, that's hard enough.

Dr. William Haskell, professor of medicine at Stanford University, supports this opinion. Speaking at a meeting of science writers I attended, he said that burning 250–300 calories a day is sufficient to substantially reduce the risk of heart attack. That translates to a brisk 30- to 45-minute walk.

In fact, you don't even have to do it all at one time. You can do that walk in short spurts of 10 minutes or so each. That means you can park your car a mile away from your appointment, walk to your destination, then walk back. Dr. Haskell believes you can divide your day's activities even further. You might want to do three or four 10-minute walks a day. Or you might prefer to do a little walking, a little gardening, a little work around the house, and then maybe a bicycle ride in the late afternoon. Another day it might be a swim. The important thing is to make that exercise a regular, routine part of your daily existence.

TAKE A WALK FOR THE HEALTH OF IT

Walking can very easily become a routine part of one's life, and well it should be. You're likely to get to a point when you'll be disappointed if anything should get in the way of your "daily constitutional" as the day's walk used to be called.

When so many goals take so much effort to achieve, it's nice to think that something as simple and easy as taking a daily walk can have so many benefits. This is something that's available to most of us.

During my media tour in London to talk about my books, I checked into a hotel that had a health club just across the street. I planned to get a short-term membership so I could keep up with my exercise program. But then I found that walking is absolutely a way of life in England. One good reason is that traffic is often so congested that one can walk to a destination faster than a taxi could get there. Before I knew it, I was walking all over the place, aided by a map and by the friendly people, who were always happy to provide directions to a "Yank." I never did go into that health club, and I never felt better.

Whether you're in a formal, structured cardiac rehabilitation program or following your doctor's exercise prescription on your own at home, walking will be a part of your recovery. A while back we used to believe that walking was the place to start a conditioning program; today we know that it very well may be all you need, now and in the future.

I happen to be lucky enough to live where the weather allows me to go out for a walk just about every day of the year. Those living in Minnesota may not fare as well when the mercury drops below zero and the wind chill factor comes into play. On those days many cold-clime residents take to the shopping malls. Today's huge enclosed malls, typically on two or three levels, offer a wonderful opportunity to walk regardless of the weather. In fact, in many cities there are mall-walking clubs, and malls often open before the shops open their doors so that walking will be unimpeded. Another alternative is the treadmill. We'll get into the pros and cons of that and other equipment in the coming pages.

A terrific way to stay on a routine walking program is to do it with a friend or two. Many couples become fellow walkers after a cardiac event. It offers a nice way to talk about the day's events when the walk is planned as the first thing to do after coming home from work. Certainly a healthier way to start the evening than with a cocktail!

What's the best time of the day to exercise? Some folks can get their exercise by simply taking advantage of opportunities throughout the day: taking a few flights of stairs instead of using the elevator; walking to put a few letters in the mail box; parking the car several blocks from the final destination.

Others find it best to have a specified time of day to get in their walk. I happen to like to get in a workout first thing in the morning. My wife prefers doing so after work. I feel that getting some exercise sets the tone for the day, providing a charge of my batteries that carries me through and helps to offset the day's stresses. Dawn absolutely hates it then, but finds it relaxing after a day in the classroom.

Investigators at the William Beaumont Hospital in Royal Oak, Michigan, compared morning and evening cardiac exercisers. They checked a total of nearly 30,000 patient sessions of rehab over a 23-month span of time. It turns out that evening exercisers missed more sessions than did their morning counterparts, even though everyone was free to choose the time of day he or she preferred. The difference wasn't that great, however, with the morning crowd attending 68 percent of the sessions and the later group coming 60 percent of the time.

I must say that on those days when I decide to exercise later in the day, I tend to come up with excuses, postponing it hour by hour until the day's over and I've not gotten my workout. For me it's best to set my workout as my day's first assignment.

That need for structure is also why I belong to a health club. I find it helpful to have to get into the car to go to the club where the phone can't disturb me and I'm not tempted to do anything other than what I'm there for. I also like working on a variety of workout apparatus, including the treadmill, stair climber, exercycle, and rowing machine. Others, on the other hand, might find it ridiculous to drive a car to a place just to do some walking.

If you need further motivation and encouragement to get out for that daily walk, there's no better way than to get a dog. We've already seen how owning a pet is a very effective stress-reduction technique that has been shown to lower blood pressure levels. You may not want to go out for a brisk walk when it's drizzling outside, but your dog won't care at all. Come rain or shine, your pet will give you your signal that it's time to get the leash and go!

If, after a while, your neighborhood starts getting a bit too familiar, you might want to expand your territory. Make a list of the places you'd like to walk. Then when you have a little extra time, get into the car and drive to a new location. Maybe there's a nice park a few miles away, or a forest preserve, or a nature path.

Or how about listening to some music? A number of manufacturers make a self-contained radio/earphone set which allows you to listen to your favorite station while walking along. Do you prefer your own music? One of the Walkman-type portable stereos might be just the thing. You'll need some tapes to set the mood for your brisk walk.

Bill Gatz of Ballwin, Missouri had a hard time doing that. He went to music stores and found that most of the tapes didn't suit his generational tastes. The "easy listening" tapes didn't keep the pace up enough. So he proceded to create his own series of four walking tapes, each orchestrated to accompany a brisk walk of three to four miles per hour. Each tape is an hour long, with invigorating and motivating music. If you're interested in getting a set of Bill's tapes, you can call or write to him at Happy Heart Productions, Inc., P.O.B. 1015, Ballwin, MO 63011-9998. The phone number is (314) 458-0810.

If you do decide to try a treadmill, you might want to set it up in front of a TV set so you can watch the news or a videotape while walking off the miles. That's another advantage of the club I joined; they have a line of treadmills facing the TV with plugs to hook up one's headphones.

Since we're really talking about making walking a way of life, don't forget to pack your walking shoes when you head off for a business trip or vacation. Consider it a terrific way to become acquainted with a new area. Just ask someone at the hotel where you can get a nice two- to three-mile walk where you can see some of the local sights.

At the beginning, you might find that a brisk walk to get your heart rate up into the target range will be just about three miles per hour. As you progress, your walking speed will increase gradually. Don't push it. You've got the rest of your life.

You might want to get in the car one day and measure out a one-mile stretch near your home. Then see how long it takes to cover that mile. Let's say you do it in 20 minutes. You're walking a 3 mph pace. If you finish in 15 minutes, you're up to 4 mph.

Once you know how fast you're walking, you can use your watch to log the miles. Start walking and note the time. If you're walking a 4 mph pace, even if you're in a different neighborhood, you can note the time, start walking, and after 15 minutes, just turn around and come back. You'll have covered two miles.

While some authorities, including Dr. Blair, discount the heart rate, most believe that patients should keep track of how fast their hearts are beating. A 60 to 75 percent target zone will give you a good cardiovascular workout. Take a look at Table 4 to see what the range would be for your age. Remember that certain medications can influence heart rate.

Gardening for Fitness. Many men and women love to work in the garden and on their lawns. If you're one of those gardeners, you probably never thought of it as being work, especially work that's good for your heart. But it can be just that.

As with any other activity during your recovery, the key is to not overdo it. During the first week you might want to spend about 15 minutes in the garden, then gradually increased both your time and your activities. At the start, avoid lifting heavy sacks and stooping, especially if you've just had open-heart surgery and your chest incision isn't entirely healed.

There's no rule saying you have to finish a given task at one time. Maybe today you can mow the lawn in the front, and tomorrow you can mow the back. Or perhaps you'd like to do a little work in the morning,

TABLE 4
Cardiovascular Conditioning Heart Rates

Age (years)	Target Zone 60–75% (beats/minute)	Average Maximum Heart Rate (100%)
20	120–150	200
25	117–146	195
30	114–142	190
35	111–138	185
40	108–135	180
45	105–131	175
50	102–127	170
55	99–123	165
60	96–120	160
65	93–116	155
70	90–113	150

and then return later in the day to do a few more chores. Raking, shoveling, hoeing all can be very aerobic activities, as well as being terrific stress-busters.

Just don't ignore the basics. Quit before you get tired. Stop immediately at the first sign of distress. If you suffer from angina, sit and rest before going on. If you go back into the house and you're feeling exhausted, you've done too much. Don't do it again. Learn your limits, realizing that your limitations will lessen as time goes on.

Pedaling for Good Health. Almost everyone knows how to ride a bicycle. Cycling can offer an enjoyable alternative to walking. Apply the same rules. Go easy at first. Take another look at the energy expenditures in Table 3 for different speeds of cycling on smooth, flat surfaces. Start off with a warm-up period of easy pedaling, then speed it up to get to your target training range. Then finish off with a five-minute cool-down.

One advantage of cycling is that you can easily increase your heart rate by increasing the speed a mile or two per hour faster or by riding over hillier terrain that gives extra challenge. But don't get yourself into trouble by biting off more than you can chew.

Another thing I like about cycling is that you can go a lot farther from home than you can while walking. This means that you can expand your territory quite easily without having to get into the car. Put some saddle-bags or a basket on the bike and you can kill two birds with one stone by using your bicycle to run errands around the neighborhood. After all, the bicycle is considered a major form of transportation in many parts of the world. And parking places for that bike are a lot easier to find.

Whether walking or cycling, try to avoid very hot days or, if you live in an urban area such as Los Angeles or Denver, days when the air quality poses a problem. On such days, a stationary bike comes in handy.

I'll admit that just pedaling and going nowhere can be mighty boring. That's the time to put the bike in front of the TV or tune in some music on your headphones.

As time goes on, you just might find that you've become a true cycling fan. A number of clubs have been formed in recent years, and you might want to look into joining one. Some hospitals even have formed cycling clubs for former cardiac patients. I met one man whose heart attack didn't keep him from becoming a cycling fanatic. Now he looks forward to each weekend when he takes off on his mountain bike, riding through some of California's roughest terrain. He takes a great deal of pride in his abilities. For him, cycling is the perfect outlet for his stressful life, in addition to providing exercise.

Staying in the Swim of Things. For those who have a pool conveniently available, swimming can be a wonderful way to get exercise. It has a number of advantages over other activities. Swimming is much less likely to lead to orthopedic injuries than jogging or running. You use both arms and legs, providing an overall workout. And there's something particularly soothing about gracefully swimming laps back and forth. Many swimmers report that they do their best thinking when in the water.

Whether swimming can serve as an adequate workout, however, will depend on your own skills. Simply paddling about, doing more standing than swimming, won't achieve cardiovascular fitness, though it can still be fun. If you've got a good stroke, on the other hand, you can put out a lot of energy.

For those who aren't as good as they'd like to be, the problem most often is a lack of skill in breathing properly. But you can still use swimming as an exercise alternative. Just get a mask and snorkle, keep your face down in the water, and paddle away. Most people find that with this technique they can do continuous laps until they achieve a target heart rate.

You might also want to look into the possibilities of "aqua aerobics" classes in your area. Many YMCA locations offer this new approach to fitness. Standing in a shallow lap pool, you use the resistance of the water to bring your efforts up to an aerobic level. A good instructor can make this a lot of fun, and you'll be pleasantly surprised at how good a workout you'll get.

Another way to watery fitness is to use a kick board. Be careful with this one, though, since it can bring the heart rate up faster than you might imagine.

As you start off doing laps in freestyle swimming or by using a kick board, do a lap or two and then check your pulse. At the beginning you might be able to do only one or two laps, with resting sessions in between. As you improve your fitness, you'll find yourself doing more and more. It's a great way to see progress quickly.

Running in the Water Let's say you've got a pool, but it's too small to do serious lap swimming for exercise. And you find running hurts your knees. The answer is to combine the two by running in the water.

Here's how it works. The Wet Vest holds you in place in the water, allowing you to walk, jog, or run. It gives you all the aerobic benefits without the aches and pains. The Wet Vest holds you firmly and comfortably in deep water, with no bobbing up and down. It's a great workout and a lot of fun. You can order one by calling the manufacturer, Bioenergetics, Inc., at (800) 433-2627 or (205) 664-0676. Their address is 2790 Montgomery Highway, Pelham, AL 35124.

Skipping Back to Health. What's an easy way to exercise that's so much fun that children all over the world love to do it? How long has it been since you picked up a jump rope and tried skipping? Here's a very inexpensive and portable approach to aerobic fitness. You can even put it into your suitcase and take it along on business trips. And don't pooh-pooh this as child's play; remember that rope skipping is a favorite training technique for prizefighters. Just 10 minutes of vigorous skipping equals the cardiovascular benefit from 30 minutes of jogging!

To get started, make sure that your rope is the right length. It should reach up to the armpits when held beneath the feet. Stand on the middle of the rope and bring the two ends up to your armpits. If too long, cut some off or wind it around the handles. Don't use a rope that's too short; you won't be able to skip well, and you may get tripped up. You can find a good-quality jump rope at any sporting goods store. Today's design makes jumping easier, especially for beginners.

If you've never tried rope skipping, start without the rope. Stand on a mat or carpet with your arms down and bent at a 45-degree angle. Then bounce from one foot to another, jumping just an inch off the floor in order to get the rhythm. (If your cardiac event was recent, this alone may be enough to get your heart into the target zone and you might want to stick with this alone for a while.) Keep your body as limber as possible, with knees and hips relaxed and slightly bent.

After you've mastered the rhythm, try it with the rope. Place the rope behind your ankles, with your arms bent and your hands just ahead of your hips. Then swing the rope, jumping just high enough to let the rope clear, about one inch.

You might also try jumping with both feet at the same time. Some people find that easier, though I don't.

Don't feel like a klutz if you don't get it right away. Do one jump at a time. Then two. Pretty soon you will put together a reasonable series of jumps. While you're working at it, take your pulse now and then to make sure you don't exceed your rate.

Once you've got the rhythm down pat, you can skip without even thinking about it. That means that you can pick up the rope and do some jumping now and then throughout the day. If you have high ceilings, try it while watching the news.

Just one word of caution about rope skipping. You may be tempted to show off your new skills to your children or grandchildren. Don't. First, they won't be impressed, since their skills will no doubt be much greater than yours. And you may be tempted to overdo it, as you won't want to take your pulse in front of the kids.

While both men and women can derive great benefit from skipping, most women are better at it. This provides women with a very convenient way to get exercise, especially for those who might be embarrassed to exercise in front of others. I'm convinced that, if done regularly, rope skipping could easily be the total exercise program for those who just don't enjoy other activities.

"Put a Little Fun in Your Life! Try Dancing!" If you remember Kathryn Murray saying that as she twirled across the floor with her husband Arthur, you're at least as old as I am! And if you are, then you no doubt enjoy dancing. In fact, the older an individual is, the more dancing has always been part of his or her social life. I'm happy to tell you that it's another wonderful way to get physically active.

Even if you just came home from the hospital, you can put a record album on and dance with your spouse for at least one foxtrot. In addition to the exercise, this is a wonderful way to bring you together. An extra hug and kiss at the end is perfectly appropriate and very therapeutic!

Tomorrow you might do two dances in a row. Tired? Take a few minutes to rest and chat, then do another dance. As your energy returns, add a cha-cha to your repertory. Don't rush the agenda, but soon you'll be doing the polka, the tango, and all your ballroom favorites. Check your heart rate to see how you do for any given dance and gauge yourself from then on. See Table 3 for a look at the energy expenditures of dancing.

One cautionary note. Avoid dancing situations where the air is thick with smoke. Unfortunately, that means most discos. Breathing in that smoke while exercising isn't a good idea.

Include Golf and Bowling in Your Program. You may have heard that golf and bowling aren't aerobic activities, and that they don't "count" for those of us trying to improve our cardiovascular fitness.

Certainly that may be true for those who drive through a golf course on an electric cart. But if you use a pull-cart, or especially if you carry your clubs, golf can, indeed, provide aerobic benefits. Bowling can also get the heart rate up, especially in the early months of your recovery.

Moreover, the reason you started golfing and bowling was to have fun. And having fun is a very important part of the recovery process. Be nice to yourself, now and in the future, by frequently doing something that's fun. All work and stress and no play make Jack (and Jill) unhappy cardiac patients instead of former patients.

Enjoy Tennis and Other Games as Well. My game of tennis is so bad that it does very little to my heart rate. I just chase the ball most of the time. But even for those of us who aren't very good, tennis can be both fun and another way to get some exercise.

If you're a very good player, you might want to limit your play to doubles until you've fully recovered. A singles game might be just too much for a while. The same applies to racquetball and handball, both of which can elevate the heart rate enormously.

A number of years ago, cardiologists told their patients to give their racquets away, since those games were forbidden for life. Aren't you glad you're living in these more enlightened times, when you can look forward to becoming a *former* cardiac patient?

The fact of the matter is that you should become a better player than you were before your cardiac event, since you'll be paying more attention to the healthy lifestyle that all athletes are following these days. Just look at Martina Navratilova. She credits her ability to keep up with the youngsters on the tour to a strict program including a low-fat diet and exercise.

RESISTANCE TRAINING: A NEW CONCEPT IN CARDIOVASCULAR HEALTH

Please don't immediately flip through the next few pages when you find out that I'm going to advise you to start pumping iron. This is not like the old days of bodybuilders sweating and grunting in places like "Al's Gym." The proper term today is resistance training, and it is a sophisticated and revolutionary addition to cardiac rehabilitation and recovery.

Until my second bypass, the last time I'd tried lifting weights was when I was 17 years old. That lasted about three weeks, and my barbells got sold to the next kid, who no doubt sold them to yet another kid.

Fast forward to my cardiac rehab program in Santa Monica. I had completed the 12-week structured program and was coming in three times a week to do my aerobic exercises when the hospital put in a circuit of machines for resistive exercise. After getting Dr. Kattus's approval I started into it, learning the proper ways to obtain the most benefit with the least chance of injury or problems.

This was a vastly different kind of strength training than I'd tried when I was a teenager. First, I wasn't trying to be a bodybuilder. Second, the use of the machines made the whole process more attractive and enjoyable. Third, the goal was to develop muscular tone which would help in day-to-day activities.

I've become a real believer. I'm still on the puny side, but that's more a matter of my genetic predisposition. My confidence has soared, and I'm frankly quite proud of my strength and capabilities. I think that resistance training should be a part of every cardiac rehabilitation program. But that's just my opinion. Here's what the experts have to say about this new development.

Cardiologists avoided strength training in cardiac patients in the past because of concern that sharp, sudden increases in blood pressure would lead to arrhythmias and to oxygen deficits to the heart. That's no longer the case, as we now have the evidence that reasonable resistance weight training is very safe. Dr. Kerry Stewart, of the division of cardiology at the Johns Hopkins School of Medicine, has reported that cardiac patients who engaged in resistance exercise had fewer ECG changes and arrhythmias during weight training than during aerobic exercise. He further explains that although systolic blood pressure may be a bit higher during resistance exercise than during aerobic activities, the lower heart rate when using weights creates a lower demand for oxygen by the heart than is the case during aerobics. Moreover, he says that the increase in diastolic blood pressure may actually facilitate blood supply to the heart, despite the apparent rise in blood pressure.

We now have years of research to back up the recommendation to include resistance exercise in the cardiac rehab formula. Maintaining muscle tone and power means the ability to keep up with all the important activities of daily living. This is particularly true for older individuals and those engaged in physical labor.

Most heart patients are more limited by their perceived lack of capability than the limitations actually placed on them by their disease. In other words, they think they're sicker and weaker and less capable than they really are. Dr. Craig Ewart, also at Johns Hopkins School of Medicine, looked at the benefits derived by such patients when they got into a program of resistance weight training. His work demonstrated that this kind of exercise contributes to emotional well-being and enables patients to perform to their full capabilities.

Once again, we're not talking about the old ideas of bodybuilding or power lifting in which one would lift huge amounts of weights while veins bulged and the face turned beet red. The approach now recommended calls for moderate weight loads with frequent repetitions. Patients are generally kept to weights that are within 30 to 40 percent of their maximum capacity, performing 10 to 15 repetitions within 30 to 45 seconds, with 15 to 30 seconds of rest between sets. For example, if someone could lift a 25-pound weight once, he or she would lift an 8- to 10-pound weight several times in quick succession.

For the most part, however, medical experts don't like to use barbells or dumbbells, today termed "free weights." Instead they recommend a circuit of resistance machines such as the ones you find in health clubs and YMCAs. These offer a number of advantages over free weights:

- easier to learn
- less injurious to lower back
- easier to grip handles
- less likely to increase blood pressure
- easier to add weight gradually.

If you've never seen or tried the new equipment, you're in for a pleasant surprise. These are user-friendly machines. You sit in a comfortable chair, often with a belt to keep you properly positioned, and simply push or pull. Adjusting the weight/resistance is a snap; just move the pin up or down the row of weights.

You'll start off with very low resistance, immediately boosting your confidence. Since it's virtually no effort, and you won't have any aching muscles, you'll look forward to the next session. Going through the entire circuit of machines to fully exercise both upper and lower muscle masses takes about 30 minutes. Because you spend so little time on any given piece of apparatus, the boredom factor is eliminated entirely.

Although the full impact of your efforts won't be seen until you've been with the program for three to four months, you'll start to actually see the differences in the mirror much sooner. The worse your condition to begin with, the faster and more dramatic the improvements will be.

I can't stress too much the idea that resistance exercise is for both men and women. A number of studies have shown that both sexes benefit equally. If anything, women might have a bit more to gain.

Men have a greater percentage of lean muscle tissue than women by nature of their sex. This gives men an advantage in weight control, since only muscle tissue not fat tissue, can burn calories. When women enroll in a resistance exercise program, they find that weight loss is much easier. One reason is the replacement of fat with muscle. Moreover, in addition to pounds lost, you'll see a remarkable change in terms of inches, which translates into smaller dress sizes.

Why not make this a family affair? Both men and women can work the circuit together, using the same machines. If one needs more weight than the other, it's a matter of a simple adjustment. Working out together can make it a lot more fun. Very often, one person can't maintain another's pace when walking or cycling. But that's not a problem at all when doing resistance exercise. Besides, don't you think both of you could use a bit of muscle toning?

Here are the ways you can pump up your physical and psychological health by pumping some iron.

Lowers blood pressure as well as drugs do. Investigators at Johns Hopkins compared the effects of resistance training and antihypertensive medications for 52 men with high blood pressure. All of them did some aerobic exercise, either walking, jogging, or cycling. Half the men got drugs while the other half were assigned a resistance exercise program. After 10 weeks, the exercise group did just as well as the drug group in terms of lowering blood pressure, reducing cholesterol, and raising the levels of HDL.

In another test, 20 cardiac patients achieved an average 12 percent gain in cardiovascular endurance. How does weight training assist endurance? By building the muscle masses in the arms and legs.

Keeps the heart strong. Most cardiac patients need to lose weight, but often that weight loss includes muscle tissue, both from the skeleton and the heart. Researchers at Emory University have demonstrated that weight training during weight loss helps keep the muscle while losing the fat.

Increases levels of "good" cholesterol. Studies have shown that HDL cholesterol levels rise with resistance exercise as well as, or perhaps even better than, with aerobics.

Keeps bones strong and prevents osteoporosis. As we age, the bones in our bodies tend to get smaller and less dense. They also tend to break much more easily. For many women, especially, bone loss can be a major problem after menopause, resulting in the bone-demineralizing disease known as osteoporosis. We've all heard a lot about how additional calcium helps to prevent bone loss, but the importance of exercise has not been as heavily stressed. And nothing does it better than weight training.

Proof comes from the University of California at Davis, where Dr. Carol Meredith worked with 46 young men. Those who lifted weights had denser bones than a control group that did not. Doing both resistance and aerobic exercise was the most effective.

Aids in controlling diabetes. The more lean muscle mass the body has, the easier it is to control glucose levels in the blood. Researchers at the University of Maryland saw that after just 18 weeks, glucose tolerance went up considerably. Many physicians believe that a program of diet, weight loss, and both aerobic and resistance exercise can virtually eliminate the symptoms of type II, non-insulin-dependent diabetes.

Improves self-confidence. All of us, regardless of age or sex, like to think that we look our best. And nothing makes us look good like a healthy, toned body. As you dress in the morning and look in the mirror, you can give yourself a well-deserved smile. And when your friends comment on how good you look, it's just fine to feel proud of yourself. It's a very nice fringe benefit of your recovery program.

Increases capabilities. You'll do more with your life in both a physical and emotional sense because you'll know that you're capable of it. If you can perform in the gym, you can do the same in life. Your actual abilities, in terms of physical strength, will grow. But more important, you will allow yourself to live your life to its fullest, without the limitations so many cardiac patients place on themselves.

Makes life easier. As we get older, things we once took for granted seem more difficult, and they are. Things like opening a jar. Or moving a potted plant. Granted, those things may not take a lot of strength and energy. But if they become too much for you, daily living becomes more of an effort. You have to ask people to do things for you, and all of us hate that feeling of dependence. Improving your strength as well as your stamina provides a new sense of independence and freedom.

Protects against injuries. The possibility of injury, especially of bone fracture, increases with age. Older people fall more frequently, and these falls can be catastrophic. Research has shown that many falls are simply the result of lessened muscular strength. Increase that strength, and the likelihood of falls and subsequent injury diminishes.

You're never too old to pump iron. No excuses! Virtually anyone can benefit from a program of resistance exercise. The ultimate proof comes from a nursing home in Massachusetts. Dr. Maria Fiatarone has been working with the Hebrew Rehabilitation Center for the Aged. There a group of nine men and women aged 87 to 96 regularly head for the weight room for a resistance exercise workout session.

In just eight weeks, the six women and three men increased the strength of their quadriceps femoris muscle in the upper leg threefold to fourfold on average. While their normal walking speed didn't change much, their speed in a heel-to-toe walking test increased nearly 50 percent.

Dr. Fiatarone reported that two of the volunteers who previously had used canes began walking without them, and individuals became able to rise from a chair without pushing off from the arms.

You have to keep up the exercise to maintain the benefits. If you stop working out, gains disappear quickly. Dr. Fiatarone says that just four weeks after the volunteers returned to their sedentary lifestyles, they lost an average of 32 percent in muscle strength. That's why these older people went back to their workouts once the study was over.

There were no problems associated with the exercise. Blood pressure and pulse showed little change during the training sessions, even though the volunteers lifted 80 percent of their maximum throughout the study with no more than two minutes between sets.

RESISTANCE EXERCISE HAS SOMETHING FOR EVERYONE

Regardless of age, regardless of sex, regardless of your physical condition, everyone can benefit from a program of resistance exercise. The time to start is after a 12-week cardiac rehabilitation program. Talk with your doctor about the benefits and appropriateness of this approach for you.

Here are some tips for when you begin your program:

- Train at a moderate intensity.
- Use light weights (or light settings on the machines) that you can lift 10 to 15 times.
- Increase weights slowly, adding small increments at a time.
- Learn proper technique from a trained professional, whether at a hospital or health club.
- Warm up and cool down before and after each session.
- Train three times a week to gain, twice a week to maintain.

GRADUATING TO HIGH-INTENSITY EXERCISE

As we've seen, all it takes to achieve a good level of cardiovascular fitness which will protect you against future problems is a solid program of brisk walking, about two to three miles five days a week. Whether you want to walk, jog, cycle, swim, dance, do aerobics, or just about any other kind of heart-quickening exercise, 30 to 45 minutes five days each week will do the trick. Add to that aerobic program some resistance exercise and you have a complete fitness program that any doctor would be proud to see. So is there any reason to go any further?

While all exercise helps to raise the levels of the protective HDL cholesterol in the blood, the more you do the higher the HDLs go up. Studies have shown that distance runners and other endurance athletes have higher HDL counts than average.

A few research projects have attempted to show an additional advantage of high-intensity exercise for cardiac patients. Most notable is the work done by Dr. Ali Ehsani at Washington University in St. Louis. His patients, in a closely supervised program, have done significantly better than those receiving typical cardiac rehabilitation. Dr. Ehsani employs an experimental regimen that raises patients' heart rates to 80 percent of age-limited maximum rather than the 40 to 70 percent levels in traditional rehab programs.

"Patients improve their myocardial work capacity, exercise ejection fraction, and plasma lipid profile," the cardiologist says. That is to say, their hearts are capable of more work and pump more blood, and their cholesterol and triglyceride counts improve. Very importantly, Dr. Ehsani reports, they have reduced exercise-induced myocardial ischemia as measured by ST segment changes on their ECGs and fewer abnormalities in their heart muscle contraction. Moreover, after a year of such intense exercise, hypotension (a drop in blood pressure that suddenly occurs when an individual exerts himself) decreases markedly.

Patients follow a routine that starts off with brisk walking and gradually increases in both duration and intensity. After several months, patients jog for 50 to 60 minutes a day four to six times a week. Dr. Ehsani has worked with more than 600 patients thus far, and deaths and complications have been rare.

But is this approach for everyone? The answer is a definite no! Only those patients who have had an uncomplicated heart attack and who have no severe heart muscle damage should be considered. The program is limited to those low-risk patients who don't have severe disease. And for those who do opt for this kind of all-out effort, close medical supervision is essential. Leaving a cardiac rehabilitation program and immediately setting off to train for a marathon is asking for trouble.

But for those who do fit all the criteria and are willing to make the admittedly tough effort, the achievement can make every minute's worth of work worthwhile. Those who "make it to the top" experience a tremendous surge in self-esteem. Levels of anxiety and depression plunge. Studies at the University of Alabama have revealed that those who complete a high-intensity exercise program do decidedly better in terms of psychological testing. They flat-out feel better about themselves.

Let's look at a parallel situation. If you do some walking on a treadmill in the cardiac rehab facility at the hospital and you realize that there's not much in the world outside that you'd want to do that would surpass that level of exertion, you feel a definite sense of security and assurance. Now imagine what it's like to be able to exercise at full-tilt for an hour, sweat pouring off your body, lungs expanding to their fullest. After your shower you feel like you can take on the world and win!

Today I have a resting heart rate of about 50 beats per minute, a blood pressure of approximately 120/80, and a cholesterol level that consistently remains in the 150 to 160 mg/dl range. Dr. Michael Lawlor at the Heart Institute of the Desert put my vital statistics through the computer program they've devised to determine the level of a person's health relative to the expected levels of performance and physiological measurements for a person of a given age. Some people may be only 50 years old, but they have the body of a 70-year-old. Imagine how I felt when Dr. Lawlor sent back the computer-generated determination that, at age 47, I was performing at the level of a 26-year-old man!

Armed with that kind of diagnosis, along with the angiogram that had shown absolutely no arterial obstruction in my heart's bypass grafts and native arteries, and you can imagine how I felt. All those little twinges, or chest discomfort, or abdominal disturbances, or other feelings that once I might have questioned of being of cardiac origin I now knew were completely benign. I was a 100-percent healthy man!

Yes, a program of brisk daily walking can keep you heart-healthy. But there's nothing like high-intensity exercise to make you feel really *alive!* And I'm not the only guy who feels that way.

Chuck Whitlock, a good friend of mine, had his heart attack and bypass surgery at age 42. His approach to recovery was much like mine, with a determination not to let this disease get him down. Today Chuck skis at breakneck speed down the slopes, scuba dives, plays a mean game of racquetball, and works hours that would exhaust a man half his age. To keep up his pace and his health, Chuck *never* misses his exercise. He belongs to a health club near his home, uses a few pieces of equipment in a spare room of his house when he just can't get away, and makes certain that he stays in hotels that have fitness equipment. Is the effort worth it to him? Chuck says without any hesitation or doubt that he's never felt better in his life, and that he'll never quit the program.

Barbara Else at Cedars-Sinai Hospital tells a wonderful story about the motivation and rationale to go that "extra mile." After one patient, Leon, had a heart attack, his wife and kids wouldn't let up. They worried about him all the time, urging him to take it easy and not exert himself. In his late forties, Leon wanted to live his life, not just exist. He knew he was just fine, that his recovery had been complete, but he couldn't convince his family. So he entered a five-kilometer race along with his sons, just to let them see that he was, indeed, OK, and that they didn't have to baby him. It worked.

Please understand that I'm not encouraging you to run a triathlon, a marathon, or even a five-kilometer race. Not everyone is physically capable of such exertion, and fewer yet would want to do so. But these men serve as shining examples of just how far one can take the concept of complete cardiac recovery.

Everyone's motivation for going all-out in terms of recovery and exercise is a bit different. I can only tell you that in my own case, the second bypass hammered home the idea that I was a mortal man with a condition that could kill me, and that if I didn't do something it would be sooner rather than later. There was a lot of living that I wanted to do, and I wanted to live that life with gusto, without limitations.

I told you about my success in the formal rehab program. If I felt that good in such a short period of time, I thought, what would I feel like if I gave it all I had? The result of my efforts, as I've said again and again, is that I feel fantastic. My exercise program has become like a drug for me; I literally need an exercise "fix" to keep feeling the physical and psychological "high" I've come to regard as the standard of living. Being just OK isn't enough for me.

Yes, a far more moderate program is all you need. But if you fit the medical criteria to allow yourself to try for a high-intensity fitness regimen, give it a try. Talk with your doctor about it. If he feels that there's nothing in your medical picture to keep you from it, go for it! There's a big difference between living and feeling really alive!

AGE IS NOT LIMITING

I vividly recall my first trip to Florida in 1961; I went there with a college classmate to visit his grandparents. We passed many retirement homes, and saw large porches with rows and rows of rocking chairs. Elderly men and women got up in the morning, went out to sit on those chairs, and left only to eat and go to the bathroom. Day after day, rocking their lives away. If that was living to a ripe old age, I thought, I'm glad I have a family history of heart disease!

Well, the times certainly have changed since then. Today my own mother lives in a retirement village in Laguna Hills called Leisure World. In reality, it's more a city than a village, with five Olympic-size swimming pools, two golf courses, lawn bowling, tennis courts, and horse stables. There's scarcely a time when you can't see men and women in their walking/jogging shoes briskly marching along the roads and paths that wind through the area, their arms pumping up and down as they log their daily miles.

A while back, doctors rather patronizingly felt that there was little reason to try to influence lifestyles of the elderly. "Let them enjoy their lives, why make them give up their pleasures or make them work," was the well-intentioned rationale. Well, bunk!

A lot of doctors (though not all by any means) have seen that the elderly are among the best patients. Maybe that's because they're more aware of life's finite limits, and maybe it's because they have more time to devote to their own care. Whatever the reason, those senior citizens are likely to take every word of advice to heart. We now know that, regardless of age, one can derive benefits—and added years of life, both quantity and quality—by quitting smoking, by eating less fat and cholesterol, and by getting more exercise.

Older people who regularly exercise also think better. Dr. Louise Clarkson-Smith of Scripps College in Claremont, California found that the more elderly folks worked out, the better their mental fitness. She surveyed 300 men and women aged 55–91 in terms of their physical activity which included heavy housework, gardening, vigorous work, and recreational exertion. Those who exercised most scored at the top in tests on vocabulary, memory, reaction time, and reasoning.

Ask any older person, and he or she will tell you that one of the worst parts of getting old is the feeling of "losing it" mentally. Here's a way to forestall or possibly even eliminate that aspect of aging by simply getting out and exercising.

Another all-too-frequent part of aging is the occurrence of diabetes. While there is a genetic component, weight gain along with reduced physical activity seem to trigger the problem. Studies done at Washington University with men and women in their mid-sixties indicates that both low-level and high-intensity exercise can do wonders by reducing triglycerides, raising levels of protective HDL cholesterol, and increasing insulin sensitivity which would limit the effects of diabetes.

Effectiveness of the exercise programs was measured in terms of maximal oxygen uptake. During six months of low-intensity training by way of brisk walking, oxygen uptake increased by 12 percent. After an additional six months of high-intensity training in which participants jogged, cycled, or walked on an inclined treadmill at least three times a week, the oxygen uptake went up another 18 percent.

"BUT I GET ANGINA. HOW CAN I EXERCISE?"

The heart send signals that it's not getting enough oxygen by generating chest pains known as angina pectoris. Episodes of anginal pain are a function of oxygen consumption by the heart muscle. The faster the heart beats, the more oxygen the muscle needs. When the blood coming through the occluded coronary arteries can't supply that stepped-up oxygen demand, angina strikes, forcing one to slow down so that the oxygen debt can be repaid.

Obviously, if that oxygen supply and demand equation were changed for the better, angina episodes would be reduced. One way, of course, is to take nitroglycerin tablets to open the vessels, allowing a greater flow of oxygen-supplying blood. Longer-acting nitrate drugs accomplish the same goal on a continuing basis. Beta-blocking drugs work by slowing down the rate of heartbeat, thus minimizing the demand for oxygen.

But exercise can be a positive factor in this equation. Physical activity can reduce the episodes of angina in a number of ways.

The end result of a continuing, regular program of physical exercise is a decrease in the episodes of angina. As time goes on, one can do more and more exercise without the interruption of angina.

Angina is one of the most obvious and painful reminders that one has heart disease. To me, the promise of reduction of such anginal episodes is reason enough to keep to one's exercise program diligently.

In fact, exercise can be just as effective in treating angina as medication. In a Scottish study, 40 men with chronic stable angina were taken off their beta-blocking medications. Doctors then tested them for physical endurance on a treadmill. The men were next divided into two groups. One group exercised vigorously for one year while the other did not.

After the year's end, the two groups were retested. The men who had been exercising were given no medication before getting on the treadmill.

Those who had not exercise received a beta-blocking agent prescribed to control angina.

Men who had exercised had lower heart rates and a much higher threshold of angina. Those effects equalled those of the beta-blocking drug. The researchers concluded that a program of exercise can replace the drugs for angina sufferers.

A note of caution at this point: If you currently take beta-blockers at your doctor's prescription, *do not* stop taking them without first discussing the matter with your doctor. He or she very likely will urge you to begin a program of exercise first, gradually building up the level of intensity, and then slowly cutting back on the dosage of medication. Moreover, there are certain instances in which the medication will have to be continued, although in a lesser dosage.

"BUT WHAT ABOUT THE PAINS IN MY LEGS?"

Many cardiac patients' disease has spread beyond the arteries supplying blood to the heart. Atherosclerotic blockage can also occur in the arteries of the legs. When physical exertion results in an oxygen deficit to the legs, the cramping pain that ensues is termed intermittent claudication. It's typically enough to literally stop someone in his or her tracks until the oxygen deficit can be repaid. The similarity to angina is obvious.

One form of treatment for this condition, also known as peripheral vascular disease, is surgery whereby a bypass is made across the blocked artery. Either saphenous vein from the leg or an artificial vessel can be implanted.

Dr. William Hiatt of Denver discussed treatment of peripheral vascular disease at the 1990 meeting of the American Heart Association. He pointed out that this condition afflicts 12 percent of the entire population, both men and women, and 20 percent of all those past age 70. He said that recovery is no better with surgery than with a vigorous program of rehabilitation. Again, it's in your hands.

The first thing to realize is that claudication pain signals no impending disaster. Unlike angina, the patient is not imperiled when claudication strikes, and there's no reason to become frightened. The treatment for claudication becomes a matter of "pushing the episodes back" further and further, thus allowing ever-increasing periods of pain-free exercise.

Let's say, for example, that you develop leg pains after a one-block walk. The pain is enough to make you stop. Fine. Rest for whatever time it takes for the pain to pass, then walk a bit more. Today you'll do just a little, tomorrow you'll do more.

A treadmill makes overcoming claudication more convenient and efficient. With a treadmill you can set the speed at a constant two-miles-per-hour rate, and increase the grade from flat to eventually 3.5 percent, moving it up at just 0.5 percent at a time.

As the pain strikes, you can step off the treadmill, sit down, and rest until the discomfort passes. Then get back on and do a bit more. Day by day, week by week, month by month, the progress will amaze you. It's important to maintain an exercise log, noting the time and distance you're able to achieve each day. As you read back through the pages from a few weeks or months earlier, you'll be pleasantly surprised.

This is about the only time in rehabilitation when one can actually say "no pain, no gain." As the pain hits, take a few steps more, walking into the pain. You can't do any harm. You're in no danger. Don't be a stoic martyr; just a few more steps will do before coming to a rest.

As you continue this rehabilitation process, the same phenomena occur in your legs as were described for your heart's muscle in our discussion of angina. Exercise will increase blood flow to your leg muscles, oxygen will be more efficiently removed from the red cell's hemoglobin, and a degree of collateral circulation will form. Some researchers believe, based on their own observations, that the blockage in the legs' vessels can also be reversed through a program of low-fat diet and exercise.

Some patients have pain in their feet at rest. Often, at night, they have to swing their legs over the side of the bed to get relief by changing position. This type of patient should *not* be exercising, and should work closely with physicians to determine the cause of the problem and best approaches to treatment.

While one can achieve claudication recovery on one's own, it's more efficient to do so in a formal, structured program. Talk with your doctor about the availability of such programs in your area. You'll work with a trained specialist on a treadmill, doing specified increases in effort at each session. The two principal advantages are that a structured program provides additional confidence and reduction of the fear element, and progress will be faster since the patient will be pushed along a bit more rapidly than he or she would if working alone.

"DOESN'T HEART FAILURE PRECLUDE EXERCISE?"

For years and years, doctors counted heart failure as one of the main reasons to restrict activity for heart patients. After a diagnosis of heart failure, patients were doomed to a life of restricted activity and progressive decline in health and attitude. But a new study has shown that even these patients can achieve excellent results with a good exercise program.

Researchers at Oxford University placed 11 patients with chronic, severe heart failure on a routine of regular exercise on stationary bicycles. Patients were rotated from an eight-week period of exercise to an eight-week stretch of restricted activity. The results were dramatic.

For those who followed their exercise prescription, both symptoms and measured physical condition improved as a result of the training. Exercise lowered the patients' increased heart rate in response to a given load of effort, lengthened the time they could exercise, and improved their ability to extract oxygen from their blood. Patients also said they felt less breathless and fatigued and that they could do more during the day.

Heart failure refers to the heart muscle's lessened ability to pump owing to the weakened heart wall. While that heart muscle isn't likely to improve back to the level of a healthy individual's, other muscles in the body become more efficient and thus require less blood and less oxygen. The entire cardiovascular system works more easily to meet the reduced oxygen demand of those trained muscles.

Yes, there are certain patients whose heart muscles are so weakened that no level of exercise may be possible. For them, a heart transplant may be the only practical treatment. But for countless others who have previously been denied the opportunity to improve via physical exercise, the British study offers wonderful encouragement.

Most of the patients were in their early sixties and were free of other complications such as severe arrhythmias. Of real importance, they were able to perform an adequate amount of exercise at home on stationary bicycles rather than having to come to a hospital. Now even heart failure has been taken off the list of contraindications for cardiac rehabilitation!

STRETCHING AND FLEXING FOR FITNESS

Did you ever see a rigid, inflexible cat? Of course not. That's because they do lots and lots of stretching, and so should you. This is one of the easiest and most pleasant of all aspects of your exercise program, yet the most likely to be ignored, especially by those just beginning to exercise regularly.

Stretching exercises can improve and maintain body flexibility, prevent injury sustained during exercise, and provide a great deal of relaxation and stress reduction. Many of the commonly performed stretches are variations on classic yoga postures which have been performed for centuries.

Here's a simple rule never to be broken: Never exercise without accompanying stretches. Don't be tempted to say that you're running late and that "just once" won't hurt. It just might. And always stretch both before and *after* your exercise sessions.

SAFE, NOT SORRY, SPORTS

Whether you like to walk, jog, cycle, do aerobics, or use various gym equipment, taking a few simple precautions can keep you out of pain and problems.

- Always warm up and cool down.
- Wear properly fitted, well-cushioned shoes with good heel and arch support. Don't go for bargains. Find a store that specializes in sporting shoes and try on a number of brands and types until you find a pair that fits just right. Tell the salesperson what you're planning to do, so he or she can custom fit the shoes to your needs.
- Avoid walking or running along congested highways where you'll be breathing a lot of smoggy air. On a really smoggy day in major cities, exercising can bring as many toxins into your lungs as smoking cigarettes.
- Avoid very hot and very cold days. If you live in an area with tem-

perature extremes, you may well want to invest in an indoor treadmill or exercycle.

- Watch for early warning signs of injury. If your ankles or knees start feeling achy, it's best to stop for the day.
- When using unfamiliar equipment, ask for directions. Instructors in any gym, health club, or YMCA will be happy to give you some instruction on safe and proper use.
- If you've been off for a while owing, say, to a cold or the flu, start back slowly. Remember it will take three days for every day off to get back into stride.

MAINTAINING YOUR MOTIVATION

We've all gone through our "deal making." Not knowing whether we were going to make it through the heart attack or bypass, we make all kinds of deals with ourselves and our Maker. Not surprisingly, once we've come through the crisis, those promises are frequently forgotten.

Those who make good their promises to make some lifestyle changes including diet and exercise experience remarkable recoveries. Those who "forget" those promises are fooling only themselves and may wind up back in the hospital making more promises . . . if they're lucky enough to survive the next event.

In a way, it's too bad that we aren't left with more of a reminder of that heart attack or bypass. Maybe if there were some sort of recurring spasm in the left toe or something like that, it would remind us of the incredible fear we had back at the time of the event. But the human mind obliterates those memories of fear and horror. And the body gets to feeling better, week after week, month after month. Pretty soon patients get the notion that they are "cured" and some even wonder whether it was really a heart attack after all. Then they go back to their old habits, and the disease insidiously progresses.

All of us who did our rehab in Santa Monica remember a friendly guy named Herb. The nurses called him Herbie. He owned a restaurant in the area and loved his own food. Herb was badly overweight; the fact is, he was quite fat. Exercise was foreign to him, and he hated every moment in rehab. He'd smile and nod his assurances when the nurses would give him advice, but that good advice was ignored. Herb never lost the weight, didn't change his eating patterns to lower his dangerously high cholesterol count, and dropped out of the exercise program. He started feeling better, and soon was working long hours in his restaurant. About two years after that time, I dropped in to his place with my family to enjoy a meal of hard-shell crabs. But Herb wasn't there. I was sad, but not surprised, to hear that he had had another, this time fatal, heart attack.

But the intention of this book is not to scare you into changing your life. That doesn't work anyway. My intention is to try to show you how you can avoid future heart problems and enjoy every step of the way.

For the next few months, you're going to have to take my word about "enjoying" every step of the way. Any time you make major changes or modifications in your life, you can expect to go through a period of adjustment.

To use the same analogy I've mentioned before, if you were in an accident, wound up in a cast for a while, and then were told you needed physical rehabilitation, you might be angry, but you'd be a fool to rip off the cast and stomp out of the hospital. Yet that's just about what most heart patients do. They absolutely refuse to make the changes in their lives that can turn those lives around entirely.

Make yourself this deal: Play this one by the rules for the next six months. If you've just come home from the hospital, rest, enjoy some reading and movies on video, and get your daily walking done without fail. Then sign up for a structured cardiac rehab program, or work with your doctor to design one to do on your own. Finally, move into a long-term program that you can continue for the rest of your life. As your fitness increases, do just a little bit more, staying within your target heart range. Eat properly, avoiding those high-fat foods that keep you heavy and raise your cholesterol levels. Get plenty of rest and relaxation. Make a particular effort to put some fun into your life.

If, after those six months pass, you can't honestly say that you feel not only OK but absolutely terrific, then feel free to go back to your old ways. In fact, you can even give it the acid test. Stop exercising for a week or two. Then try to go back to it. You'll find that in just that short period of time you can't perform as well. And you'll most likely start feeling a bit more fatigued and less energetic.

If you keep up your good efforts for a year, you'll be hooked for life. I can honestly say that I've never met a single man or woman who got actively into a solid diet and exercise program who quit. If this is addiction, I love it!

THE FIFTH STEP:

Quitting Those Cigarettes

CHAPTER 12

Saying Goodbye to an Old Friend and Enemy

Imagine what it would be like if every time you got on an airplane you were struck with the realization that three fully loaded jumbo jets crashed daily, killing all aboard. Needless to say, there would be much more fear of flying. Yet those are the statistics for deaths directly caused by smoking cigarettes, with a total of 390,000 Americans dying each year, the equivalent of three jumbo jets every day.

If you're a smoker, or even a former smoker, you and I provide more statistics. Cigarette smoking is one of the Big Three risk factors for a heart attack, along with high blood pressure and cholesterol. I know in my own case that it was the real reason for my heart attack at age 35.

As I've already told you, I have a family history of heart disease. Yet my Dad didn't have his attack until he was 57. The big difference was that he didn't smoke. By the time I entered college, I was a confirmed smoker, and soon I was smoking two packs a day. And I do mean I smoked them all, I didn't just light them and leave them to smolder in an ashtray. I sucked that smoke down to my toes, 40 times a day, every day.

Of course we've all heard over and over that smoking is bad and that everyone should quit. But this takes on a whole new meaning for those recovering from a heart attack or bypass, or for those who have confirmed heart diesase. It's now a matter of secondary prevention, making sure that we don't have another attack or need another bypass.

If you've already quit, congratulations. I know it can be one of the most difficult things in life to do. If you haven't quit yet, don't feel too ashamed. You're in good company. It's a sad but true fact that fully half of all of us who have a heart attack continue to smoke. Anywhere between 40 and 75 percent of patients will go back to smoking after a bypass, even if they quit for a while after getting back from the hospital.

Those most likely to quit are those who have a really close call, a really major heart attack. Then there are those who realize that this is a truly serious matter, and that quitting can be a matter of life or death.

I must admit that I continued to smoke after my heart attack and first bypass. First there was the matter of my mental attitude. I was mad at the world and furious with my own body for failing me. I'd be damned if I was going to give up all my pleasures. And, down deep inside, I didn't admit that the disease was bigger, "badder," and meaner than I was.

To make matters worse, my cardiologist at the time did little to discourage my habit. I had cut down to about eight cigarettes daily, and he asked whether those helped me to relax. I said they did, and he reassured me that the relaxation I derived probably balanced out the damage done. So I kept on puffing, staying in a state of perpetual withdrawal since I really wanted to smoke more than that. But the doctor said it was OK, and that was OK with me. Remember, however, that this was in 1978. We've learned a lot since then, and I don't imagine one could find a single physician today who would counsel heart patients that it was acceptable to smoke even a few cigarettes daily.

Unfortunately, while those doctors might intellectually recognize the dangers of smoking, especially for heart patients, they don't always do everything necessary to help those patients quit. Too frequently, doctors mention it only in passing, but don't press the point. Yet those who do quit most often are those who have been given very strong encouragement from their doctors. Some physicians actually refuse to continue to treat patients who won't try to quit. But most take a far more passive role, at most giving out little brochures pointing to the dangers.

Why is quitting such an important step? By doing so, you cut the risk of sudden cardiac death in half in just two days. Immediately following a heart attack, and for the ensuing weeks, the risk of another heart attack, and potentially a fatal one, is highest. You can cut that risk in half by quitting now.

Moreover, you'll halve the rate of all morbidity and mortality that may occur after heart attack. This is true no matter how severe that heart attack might have been.

The converse is just as true. You cut your chances of survival by 50 percent if you continue to smoke.

And it's never too late. Many patients erroneously believe that the damage is done, and that there's no point in quitting after the heart attack. Kind of like closing the barn door after the horse has run away, they feel. But it's not true. Those statistics above apply to everyone, young or old.

The importance of quitting applies to women as well. For women, *nothing* raises the risk of heart attack more than smoking. Want proof? Researchers at the University of Pennsylvania and Boston University schools of medicine studied 555 women who had survived a first heart attack. There was a distinct increase in risk of having a second heart attack as the number of cigarettes went up, even after considering the effects of other risk factors such as blood pressure and cholesterol.

Unlike men, women are at risk of a heart attack when they smoke even if their coronary arteries aren't all that clogged. British researchers have found that women smokers are twice as likely to die from a heart attack, regardless of the state of their arteries. For women, smoking may have a more immediate influence, involving the clotting and clot breakdown processes rather than just contributing to the long-term atherosclerotic process as with men.

On the plus side, women can reduce their risk quickly when they give up the cigarettes. On the other hand, they often find that even more difficult to do than men. Regardless of difficulty, however, it's worth every bit of effort.

After a heart attack, both men and women hate the notion of having to give up all their pleasures. Smoking appears to provide the comfort and solace not found elsewhere. This is particularly true for those who become depressed after their heart attack. Here we have a vicious circle. Depressed persons are more likely to smoke cigarettes, yet smoking contributes to guilt and further depression, and the act of quitting can lead to depression itself.

For some heart patients, there seems to be so much to be done at once. You want to quit smoking, but you're also trying to control your weight, and you're avoiding fatty foods to keep cholesterol levels down. Moreover, the chance of failure looms, and the last thing you want is something else to fail at.

If anything, the mind rationalizes, this is the time you really need a friend, and that cigarette is a friend indeed. After all, it was the cigarette that was there for every time of trouble and for every time of triumph for just about as long as you can remember. Is it even possible to think about living life without the cigarette?

Yes, it *is* possible. Although that cigarette has been your "friend," it is also your deadly enemy. Compare it with the black widow spider that eats its partner after mating. You lived for quite a few years before you began to smoke and you'll live a lot more years if you stop. It's tough, yes, but 40 million Americans have done it, and you can too.

REASONS TO QUIT NOW!

Just in case surviving isn't reason enough to throw that butt away forever, I have quite a few additional reasons for you to think about:

- Cigarette smoking can mask angina, the chest pain which is an important sign of heart disease. This may be why smokers have such a high rate of silent ischemia; that is, oxygen deficit to the heart muscle without feeling pain. Without the warning sign of angina, patients may not be aware that they must curtail activity and thus are more vulnerable to heart attack.
- Cigarette smokers are two to three times more likely to have strokes than nonsmokers. Quitting cuts your risk of stroke in half.
- Regardless of the number of cigarettes smoked, lifelong smokers have a much greater incidence of clogged arteries in the neck. The longer you smoke, the greater the risk. But, again, quit and the risk gets cut in half. *Here's a reason to quit entirely rather than just cutting down.*
- Smokers' coronary arteries have smaller lumens, with less blood flow, regardless of development of atherosclerosis. Couple the reduced flow with a spasm of the artery, from stress for example, and one could face total shutdown, perhaps resulting in heart attack.
- Smokers have a lower level of the protective HDL cholesterol; this is now known to be an independent risk of heart disease. Smokers' children, and others around them as well, also have lower HDLs. Quit and everyone's HDLs will go back up.

- Smokers are more susceptible to claudication, the leg cramps that come on during exercise owing to clogging of the leg arteries. Those who quit smoking, watch their diet, and get into a regular program of walking can frequently totally eliminate those pains.
- Cigarette smokers are lousy lovers, and not just because their breath smells like an ashtray. Blockage in blood vessels in the penis—even as little as 25 percent—can prevent an erection. Those who quit often find their problems with impotence go away with the smoke.
- Cigarette smokers have a significantly greater number of sick days every year. Those who are sick and tired of being sick and tired should quit.
- Smoking puts you at risk of other degenerative diseases as well, including lung cancer and emphysema. If you've ever known anyone in the last stages of emphysema, unable to even walk across the room without panting for breath and needing an oxygen tank with tubes running into the nose, you know that this is a terrible way to die. Lung cancer's no day in the park, either.
- Smokers flat-out don't feel as well as nonsmokers. You just have no idea what it's like to breathe normally, to have greater stamina than you can remember for years, and to receive a sudden gift of vitality. It's all yours in trade for a couple of weeks of withdrawal and a real effort in the willpower department. I know what it's like, having been there myself. I never knew just how well I could feel until I finally beat my habit. It's hard to explain; you've got to feel the difference to understand it.

WE'VE COME A LONG WAY, BABY

Athletics coaches, little old ladies, and some others knew instinctively and by experience that cigarettes were "coffin nails" many years ago. Yet it was only in January 1964 that Dr. Luther Terry, then Surgeon General of the United States, announced that smoking was dangerous to health. Today we know that one out of every six deaths in the United States is related to smoking.

Americans have taken the message to heart. In 1965, 40 percent of the population smoked cigarettes. By 1987 that number had dropped to 29 percent. Two years later it was down to 27 percent, and the trend continues downward. Half of all smokers who once smoked, that's a whopping 40 million Americans, have now quit.

The percentage of smokers today is greatest among blacks, blue-collar workers, and the less educated segments of our population, and advertisers know it, targeting those individuals with their messages. It's sad to think that such persons, beset with enormous social and financial problems, are hunted down by the jackals in the tobacco industry.

When you and I began to smoke it was the "in" thing to do. If you didn't smoke, you were somehow different from the fun-loving young people of the day. The pressure to smoke was tremendous, coming from peers, advertisers, and our heroes in the movies. Today the tables are turned, and smokers are fast becoming social pariahs. It's "in" not to smoke. In fact, in many instances it can be detrimental to one's career. Some employers refuse to hire smokers. And restaurants, airlines, and public places can make the smoker feel like a leper.

Despite their protests and their demands for their "rights," most smokers actually want to stop. Most have tried to do so a number of times and have failed. It's a rare individual, indeed, who wouldn't opt to quit if he or she could do so painlessly—could wake up one morning a nonsmoker with no desire to light up.

Well, no "magic pill" has been invented yet, but the prognosis for your successful quitting is really better than ever before. Consider the following markers for success in your own case:

- All those who want to quit eventually do so. Study after study has shown that, while difficult for most and seemingly impossible for others, it can be done.
- Older smokers are more successful than younger puffers.
- Those who have failed in the past are *more* likely to succeed than those who never gave it a try. Seems that we learn from past failures.
- More help is at your disposal than ever before. We have nicotine gum, drug patches, hypnosis, acupuncture, aversion therapy, and group counseling at our disposal. We'll discuss those options, and you can decide if one is right for you.
- This is historically the best possible time to quit. You'll have support from everyone around you, encouraging your efforts.

FACE IT, YOU'RE ADDICTED!

Why is it so tough to quit smoking cigarettes? Over the years during my career as a medical writer I've had occasion to write about alcoholism and drug addiction and to visit rehabilitation centers. Talking with recovered and recovering alcoholics and addicts, I heard again and again that it was easier to give up the booze or heroin than it was to quit smoking.

Yet for many years nonsmokers scoffed at those of us who told of horrible problems with withdrawal, and the irritability that inevitably occurred. I've known nonsmokers who have bought cigarettes for friends or relatives to end the mutual suffering, rather than putting up with and encouraging those trying to quit. All of us smokers who tried to stop and failed were branded as having no willpower.

It wasn't until 1988 that Surgeon General C. Everett Koop, M.D., declared cigarette smoking to be an addiction, as much so as addiction to heroin or cocaine or any other drug. The addicting substance, he said, based on much research, was nicotine. Occurring naturally in tobacco leaves, nicotine is found nowhere else. It has amazing effects on the brain and nervous system.

Used in low dosages, nicotine can produce a feeling of alertness. Light up a cigarette to get started in the morning, puff away to keep going late at night. At higher doses, the drug can have a calming effect. And we control those doses by drawing more or less smoke into our lungs. Within seven seconds, that nicotine has entered the bloodstream and hit the brain. That's faster than a drug can act when injected into a vein!

Here we have a perfectly legal drug that's used with no social objections for the most part. Smokers give themselves a "fix" again and again throughout the day. This is a drug that increases the alpha waves of the brain associated with relaxation and triggers the release of beta-endorphins, the body's natural tranquilizers.

Try to switch to low-nicotine cigarettes and you're just going to smoke more of them and to suck deeper. Pick up a Carlton and there's no satisfaction unless you block those tiny holes in the filter. Right?

But if it's just a matter of addiction to nicotine, why do we enjoy those cigarettes so much? Why are they so good with a cup of coffee, after a meal, and especially after a period of deprivation such as during a movie or church service? In fact, the three most enjoyable things in life are a drink before and a cigarette after. Right?

Well, that's actually wrong. What you feel as pleasure is actually the elimination of pain. After a period of deprivation, even a short period such as 15 to 20 minutes, you enter withdrawal. Receptor sites in your brain begin to scream for a nicotine "fix." You provide it by lighting up, and the withdrawal is gone in seven seconds flat. You're at peace. For a while.

Even when your body begins to feel the adverse reactions from sucking in all the tars and crud from the burning tobacco, your throat is sore, you cough in the morning or throughout the day, you still crave the nicotine. You might have a cold or the flu, and smoking makes you feel worse, but you still need that fix on a regular basis to keep your brain's receptors from giving you grief.

As with heroin, a little goes a long way at the start. But then you need more and more, until you settle into your own daily maintenance dose. That might mean a pack, a pack and a half, two packs, or more. When the nicotine level goes too low in the brain, you're painfully aware of it.

Imagine having a lover whose idea of giving you pleasure is relieving you of the pain that he or she inflicts! Hard to believe, and hard to come to grips with, isn't it? But that's the reality of the pleasure of smoking.

Of course, there's far more to it than the nicotine addiction. The withdrawal from nicotine lasts only about two weeks, and with the aid of nicotine gum or drug patches, even that agony can be lessened significantly. So why doesn't everyone quit? And why do so many go back to the habit? Now we enter the realm of psychological addiction.

Smokers have allowed cigarettes to become inextricably entwined in each and every aspect of life. Virtually anything and everything is a cue to light up. For some smokers, life is unimaginable without cigarettes. One man told me that he really believed he'd rather die. He came close to dying, but eventually he did quit. Now he wonders how he could have thought that way.

I was just about as bad. At work I couldn't leave the office without my pack of cigarettes, even to go to the men's room, because I might run into someone who'd start a conversation. Can't talk without smoking, of course, because that would mean the jitters. The phone rings, light a cigarette. Coffee, drinks, meals, snacks, all meant a cigarette or two. Start the car, light a cigarette. Read a book, light a cigarette. Forty times a day.

I couldn't buy a shirt that didn't have a pocket. I planned my vacations in terms of how many cartons to pack. I kept a "stash" in the office, in the car, and at home. The idea of running out was unthinkable.

I had *learned* through many years of experience to associate all my waking experiences with cigarettes. It took a long time to *learn* to live without those cigarettes. As I'll discuss a bit later, you learn to do that one cigarette at a time, one day at a time. But I did it, anyone can do it, and you can do it, too.

ALTERNATIVES TO CIGARETTES

Well, if cigarettes are so bad, what about pipes and cigars? For cigarette smokers, especially, switching is just fooling yourself. You'll inhale the smoke to get the nicotine effect. Besides, pipe and cigar smokers have their own health problems, including cancer of the lip, tongue, throat, and esophagus.

How about smokeless tobacco such as snuff or chewing tobacco? These provide "satisfaction" by giving a shot of nicotine. It just takes a bit longer to get the hit, but then if one keeps the stuff in the mouth, there's a constant flow to the brain. And the nicotine, regardless of the source, still has the effects on the cardiovascular system that can kill. Moreover, smokeless tobacco has been well established as a deadly cause of cancer of the mouth, and it also leads to gum disease that can mean tooth loss.

There are other things that can substitute for the oral satisfaction you'll crave, and for the fiddling around that you do with the cigarette in your hand. I'll detail a number of options.

A NOTE TO SPOUSES AND NONSMOKERS IN THE HOUSEHOLD

Once upon a time people complained about secondhand smoke because it stunk up the house and was a general annoyance. Today we know that "sidestream" or "passive" smoke poses a real danger to those around the smoker. A nonsmoking woman with a smoking husband has twice the likelihood of dying of a heart attack than if the spouse didn't smoke; that's based on data from a 10-year study at the University of California at San Diego. And in 1985 an American Cancer Society study showed that wives of smokers have an extra 20 percent cancer risk.

Passive smoking results in lower HDL levels than are found in families without smokers. That's true for children as well as for spouses. Women whose husbands smoke are likely to enter menopause earlier also.

According to an article in the journal *Circulation* (January 1991), secondhand smoke causes an estimated 53,000 deaths annually, making it the third leading preventable cause of death in the United States today.

Nonsmokers exposed to other people's smoke are in danger of both cancer and heart disease. The carbon mononoxide in the smoke appears to be the culprit.

Heart patients already have a limitation on the amount of oxygen getting to their heart muscle. Increasing the level of carbon monoxide in the blood further cuts the oxygen supply. There's also evidence that passive smoking makes blood platelets abnormally "sticky" and more likely to form clots. The aggregation of platelets plays a role in heart attacks as well as in the development of atherosclerotic plaques that block the arteries.

If you're a man whose wife has had a heart attack or bypass surgery, please quit, both for her sake and yours. If you're a woman whose husband has had a heart attack, please quit, again, for your sake and his.

But what if you both smoke cigarettes? Don't quit at the same time. This is no time for togetherness. Both of you being nasty and irritable simultaneously will undermine the chances of success. And if one of you slips, he or she is likely to sabotage the efforts of the other in order to share the failure and thus lessen the feelings of guilt.

The first spouse to quit should be the one who's had the heart attack. The smoking spouse should make every effort to support the other's efforts, and should keep from smoking in his or her presence. Certainly, in terms of the dangers of passive smoking, don't smoke in the house. After a reasonable period of time after the heart patient has quit, you can join your spouse in a life free of tobacco. Then you can become mutually encouraging, supportive, and capable of contributing to each other's success on a long-term basis.

If you're not a smoker, and your spouse must quit to ensure his or her chances of a complete recovery from heart attack and heart disease in general, please be as sympathetic as you possibly can without being a nag. As a nonsmoker, there's just no way to make you understand just how hard it is. You'll just have to accept it on faith. Remember, even the Surgeon General has called it a major addiction, as difficult to overcome as any other drug addiction. It's not just a "dirty habit."

Your spouse will undergo a period of withdrawal. That is a painful and difficult experience, with symptoms of irritability, jitteriness, difficulty in sleeping, and sometimes even flu-like symptoms. You may even think your spouse is behaving "like a caged animal." Withdrawal lasts about two weeks, and then starts getting easier and easier. As each day passes, the urge to smoke will come less and less often and will strike with diminishing intensity.

There's no doubt that stopping the smoking is *the* most important aspect of recovery during the early stages, even more important than being 100% perfect in making dietary changes or getting regular exercise. Helping your spouse to quit smoking is the best thing you can do to help him or her to recover.

You might even wish to read some of the material dealing with stress management and relaxation techniques for your own needs during this trying period of time. When your spouse acts particularly irritable it's best to simply leave the room, go to a quiet place, and do some deep breathing exercises. At those times when the irritability factor isn't too bad, and you can bear to be with your spouse, you might like to get into the habit of doing those breathing exercises together. You'll both derive real benefits from this, and it's a wonderful thing to do as a couple.

You can help your spouse "get the monkey off his or her back" in other ways, too. Help him to avoid smokers and smoking situations. Ask visitors to please not smoke in her presence. After dinner, get up from the table rather than lingering over a cup of coffee. For a smoker, that's agony for the first weeks of going without nicotine. Suggest a number of nonsmoking activities such as movies and theater, places where no one is allowed to smoke. To further assist your spouse, read the section on coping strategies on page 268.

Your contribution will be unsung, but it will be enormous in terms of short-term recovery and potential for a longer, healthier life.

THERE MUST BE 50 WAYS TO LEAVE YOUR LOVER . . .

It was Mark Twain who first said, "It's easy to quit smoking . . . I've done it hundreds of times." All of us have known the resolve to get rid of the cigarettes, but we keep going back to them. I personally "quit" hundreds of nights as I stubbed out the last butt of the day, only to light up again in the morning.

But, to use the refrain of Paul Simon's song, "There must be 50 ways to leave your lover" when that lover is the cigarette habit. All of them work—for some people. There's no magic pill, though certain approaches seem to be just that when you hear the testimonials or the advertising.

All methods work for those individuals who really *want* to quit. In a way, those who eventually do get rid of the habit have hit bottom in very much the same way as alcoholics do before they will admit to their disease and seek help. For me, it became the realization that I was no longer in control. The cigarettes, in effect, were smoking me. I was no longer enjoying most of them. And when I tried to cut back I was in a constant state of withdrawal, yearning for the next "allowable" smoke.

I hit bottom the morning I woke up with a throat so sore that I could scarcely swallow. I lit a cigarette and it was like acid hitting my throat. Now, I'd smoked through dozens of colds, coughs, flus, and sore throats before, but this one was a real doozy. I decided that I'd not smoke that one day, threw the butts I had on hand away, and somehow made it through the day. The next morning I bought another pack, but the pain was as severe. So I decided on one more smokeless day, just one more. Those days got linked together, one by one, and I've never smoked since. But as you and I know, it wasn't nearly as simple as that, and I'll share some of the ways I got through it in the coming pages.

Yes, there are many ways to quit, but the best method remains "cold turkey." Ninety percent of those who do kick the habit do so on their own, with no outside help at all. And cold turkey means just that: no cigarettes at all. Cutting down may seem like a less painful way to do it, but it's just not as effective. It comes down to the period of withdrawal.

Nicotine's effects on the body take about two weeks to dissipate. But if you have a cigarette here and there, and a puff of someone else's now and again, you maintain a low level of nicotine in the bloodstream. Enough to keep you hooked but not enough to keep you satisfied, so you're in that horrible limbo state of permanent withdrawal. Most smokers who try to cut down fail miserably and are miserable in the process.

The addiction to cigarette smoking takes two forms. First you have the physical cravings for nicotine. The fact remains that within two weeks those cravings largely subside, as the level of nicotine decreases in the bloodstream and the body is finally rid of it. By the end of the two-week period, the nicotine addiction will have gone.

But now you have to deal with the psychological addiction. As you know, there are seemingly endless social and personal cues for you to smoke. You've relied on cigarettes to pick you up, calm you down, celebrate your victories, and console you during life's tougher moments.

For some, the thought of going through the process of quitting on one's own is enough to create the stress to light up another cigarette. You might not be up to doing it cold turkey. For you there is help, and you might want to consider some of the possibilities.

Clinics and Support Groups. If you listen to the advertising and read the brochures, every organization has *the* perfect program to virtually guarantee that you'll quit. And each one of them *can* make it happen for you, but only if you really have made the commitment.

There's a bit of controversy surrounding all the groups and clinics. Some authorities dismiss them out of hand, with the conclusion that the failure rates are horrible and that claims to the contrary are statistically inaccurate. Others feel that formal programs can provide the additional impetus some smokers need.

One possible reason for the less-than-perfect success rate of all the programs is an exaggerated level of expectation smokers might feel as they plunk their money down. It's as though by writing the check one delegates responsibility for success to the program rather than keeping that responsibility for oneself. It may well be that groups and clinics attract those who are least likely to succeed, since they want someone else to do it for them. Bear in mind that ultimately you must want to quit, and must go through the physical withdrawal that inevitably occurs. Moreover, you'll have to make the lifestyle adjustments that allow you to live your life without cigarettes.

Who might benefit from joining a clinic? Women are likely to get more out of support groups and outside assistance than men. That's because women are more able to open themselves up to help and suggestions. They go along with the program, following the ideas and tips to the letter, rather than fighting it as men tend to do. Women also have less need to show how tough they are in terms of going it alone. That, in fact, makes women *less* likely to succeed in going cold turkey.

A report from the Surgeon General's office indicates that on-the-job stop-smoking programs are more successful than community-based clinics. When you participate in on-the-job programs, you're likely to be in greater contact with others making the same effort. You reinforce and support the resolve of others, and they provide the same for you. This is particularly important during the crucial first weeks after quitting.

If you have a stop-smoking program where you work, you might want to give it a try. About 15 percent of companies in the country provide this benefit, and more are adding the programs annually as they realize that healthier employees will lose less time from work and make fewer insurance claims.

Both the American Cancer Society and the American Lung Association offer smoking cessation clinics in communities across the country. A report published in the American Journal of Public Health in May 1990 indicated that the ALA's Freedom From Smoking program has a better success rate than ACS's FreshStart program. On the other hand, both approaches have worked for many former smokers.

Of all the commercial programs, the best known probably is Smokenders. This was started in 1969 by Jacqueline Rogers, a dentist's wife who was herself a compulsive smoker. It is a six-week program which forms groups of 15 or more men and women who meet in hotels or other public places. The fee is about $300 per person.

At Smokenders you continue to smoke for the first four weeks, during which time you learn behavior modification techniques designed to make the final quitting easier and more successful. You're taught to think about how, when, and why you smoke, cigarette by cigarette, and how to deal with each situation in which you're tempted to light up.

During those first weeks you switch brands to those you enjoy less and which provide less nicotine. You learn to postpone lighting a cigarette after a meal, and to avoid situations likely to trigger a craving. The idea is to learn how to live without smoking, in the same way you learned to live with cigarettes.

Certainly there are advantages to Smokenders and other similar programs for those who like structure. The concepts taught are sound, though certainly not exclusive to Smokenders. Their claims of success have been challenged, however, and there is no guarantee that the program will enable you to stop. Again, it comes down to your own commitment to quit.

The Doctor's Stop Smoking Clinic was developed by psychologists and physicians to be implemented in doctors' offices. The clinic offers groups of 10 to 30 patients a five-week program including testing, behavior modification, exercise, stress management, coping skills, nicotine gum, and supervision by a physician. The biggest difference here is the use of nicotine gum, which I'll get to in just a moment. Fees charged will vary from office to office and community to community. The program was developed largely to attract new patients to physicians' practices.

Nicotine Gum. Remember that the first aspect of quitting is getting over the physical discomfort of nicotine withdrawal. Your body will crave that nicotine during the first two weeks after you quit. Nicotine gum has been developed to alleviate that physical craving by supplying nicotine during the day, with the idea of allowing the smoker to focus on the psychological aspects of tobacco addiction.

While the concept has definite merit, two things tend to lessen success. First, patients may come to think that by writing the prescription for the gum, the doctor has magically taken away responsibility for quitting. Second, physicians may not properly educate patients as to the proper use of the gum.

Nicotine is absorbed through the mucosa in the mouth, not through the stomach. The gum, then, must be chewed slowly to allow absorption, and you should not swallow the juices as you chew. Use a new gum every time you begin to think about having a cigarette; don't wait until the desire is overwhelming. How many you'll need during the day depends on your own addiction. Some will need 20 gums a day, others only eight or ten. Each 2-mg gum has the nicotine equivalent of a half cigarette. Don't worry about overdosing.

The need for using nicotine gum will gradually reduce. The total time may be from six weeks to six months. Why so long? Remember that you're not going cold turkey, cutting off all the nicotine at once. This spreads the process out. Some like that idea, others want to get it over with and will prefer to just quit and not use the gum at all.

If you do begin using the gum and you still feel severe cravings, simply chew more. Remember that you really can't overdose. Better to chew another gum than to give in to a cigarette.

As the physical cravings subside, you can work on the idea of not fiddling with those cigarettes. Follow the suggestions I provide on page 270.

You may experience some ill effects from incorrect use of nicotine gum. Chewing too quickly can produce feelings of nausea; take an occasional bite rather than chewing as you would ordinary gum. If you still have cravings even though you're chewing a sufficient number of gums, your physician may need to increase the prescription to 4-mg gums.

The effects of nicotine gum and cigarettes are the same in terms of heart disease and contraction of arteries. Don't feel that you can simply chew the gum permanently. It is a temporary bridge, a crutch to help you quit entirely.

Nicotine Patches. Since 1992, four brands of nicotine patches have been approved by the FDA. They help one quit by easing the withdrawal from nicotine addiction, and have been found to be quite effective when used properly. It is important not to smoke while wearing a nicotine patch, as the combination of the two sources of nicotine can and has resulted in heart attack.

Drug Patches. A drug used to treat high blood pressure might help you quit smoking. By prescribing the drug clonidine, your physician can prevent the irritability, anxiety, and insomnia that often accompany withdrawal from nicotine. As with all help methods, this is not a panacea but must be used with your own commitment along with efforts at behavioral modification.

It appears that clonidine works best when administered through a skin patch rather than orally. The patch is skin-colored, postage-stamp sized, and is worn on the chest or shoulder. A month's supply costs less than $30. Physicians feel that 30 days will be enough for quitters to get over the nicotine effects.

Clonidine has been used for more than 20 years without significant side effects. However, you might experience a bit of drowsiness, dry mouth, and a slightly woozy feeling.

Aversion/Rapid Smoking. "Too much of a good thing." Could that apply to smoking as well? It's the concept behind a form of aversion therapy used in some smoking cessation programs. The idea here is to have the smoker take drags off his or her cigarettes every six seconds for as long as possible, usually four or five cigarettes in a row. After a rest period of about five minutes, the smoker repeats the process. Sometimes there is a third rapid-smoking session the same day.

The result of such rapid-smoking is nausea and sometimes even vomiting. The goal is to associate the sickness with cigarettes such that the smoker is turned off to the idea of smoking for the rest of his or her life.

As with all stop-smoking programs, the success rate cannot always be validated, and the results may be exaggerated by those who profit from the program. There's no doubt, however, that rapid-smoking aversion does work for many people. Long-term effectiveness has been documented.

All of us have the capacity to associate a negative reaction with a previously positive experience. I recall one evening having a particular brand of gin in my martini before dinner. Later that evening I became ill and, while it had nothing to do with the gin, I've never been able to drink that brand again.

Doctors call this the "béarnaise sauce syndrome," referring to the notion of becoming ill after eating that particular sauce. Patients frequently will never eat that food again. Almost everyone has experienced a similar situation.

The problem with rapid-smoking involves its safety, especially for heart patients. Researchers at Pennsylvania State University questioned the concept back in 1978. They found that subjects' heart rates jumped considerably, as did their blood pressures and levels of a chemical in the blood called carboxyhemoglobin. Worst of all, there were signs of heart irregularities on the electrocardiogram, although all the subjects were perfectly normal before the rapid smoking.

The Penn State researchers noted that the symptoms of rapid smoking, including dizziness and nausea, are the same as those for nicotine poisoning. The later could be a significant hazard for a person with a recent history of heart disease.

On the other hand, a 1984 publication stated that the use of rapid smoking was "safe and effective with mild to moderate cardiopulmonary disease and those who have had previous, uncomplicated heart attacks." The researchers, from three major medical centers, also found a high level of long-term success with the approach after two years.

Is this the approach for you? Before giving it a try, you might want to discuss it with your physician to be certain of its appropriateness in your own case.

Acupuncture. When acupuncture was first introduced to the western world by Oriental practitioners in the early 1970s, medical authorities scoffed. The idea of inducing anesthesia, lessening pain, and treating illnesses by inserting needles into specified points of the body was foreign to our way of thinking, and not easy to accept. In the intervening years, however, this approach has been shown to have widespread value in a number of applications including weight loss and cigarette cessation.

Either a straight needle or a staple is inserted into either the nose or the ear to effect a lessening in the desire to smoke. Different practitioners' techniques will vary enormously. Success rates, as usual, are exaggerated but have been documented to a certain extent.

Does it work for everyone? No. Could it work for you? Perhaps. Once again, you must really want to quit. And for the method to work best, you must believe in it. To help ensure effectiveness, most practitioners instruct subjects in coping techniques, since withdrawal will be alleviated but not eliminated in most cases.

If interested, you can find practitioners listed in your area's yellow pages under acupuncture. It definitely is not quackery, and it may be just what you need.

Hypnosis. The art of the skilled hypnotherapist or other health practitioner trained in the use of hypnosis is a far cry from the parlor tricks portrayed by Hollywood. Hypnosis is considered a legitimate therapy, with a number of well-documented applications. By almost all estimates, virtually everyone is capable of being hypnotized, though some may be more suggestible than others. Two schools of thought exist as to the best use of hypnosis to help someone quit smoking.

Dr. Herbert Spiegel, a New York psychiatrist with an excellent reputation in the field of hypnotherapy, developed one recognized approach. In a session utilizing his technique, the subject sits in a comfortable chair and, with eyes closed, tries to roll the eyes up as though looking up into the head. The therapist then tells the subject to imagine an arm being very light and capable of floating. Though in a trance, the subject remains conscious of what is happening.

The next step is to imprint a positive message in the mind. "Cigarettes are poison to your body." "You owe your body respect and protection." "You need your body to live."

The subject next learns self-hypnosis and is instructed to use the technique, which lasts about 20 seconds, whenever the urge to smoke comes on, usually about 10 times a day. A card reminds the subject of the positive messages about smoking and the body.

The entire process takes about 45 minutes. For many former smokers, it's the last time they ever wanted to smoke, and they've never lit another cigarette.

More typical is the hypnotherapist who uses a straightforward approach. My good friend Rick Reinert, a well-known animation artist and a smoker for 36 years, says that after just one session it was as if he never had smoked. He walked out of the office without any cravings and hasn't smoked another cigarette since.

I mention Rick specifically because I really thought he would never quit smoking. A cigarette burned at his drawing table or desk almost constantly, and his voice has been permanently lowered by the smoke. He learned about the hypnotist from a friend who swore the method made quitting a snap. Rick had wanted to quit for years, and his family and I had urged him to do so again and again. But he feared withdrawal. When he decided to go to the hynotherapist, he threw his last pack of cigarettes into the trash as he entered the elevator going to her office.

In the approach that worked so well for Rick, the therapist places the subject in a trance and records the session. Positive messages are implanted in the mind. The subject receives the tape and is encouraged to listen to it whenever cravings develop. A follow-up session is included in the fee if it is necessary. Rick didn't need the follow-up and never even bothered to listen to the tape. He never wanted another cigarette. A truly amazing case history, but not an isolated one.

Rick had something special going for him. He really wanted to quit, and he really believed that the hypnosis was just what he'd been waiting for to give him the assistance he needed. Another friend of mine did not fare so well.

Dan Lescoe didn't really want to quit, and he thought the idea of going to a hypnotist was "a crock." Still, friends and family urged him to quit, and Dan says that he knows it would be better if he didn't smoke. On the other hand, he justifies his smoking by pointing out that he smokes only a half-pack a day, and he often makes it through a whole weekend without lighting a single cigarette.

The outcome of his experience was predictable. Dan went into the session and came out a smoker. "I might go back," he says, "when I really want to quit."

The costs vary for hypnosis sessions but are typically less than one would pay for commercial stop-smoking programs. The chances for success will be much better for those who really want to quit, who believe this will work, and who follow the coping strategies I've mapped out in the coming pages.

If you're interested in this approach you can get a list of hypnotists in your area from the American Society of Clinical Hypnosis, 2250 East Devon Avenue, Suit 336, Des Plaines, IL 60018. Their list will include psychologists and psychiatrists as well as those practicing hypnotherapy exclusively.

You might wish to speak with two or three practitioners before deciding which would be the best for you. Perhaps they can answer specific questions you might have.

Those who succeed with the assistance of hypnosis have two things in common. First there's a real desire to quit smoking, a true commitment. Second there's a belief that this approach will be just the ticket to making that desire a reality.

GOING COLD TURKEY—THIS TIME FOR SURE!!!

Yes, there are all sorts of testimonials for this and that method of quitting. And one of those approaches might just work for you. But when it comes right down to it, the majority of men and women who successfully kick the habit do so on their own. There's even proof.

Dr. Michael Fiore headed up a University of Wisconsin study that questioned about 13,000 men and women about their smoking. Of those who hadn't smoked for over a year, almost 85 percent went cold turkey. Only 13 percent succeeded by gradually cutting back on the number of cigarettes smoked daily.

About 48 percent of those who tried to quit on their own did so, while only 24 percent of those who used various other approaches succeeded. Of those who did succeed, certain characteristics jumped out. Successful quitters were more likely to have had strong encouragement from their doctors. Those who manage on their own tend to smoke fewer cigarettes than those who succeed best in groups or clinics.

So now you've made up your mind. You want to quit, you know you have to quit, and you know you're going to succeed this time for sure. It's not going to be easy, but you'll get the job done. Very soon you'll look back, as so many of us ex-smokers have done, and wonder why you didn't do it sooner.

The first thing to do is to set a quit date. Mark your calendar for a few days from now. Tell your spouse, your family, your friends, and your coworkers that this is it. Ask for their help and understanding, since you just might get a bit irritable. Then start making plans.

For openers, you might want to talk with your doctor about the use of nicotine gum or the clonidine or nicotine patches. They might get you through the withdrawal stage a bit more easily. Your doctor might also suggest the use of a mild tranquilizer during the first days, or a sedative to help you get a good night's sleep.

Make a list of the times you smoke. Work on that list for a while. Put it down and review it later, adding some cigarettes you forgot earlier. Don't omit those once-in-a-while situations as well as the day-to-day cues for smoking.

Next think about how you'll deal with each of those times you'd normally smoke. After meals, for example, you will want to get up from the table immediately after the last bite rather than lingering over a cup of coffee. In fact, during the first few weeks it would be best to forego drinking coffee, tea, and alcohol, since one normally smokes along with those beverages. What will you do when the telephone rings? A supply of toothpicks near the phone might help. Or a pencil and pad to fiddle with to keep your hands busy. While watching TV you might plan to have carrot sticks to nibble on. Match your list of smoking encounters with alternative strategies.

Arrange your calendar so that you'll avoid smokers and smoking situations during the first few weeks after quitting. As time goes on, you'll get back to them little by little as you're able to cope more effectively and the initial nicotine withdrawal cravings have passed.

In place of those smoking situations, plan on doing a number of activities in places where smoking is impossible. Go to movies, museums, church, and other locations with smoking prohibitions.

Start working now on the very positive attitude that will make you a success. Don't focus on the negative, on how you miss that cigarette. Instead concentrate on how good you're going to feel, how wonderful flowers will smell and food will taste, and how nice it will be not to have to carry the pack around with you, always looking for an ashtray.

By now you should be doing regular deep breathing as part of your routine stress reduction and relaxation program. This activity will make quitting a lot easier. When those cravings hit, deep breaths will help them pass.

Plan to start your first smokeless day in the morning, not later when you've smoked even one cigarette. It's a bit easier to get started when you've had a good night's sleep.

If your spouse smokes, ask him or her not to do so near you, at least during the first few weeks of going smoke-free. Good friends will also be willing to accommodate you in this way.

One Day at a Time. No one can deal with "forever." Don't dwell on the idea of never having another cigarette as long as you live. That can lead to obsession and can be self-defeating. Instead, concentrate on making it through just this one day. Tomorrow will take care of itself.

Get rid of all your cigarettes and all reminders of smoking, such as matches and ashtrays. The worst thing to do is to keep a pack of cigarettes nearby to "prove" that you don't need them any longer.

Recognize that there will be some very difficult times, and keep to your game plan of coping strategies for situations in which you'd normally smoke. You're going to take it one step, one day, one craving at a time.

In a very real way, you're like the alcoholic who must recognize his or her own weakness in this regard. You are addicted to a deadly drug. The withdrawal period is a very real physical condition. But don't panic. Many millions of others who have become ex-smokers have gone cold turkey and they did it the same way, one day at a time.

During those first few days, you may well notice that your mind wanders and it's more difficult to concentrate. That's a natural reaction, a part of the withdrawal process. It's *not* a sign that you are unique and that you need nicotine to function properly.

Be aware of a disturbing paradox. As you stop smoking, your lungs will begin to regenerate, and to slough damaged tissue. You're going to cough more now than when you smoked. Again, this is natural and it affects just about everyone in the same way.

The only truly terrible mistake you can make is to smoke "just one" cigarette to get you through a particularly tough craving. Don't even take "just one" drag on someone else's. Logically, you think it would make it easier, but in truth it just makes it more difficult and could destroy your effort.

You may find yourself literally pacing the floor like a caged animal. You'll experience a kind of inner explosive force that begs to be released. So release it. But not by giving in to having a cigarette. Take a walk around the block. Do some serious deep breathing. Meditate. Take a bath or shower.

Be aware that cravings are transient. Each one passes. No craving goes on indefinitely. Recognize that fact as the craving hits, and work your way through it. As time goes on, those cravings will be less intense and will become more and more infrequent. Each day will be easier than the day before. But concentrate on this day. One day at a time.

Here are some coping strategies to help you make it through this particular day:

Meals
• Get up from the table immediately after eating

- Start washing the dishes and cleaning the table
- Avoid coffee, tea, and alcohol
- Brush teeth frequently. Floss often.

Coffee Breaks
- Practice deep breathing instead of taking a break
- Go for a walk
- Do some stretching exercises
- Drink water or juice instead of coffee
- Fiddle with a pencil, toothpick, or swizzle stick

Telephone Calls/ Conversations
- Keep supply of pencils, swizzle sticks near by
- Work a rosary or worry beads through your fingers
- Suck on hard candies
- Keep conversations short

Television
- Go to the movies instead
- Nibble on carrot sticks and pretzels
- Sit on the floor rather than in a regular chair

Driving the Car
- Spray deodorizer to scent the air in the car
- Keep both hands on the wheel (a good idea anyway)
- Concentrate on the road ahead
- Do stomach-tightening exercises

There are also some general strategies that make those first critical days easier:

Drink Lots of Water
- Enjoy ice tinkling in a glass of cold water
- Celebrate yourself by using a nice wine glass
- Visualize the poisons of smoking being voided in your urine

Develop Hobbies Using Both Hands
- Knitting, crocheting, needlepoint
- Gardening and fix-up work
- Building model ships and planes

Alternative Activities and Thoughts
- Walking
- Stretching

- Deep Breathing
- Meditation
- Prayer: This is a great time to ask for help!

Frequently Review Reasons to not Smoke
- Improved health
- Recovery of your heart
- Feeling terrific
- Improved athletic performance
- Improved sexual performance
- Freedom from matches and ashtrays
- Fitting into the Smoke-Free Society
- Saving money
- Self-control
- Feeling of pride in accomplishment

Reward Yourself. Let's face it, this is not the easiest thing in the world to do, and you deserve a reward. In fact, you deserve lots of rewards. So starting planning some. What would you like to do with the money you save by not buying those daily packs and weekly cartons? Make a list of little things, and maybe some bigger things. Then, on a regular basis as you remain smoke-free, treat yourself. Do something nice for yourself each and every day.

Announce your achievement in terms of a progress report to your friends now and then, and tell them about your rewards.

Is this just silliness? Much to the contrary, you'll be enhancing your chances at being successful in your efforts. In a research study to determine what separated the quitters from the failures, psychologists found that use of rewards and positive reminders made the difference. Unsuccessful individuals tended to use negative reminders, such as how they would appear weak and lacking in willpower to others. These findings are backed up by other research which similarly indicates success in weight loss using these techniques.

Trouble Shooting
- Dry mouth: sip cold water, suck on hard candies, chew sugarless gum
- Insomnia: avoid alcohol and caffeine; take a warm bath before retiring; meditate
- Irregularity: drink lots of water, increase soluble fiber in the diet

- Hunger: keep lots of low-calorie snacks in the refrigerator, eat more frequently
- Coughing: sip warm decaf beverages; suck on cough drops or hard candies.

Weight Control. It is absolutely not true that everyone who quits smoking automatically gains weight, any more than everyone who has a baby remains heavy for the rest of her life. On the other hand it *is* true that nicotine has an effect on the metabolism and that one has a tendency to gain weight. But one can very easily counter that tendency by increasing the amount of daily exercise. Since extra walking is one of the best alternative activities to smoking, especially when those cravings hit, you should have no trouble at all.

Moreover, as part of your overall program for complete cardiac recovery you're already cutting back on the fatty foods that led to the clogging of your arteries. Without that fat in the diet, you can eat lots more of the kinds of foods that you'll want to snack on during those first weeks without cigarettes.

Stock your cabinets with pretzels, especially the low-salt or saltless kinds. Keep a platter of freshly cut carrots, zucchini, celery, green peppers, and so forth in the refrigerator so you have something to nibble on through the day.

Drink lots and lots of water. I can't emphasize it too much. Shoot for at least eight 8-ounce glasses of water daily. You can replace some of the water with decaf beverages including club soda, mineral water, and diet sodas.

Eat more frequently, rather than having fewer and larger meals. You'll be more satisfied, and you'll actually consume fewer calories in total.

Weigh yourself every other day. There will be some normal fluctuation from day to day, with a pound or two gained or lost. But if the weight remains up even by one or two pounds after a few days, cut back on the food and increase the exercise.

Concentrate on alternative oral habits such as using a toothpick, chewing on a swizzle stick, chewing sugarless gum, and frequently brushing and flossing your teeth.

Even if after following all this good advice you do gain a few pounds, remember that it's far more important to quit smoking. You can always shed those extra pounds when you've gotten the cigarette situation under control.

Falling Off the Wagon. I really hope that from quitting day on, and for the rest of your life, you'll never smoke another cigarette. But it's possible that you'll slip. IT'S NOT THE END OF THE WORLD. This does not mean that you're a worthless person who has no willpower and deserves all the rotten things in life. It simply means that you've slipped, nothing more and nothing less. It's time to start again.

Don't let that one cigarette lead to buying a package. You've lost a battle, not the war. Go back to all the good reasons to quit. Remember how you made it this far, and strengthen your resolve to make it all the way the next time. Then start that "next time" right now!

When the Smoke Clears. You and I and everyone else who calls himself an ex-smoker is really nothing more than a smoker under control. We're just like the alcoholics who are "recovering" rather than "recovered." Once a smoker, always a smoker. The worst thing you can do is falsely believe that you've "beaten" the cigarettes and that you can have one once in a while.

Recognize the mind's ability to rationalize a return to old habits. Having one cigarette can lead to another, and another, and another until you're hooked again. Don't allow yourself to light that first cigarette, regardless of the situation, either good or bad.

A good friend of mine had been off cigarettes for a full six years. Then one day he was on a long-distance trip through the desert and his car's engine broke down in the middle of nowhere. Angry and frustrated when he finally got to a service station, he bought a pack of cigarettes which led to another three years of smoking.

Then there was the actor who landed a role that required him to smoke a cigarette. Of course that scene had to be reshot several times. After ten smoke-free years, he was hooked all over again.

When tempted to smoke, try to remember just how hard it was to quit in the first place. You don't want to have to go through all that again.

Concentrate, too, on all the reasons you wanted to quit. Focus on how much better you feel now. Recall the frustrations of wanting to quit but being unable to do so.

In my own case, I remember how I used to smoke during meetings. There was nothing else to do with my hands, and I'd light one after another. Now when I attend such meetings I call to mind how my lungs used to feel and how powerless I felt to keep from lighting the next one.

Every former smoker has a recurring dream with just a variation or two. You dream that you reach for your pocket and discover a pack of cigarettes there, realizing that you've started in again. There's a sense of panic. When did I start? How did this happen? How am I going to quit again? You wake up in a sweat, eminently thankful that it was just a dream. Talk with some former smokers and you'll find that almost everyone has had that dream. I think it expresses the strong psychological hold cigarettes can exert over us.

During the first days and weeks, the desire to have a smoke seems to strike every few minutes. As time goes on, those cravings will be spaced further and further apart. Moreover, the intensity of the craving will lessen.

But don't be surprised when, months later, you find that you'd really like a cigarette. Bear in mind that it's been quite a while since such a craving struck, and realize that the desire will pass quickly. Speed it along by doing a few deep breaths.

Sometimes those cravings will strike, it seems, out of the blue. Often that's because you find yourself in a situation in which you used to smoke but which you haven't learned to deal with as a nonsmoker. My wife Dawn had that happen to her just recently.

When we first met, Dawn and I were heavy smokers. At the time, I had an apartment in Chicago with a commanding view of the city. We loved to have dinner together, the electric canyon of lights spread out for miles below us, and to finish off the meal with a cigarette.

Fast forward many years. We'd moved to California, both of us had quit smoking for years, and we lived far from the high-rise lifestyle we'd enjoyed before having our children. Then one day we had dinner in one of L.A.'s few hotel-top restaurants. Dawn fidgeted in her chair, nervously toying with her glass of wine. She said, "Bob, I can't believe it. I want a cigarette so badly I can hardly stand it!" I explained to her that this was a kind of "flashback" to our high-rise dinners during our smoking days. Understanding this made it easier, the craving passed, and neither of us is tempted to smoke in that situation anymore.

Even if you started smoking at a very young age, you spent many years without cigarettes. You lived without them quite well. Then you spent years learning how to live with cigarettes, one situation, one setting, one cue at a time. It will take some time, but you'll learn how to not smoke in those same situations and settings.

No one will tell you that quitting is easy. It can be one of the most challenging things you can do. But it's worth the effort. Millions of Americans have quit. Welcome to the "in" crowd of the Smoke-Free Society! And congratulations!

THE SIXTH STEP:

Enjoying a Heart-Healthy Diet

CHAPTER 13

Eliminating the Cholesterol Confusion

Just a few years ago, cholesterol was a word that few could pronounce or spell, much less have any regard for in their own lives. Today that's all changed. So much so that when Vanna White spelled out CHO-LESTEROL on "Wheel of Fortune" the category was "common household term." And my wife and children were delighted when the question for "Best-selling health book of 1988" on "Jeopardy!" was "What is *The 8-Week Cholesterol Cure?*"

A tremendous amount of publicity aimed at both doctors and their patients resulted in massive public awareness of the need for cholesterol testing and control. Still, the average American doesn't completely understand what all the terms really mean. Now that you're on the road to recovery from heart disease, it's particularly important that you fully understand cholesterol and what you can do about it.

Actually cholesterol isn't all bad. We need some of it for a number of the body's functions: to manufacture adrenal and sex hormones, to produce bile acids used in digestion, to build cell walls, and to form the protective sheath around nerves. Because cholesterol is so important, the body makes its own supply in the liver. In fact, if we never ate a single bit of cholesterol, we'd make all we need. Unfortunately some of us make more than we need, and we add fuel to the fire by eating a high-fat, high-cholesterol diet.

The result is an elevated cholesterol level in the blood of more than half of all Americans. We'd like to see levels at no more than 200 mg/dl, and more ideally at between 160 and 180. The "mg/dl" stands for milligrams of cholesterol per deciliter of blood. From now on, I'll drop that designation and just provide numbers.

While the total amount of cholesterol in the blood is important, it's also essential to know about individual constituents. A number of years ago, researchers found that the total cholesterol in the blood could be broken down into a number of fractions, determined by the lipoproteins which carry cholesterol through the blood. These lipoproteins can be likened to transport ships, since cholesterol itself does not dissolve in blood and needs to be shuttled around.

Low-density lipoprotein cholesterol (LDL) is the real culprit in heart disease. This is the "bad" cholesterol we hear about. For those who have had a cardiac event and hope for disease regression, LDL should be no more than 100. LDL carries cholesterol through the blood and deposits it in the arteries in a solid mixture of calcium, fibers, and other substances collectively referred to as plaque. The formation of such plaque is called atheroma, and the disease is atherosclerosis. It is this atherosclerosis that we commonly call heart disease. Actually, the heart is usually healthy, but the arteries are blocked. So a more proper term is "coronary heart disease" (CHD), with the word coronary referring to the coronary arteries supplying the heart with blood. The higher the level of LDL in the blood, the greater the risk of heart disease.

Very-low-density lipoprotein cholesterol (VLDL) is the substance that the liver uses to manufacture LDL. Scientists refer to VLDL as a precursor of LDL. In other words, the higher the level of VLDL, the more LDL can be produced by the liver.

High-density lipoprotein cholesterol (HDL) is the protective fraction of cholesterol. HDL actually acts to draw cholesterol away from the linings of arteries. The higher the level of this "good" HDL cholesterol, the more protection against heart disease. Levels of HDL should be no lower than 50 to 55 in women and 45 to 50 in men. Levels of less than 35 are considered to be an independent risk factor for heart disease. That is to say, even if total cholesterol levels are in the desirable range, if the level of HDL is less than 35, heart disease can occur. In fact, it is estimated that about 20 percent of all men suffering a heart attack have a perfectly normal cholesterol level of 200 or less; but their HDL falls under 35. Conversely, women tend to have a higher level of HDL, and even if their total cholesterol counts are high, they can be completely free of heart disease risk.

You may hear your doctor talk about a cholesterol risk ratio. He's referring to the ratio between either total cholesterol or LDL cholesterol and HDL cholesterol. This is an excellent index of heart disease risk. Let's look at some examples.

If total cholesterol is 200 and HDL cholesterol is 50, the ratio is 4:1 or 4.0. A total of 250 with an HDL of 40 gives a ratio of 6.25. Ideally that ratio should be no more than 4.0 for women and 4.5 for men. The difference reflects women's greater production of HDL as a rule.

If using the LDL to HDL ratio, the numbers should be no more than 3.0. As an example, if the LDL were 140 and the HDL 35, the ratio would be 4.0. In this case we'd like to see the LDL come down and the HDL go up. We'll discuss just how to achieve those changes in this chapter.

Blood tests prescribed by doctors will usually include information about levels of triglycerides. These are another category of fats in the blood, although their involvement in heart disease remains in question. Some doctors feel that elevated triglyceride levels have nothing to do with heart disease. Others believe that levels should not exceed 250. Still others are more stringent, calling for triglyceride counts of no more than 150. The concern here is that triglycerides are the major components of VLDL, which in turn can lead to increased LDL in the blood. An international expert panel upgraded the risk of elevated triglyceride levels at a 1991 meeting in New York. Those with levels of 200 or more are now considered to be at increased risk, especially when other risk factors are present.

Dietary fat, especially saturated fat, and cholesterol raise levels of cholesterol in the blood. Triglycerides are influenced by simple sugars and alcohol. The ideal dietary prescription, as we'll see in more detail, calls for reduced amounts of fat, cholesterol, refined sugars, and alcohol. But you've heard that before! Now it's a matter of putting it to practice as you make your recovery.

The National Cholesterol Education Program, a joint effort of the nation's medical organizations in concert with the National Institutes of Health of the federal government, radically altered its guidelines for cholesterol management. While the general population should ideally have a cholesterol level of no more than 200, and a level of LDL cholesterol of no more than 140, those with existing heart disease should strive to get those numbers down to 160 and 100 respectively.

Doctors were urged by the NCEP Adult Treatment Panel to use "aggressive" management to achieve those goals. A diet with no more than 20 percent of calories coming from fat and no more than 200 mg of dietary cholesterol was recommended. And if diet alone is not completely effective, treatment with niacin or prescription drugs should be implemented.

I was, of course, elated to hear those changes in medical philosophy announced, as they are exactly the recommendations I've been making—and personally following—since 1984. But beyond personal pride, I'm pleased that patients will finally receive the treatment they desperately need from the physicians who will heed the experts' recommendations.

STILL A CONTROVERSY

Especially since 1987, with the establishment of the National Cholesterol Education Program, public attention has been drawn to the importance of cholesterol as a risk factor. Unfortunately, the mass media also provided a forum for a few nay-sayers who maintained that diet and cholesterol reduction would do little to prevent heart attacks. With the evidence we now have at our disposal, that was akin to saying that the earth is flat!

The controversy in 1989 and spilling over into 1990 made for sensational journalistic coverage, but lacked any scientific credibility. The fact remains that elevated cholesterol levels are one of the major risk factors in the development of heart disease, and a principal contributor to the leading cause of death in this country.

The authors of the books and magazine articles which made some people question the value of giving up their bacon and egg breakfasts and their cheeseburgers for lunch simply chose to ignore some of the more recent and dramatic data. They concentrated on pointing to early studies in which the results were not convincing.

Why did those older research projects fail? For the most part, it was a matter of not going far enough in intervention efforts. The average American consumes about 40 percent of his or her calories as fat and about 500 to 600 milligrams of cholesterol daily. Simply cutting down the fat intake to 35 percent and the cholesterol consumption to 300 milligrams wasn't enough to achieve a significant cholesterol reduction in the blood. Today we know better.

The evidence begins in early childhood. Researchers in a number of centers throughout the United States have correlated children's diet with their cholesterol levels. Dr. Gerald Berenson at Louisiana State University studied the children in the town of Bogalusa outside New Orleans for 16 years.

During that time, a number of children died as a result of accidents, homicides, and suicides. Upon autopsy it was learned that children as young as 10 and 11 years old already had fatty streaks of cholesterol buildup in the aorta and arteries. The higher cholesterol levels were, the greater the signs of early atherosclerosis. Dr. Berenson concluded that heart disease begins in childhood and often relates directly to the diet.

Misfortune provided additional evidence during the Korean and Vietnamese wars. Soldiers who fell in battle were autopsied, and doctors found their arteries significantly blocked with cholesterol-laden plaque. Researchers also autopsied Korean and Vietnamese soldiers who, obviously, consumed a much different diet. Their arteries were clear.

Reducing cholesterol levels can have an impact on the rate of heart disease. The Lipid Research Clinics Coronary Primary Prevention Trial in 1984 proved that. Patients achieving an average 22.3 mg/dl drop in the levels of the "bad" LDL cholesterol demonstrated a 17.2 percent reduction in the actual incidence of coronary heart disease.

The authors of the published study state that for subjects following the program to the letter, LDL levels fell by 35 percent. Total cholesterol levels dropped 25 percent. This much of a difference, they say, would reduce the incidence of coronary heart disease by 49 percent. The practical implications are clear: The risk of heart disease drops two percent for every one percent decline in total cholesterol levels.

Virtually all the early cholesterol studies focused on preventing heart disease in healthy individuals or those at risk of developing the disease. This approach is called *primary prevention.* But what about people like you and me, those who have already had a heart attack and, obviously, have heart disease already established? Our goal is to prevent another heart attack, and to extend our lives. This kind of intervention is termed *secondary prevention* and we have a tremendous amount of evidence to prove that it really works. Not only can we stop heart disease dead in its tracks, but we can actually reverse the process.

The first carefully controlled study was done at the University of Southern California by Dr. David Blankenhorn and his associates. He has studied 162 coronary bypass surgery patients, each of whom under-went angiography to carefully measure the amount of blockage in his or her arteries at the beginning of the project and at intervals thereafter. Half the patients were given a fat-modified diet in which fat comprised about 20 percent of total calories, and were given the bile acid-binding drug colestipol and niacin. We'll discuss those and other cholesterol-lowering substances later. The other group was placed on a modified diet, about the same as the American Heart Association recommendations, and given a placebo in place of the colestipol and niacin.

At the end of the two-year period, the first group showed a 26 percent reduction in total plasma cholesterol, a 43 percent drop in LDL, and a 37 percent rise in HDL. Looking at the angiograms done at the end of the study and comparing them with those done two years earlier, re-searchers found that not only was the progress of the disease stopped in those on the diet–colestipol–niacin program, but also there was reversal of the atherosclerotic plaque buildup in more than 16 percent of patients, as compared with 3 percent in the placebo group. Those in the other group, however, exhibited a worsening of their disease, with arteries more seriously blocked.

Those patients were then tracked for another two years. Again, the treatment group improved significantly while the control group showed deterioration.

Dr. Blankenhorn has been adamant in his presentations of these data that everyone having a bypass operation should receive *aggressive* therapy to reduce cholesterol in order to prevent the need for a second surgery. Unfortunately, only about 20 percent of bypass patients currently receive this kind of advice and treatment.

Another study demonstrating the value of secondary prevention was done at the University of Washington. There Dr. Greg Brown studied 146 men 62 years old or younger who had a family history of heart disease, high levels of total and LDL cholesterol, and evidence of block-age of the arteries on an angiogram. Of those men, 120 completed the study.

At the end of two and a half years, atherosclerosis worsened in 46 percent of patients treated with diet and placebo. In the groups receiving either niacin and colestipol or Mevacor and colestipol, half as many patients showed progression of disease and 35 percent showed improve-ment. In addition, Dr. Brown said, the aggressively treated patients showed a 75 percent reduction in clinical events such as heart attack or death.

Using a program that calls for no drugs, but that does require dramatic lifestyle changes, Dr. Dean Ornish at the University of California School of Medicine in San Francisco has demonstrated that even severe heart disease can be reversed. Half of his group made extensive modifications in diet and lifestyle. They ate a low-fat vegetarian diet that allows no animal products other than egg whites and skim milk and uses no fats or oils whatsoever. The patients also practiced yoga stress reduction techniques and engaged in daily exercise. The other group received standard advice calling for less fat in the diet.

After one year, 82 percent in the treatment group showed some overall regression of disease as measured on angiograms. For those getting usual care, 53 percent showed progression of disease. There's no doubt that this approach works, and we'll discuss it further in the treatment section of this chapter.

How low must cholesterol levels fall? Dr. Jeremiah Stamler at Northwestern University in Chicago has observed that while shooting for a cholesterol level of 200 is a step in the right direction, the incidence of heart disease begins to appear at 160 and slowly increases to 180. After 180 there is a dramatic surge in heart disease, and after 200 it soars. His recommendation, then, for the entire population is to aim for the 160 to 180 range.

What does it take to completely remove the risk posed by cholesterol levels? Dr. William Castelli, medical director of the Framingham study in Massachusetts, has said that he's never seen a heart attack in a patient whose cholesterol is 150 or less, even when HDLs are low. To reverse the disease that's been getting worse throughout a lifetime, Dr. Castelli proposes "membership" in what he calls the "150/5" club. He believes that getting cholesterol levels down to 150 for five years will lead to reversal of heart disease.

In Dr. Ornish's reversal program, total cholesterols fell from an average of 227 to 136. In the control group there was no significant change in cholesterol levels and, as noted, the disease worsened.

The handwriting is on the wall and on the pages of the medical journals. Get those cholesterol levels way down, much lower than 200. That number might be just fine for the general population, especially for those without other risk factors such as family history or cigarette smoking or high blood pressure. But for those of us with heart disease already present—and having a heart attack or bypass surgery is proof of that, even without an angiogram to back it up—we need to work a lot harder.

I must say, however, that as strongly as I feel about cholesterol reduction, we can never forget that it's just one of the steps to be taken for total recovery from heart disease. All those other steps play important roles: controlling high blood pressure, quitting the cigarettes, losing extra weight, and playing the "inner game" of stress control and relaxation.

In discussing this with Dr. Ornish at a heart association meeting, I found that some of his patients did not achieve as dramatic cholesterol reductions as others. Yet they did manage to control their disease. He said that might be because they didn't eat the foods which clog the arteries, even though their cholesterol levels didn't come down appreciably. He also believes the element of mental control cannot be over-emphasized as part of a reversal program.

I can add my own personal experience to underline his feelings. My own cholesterol level at the time of my second bypass surgery was 284. With the program I described fully in *The 8-Week Cholesterol Cure*, and which I'll outline in this chapter, I brought that number down to levels that have ranged between 160 and 180 for the past several years. But I also do my exercise religiously and practice a number of stress control and relaxation techniques. The angiogram showing my clear arteries demonstrates that the program works very well.

There's no doubt, in any case, that cholesterol control is an essential part of any recovery program. You'll want to have your level measured on a regular basis to be certain that you're keeping your numbers down.

WOMEN BENEFIT AS WELL AS MEN!

While most studies have focused on male heart patients, women can expect the potential for reversing heart disease as well. We now have the proof! In a trial lasting 26 months, Dr. John Kane and his colleagues at the University of California at San Francisco studied 41 women and 31 men with dangerously high levels of the bad LDL cholesterol. At the start of the project, all patients had plaque clogging their coronary arteries.

The researchers encouraged the entire group to consume a low-fat, low-cholesterol diet. Half the men and women got aggressive drug therapy to lower their blood cholesterol, while the others remained on diet alone.

The doctors compared "before and after" angiograms of the patients' coronary arteries.

Those who dramatically lowered their cholesterol levels were rewarded with regression of blockage, while those who did not saw a progression of the disease. Very importantly, women did just as well as men. The proof was published in the December 19, 1990 issue of the *Journal of the American Medical Association.*

TESTING FOR CHOLESTEROL

It's important to realize that your cholesterol level can vary considerably from day to day and month to month, even if you don't change a thing in your diet. Unlike an absolute number such as your body temperature at exactly 98.6°F (unless you have a fever), cholesterol levels represent a range from the low end to the high end.

Daily variability may range a full five percent in either direction. Thus if your cholesterol reading comes in at 200, it might mean that it could be 210 or 190 tomorrow. Or, of course, that number could represent the high or low end of your particular range.

Moreover, a number of things can influence your count. Stress plays an important role. Accountants demonstrate a higher cholesterol level prior to the April 15 tax deadline; it drops back down once the deadline passes. Medical students have shown a cholesterol increase just before major examinations. Even world-class athletes concerned about an upcoming event will experience a rise in cholesterol levels.

An illness can cause fluctuation, so it's best not to have a test done when you're suffering from the flu. Women will show a variation during their menstrual period. Your level will be higher in the winter than during summer months.

But don't throw your hands up in despair. All this means that you shouldn't trust a single number. That's especially true for those who've just had a heart attack or bypass surgery, both of which can result in an abnormally low count. To have an accurate assessment of your cholesterol level, you should consider the average of at least three separate tests. If your cholesterol test comes in at well over 250 each of those times, it's quite certain that you have a problem to contend with.

There's been a bit of media publicity regarding testing accuracy. So how can you be sure of your own measurements? The most accurate cholesterol tests are performed in hospital laboratories, where the equipment is regularly serviced and calibrated for both accuracy and precision. Fingerprick tests such as you might see at a shopping mall or supermarket are fine as a way to monitor your levels, but you must realize that they will probably not be as accurate as those processed at a fully equipped laboratory. On the other hand, if the equipment is properly maintained and the personnel are well trained, one can expect a quite accurate measurement from a fingerstick test.

Regardless of the site or method of your test, you can take certain steps to ensure accuracy. If your doctor orders a laboratory test, he'll probably want a full lipid profile; that is, a complete breakdown of total cholesterol, HDL and LDL cholesterol, and triglycerides. Fasting 12 to 14 hours prior to the test ensures an accurate measure of the triglycerides, and that number is used to calculate the level of LDL in your blood. Fasting is not required if only the total and/or HDL cholesterol will be measured.

Foods eaten the day before a cholesterol test will have little effect on the results, as long as the 12- to 14-hour fast is observed. The effect of a high-fat, high-cholesterol meal takes two to three days to show up in the cholesterol count.

If you have a fingerstick test, rest seated for about five minutes prior to blood drawing. Make sure your hands are warm so that the technician will not have to "milk" a drop of blood from your finger. Such milking results in inaccurately low results. If cold hands are the result of inclement weather, keep your hands in your pockets during your five-minute rest. If they are cold as the result of stress, take those five minutes to do some deep breathing or biofeedback.

A remarkably accurate and precise cholesterol testing device was approved in 1991 for use by physicians. The AccuMeter is a small, self-contained disposable cassette that reads the total cholesterol level from a fingerstick blood sample. I tested it along with Dr. Charles Keenan in Santa Monica, and we found it to be both accurate and easy to use.

I see a very important role which can be played by the AccuMeter for those of us trying to control our cholesterol levels. Have you ever come back from a vacation wondering whether your splurges boosted your count, but didn't want to go to the doctor's office or laboratory to find out? Maybe you were too embarrassed or didn't have the time. Or perhaps you've been trying something new and would like to see whether the cholesterol level has come down. The AccuMeter will be able to satisfy your curiosity at any time, right in your own home. It's also a terrific way to monitor your count on a regular basis.

Through your physician you can get a supply to keep on hand at home. For more information, call the manufacturer, ChemTrak, at (800) 927-7776.

How do your cholesterol levels match up with others in the population? Compare yours with the tabulations in Tables 5A–5F (pages 316–19).

Women should note that their HDL levels typically are much higher than those for men. While a high total cholesterol count may be an initial cause for alarm, it may be balanced out by a very high HDL level. It is an unfortunate reality that many women today are being treated aggressively, perhaps even with drugs, for elevated cholesterol measurements when those elevations may be largely due to high levels of the protective HDLs.

Why might your cholesterol level be high? While we've heard so much about diet during the past few years, your eating habits may not be the only reason for cholesterol elevations.

Indeed, a significant part of the problem was inherited from your parents and grandparents. Some people are simply more genetically programmed to produce large amounts of cholesterol in their livers. Eating a high-fat, high-cholesterol diet just makes matters worse.

Other medical conditions also play significant roles. Hypothyroidism can result in cholesterol elevations. So can diabetes and menopause. Moreover, certain medications, such as antihypertensive drugs, can raise cholesterol levels. Your doctor will want to take all of these into consideration in diagnosing your own condition. But to effectively control your cholesterol, you have to play the principal role.

THE DIETARY FOUNDATION

The same dietary modifications that you'll need for controlling your cholesterol will pay off in additional dividends. Without even thinking about calories, cutting back on fat will help you lose those pounds you've been meaning to shed. If you're diabetic, you'll find it a lot easier to keep your glucose levels controlled. In the long term, a low-fat, low-cholesterol diet can also provide protection against cancer.

The best news is that the dietary changes necessary for good health don't mean deprivation. You'll find yourself eating as much as you want, never feeling hungry, and indulging in tasty treats that you'll find mouth-wateringly delicious.

Hearing numbers regarding your foods can be bewildering. What does it mean to eat 30 percent or 20 percent or 10 percent of your calories as fat? Some nutritionists and certain publications have tried to illustrate such numbers in terms of teaspoons of fat. But have you ever seen fat listed in teaspoons on a package of food? There's an easier, far more practical way to deal with all this.

First let's assume that like most Americans you now consume about 40 percent of your calories as fat. That means that an awful lot of your food has a significant amount of fat in it. Compare that with populations in the world who eat much less fat, about 15 percent, and have virtually no heart disease. The American Heart Association has long recommended a 30-percent-fat diet for Americans; but while that may be fine for others, it's just not effective for those of us who already have heart disease. On the other hand, a diet calling for only 10 percent fat will be unacceptable for most people to follow for any length of time. While that may be very effective, it's just not very practical.

I propose a 20-percent-fat diet. This comes close to the levels of fat intake in countries which are nearly free of heart disease. It allows a delicious choice of foods which can be enjoyed not only at home but while dining out in restaurants and at the homes of friends and relatives. This level of fat intake is endorsed by the American Health Foundation as well as by the American Heart Association for those with a compelling need for cholesterol control. That means you and me.

But, again, you won't see percentages of fat listed on food packages or in magazine recipes. What you will see listed is the amount of fat measured in grams. That's something we can all get a practical handle on for our own purposes.

Bear with me for the next few paragraphs and you'll have your personally tailored prescription for gram intake to achieve a 20-percent-fat diet. We'll start with the calories you need daily.

The average, moderately active man needs about 15 calories to maintain each pound of body weight. A very active man may need more calories to maintain his weight. Less active men, and most women, will require fewer calories. A middle-aged, moderately active woman, or a less active man, may need only 12 to 13 calories to keep weight at the current level. Thus to determine your daily caloric needs, multiply either

15 or a greater or lesser number by your ideal weight. Notice that I say *ideal* weight. We'll discuss that in a moment.

Let's take an average man who weighs 150 pounds and is moderately active. He walks regularly, plays an occasional round of golf, and engages in leisure activities other than just watching television. He needs 15 calories per pound to maintain his weight. Here's his calculation:

$$150 \times 15 = 2{,}250 \text{ calories/day}$$

What if you'd *like* to weigh 150 pounds, but right now you tip the scales at 170? By consuming 2,250 calories daily you, our reference man, will feed only your ideal 150 pounds. Little by little, but in a very satisfying process, those extra pounds will come off. You'll feed only your ideal weight; those extra pounds will be starved away.

Now that we know that our male example needs 2,250 calories daily, let's assume that he's going to get heart-healthy and consume 20 percent of those calories as fat. The calculation is simply to multiply the daily calories by 20 percent.

$$2{,}250 \times .20 = 450 \text{ calories consumed as fat}$$

While carbohydrates and protein supply only four calories per gram, fat provides a full nine calories. Thus to translate those abstract calories into practical grams, we do the next calculation of dividing our calories consumed as fat by nine, the number of calories in each gram.

$$450 \div 9 = 50 \text{ grams}$$

There we have it. Our reference male example will want to consume no more than 50 grams of fat daily. That's something he (and you and I) can easily keep track of regularly.

Of that total amount of fat, no more than one-third should be saturated. The balance should come from polyunsaturated and monounsaturated fats. More about that in the coming paragraphs.

Of course, you're not yet familiar with the number of grams of fat in foods. Begin by reading the labels on packages. Look at the labels on milk cartons, bread packages, TV dinners, and almost every food that's processed by a manufacturer. Next, familiarize yourself with the number of grams of fat found in commonly eaten foods including meats, fish, cheese, and the like which are not processed when you buy them in the supermarket. Take a look at Table 6 (page 321) for a brief overview. For a complete listing of the fat, cholesterol, caloric, and sodium contents of foods, I'd recommend the book *Food Values of Portions Commonly Used* by Jean A. J. Pennington; it's available in most bookstores in paperback.

When I first began to control my own cholesterol by keeping tabs on fat grams, I knew no more about those numbers than you do now. Within a remarkably short period of time, however, this all becomes second nature. You may not know that cheddar cheese packs about 9 grams of fat per ounce versus the 6 grams for mozzarella or the 7 grams for Swiss, but you'll have a general idea that cheese has a lot of fat and that eating just one ounce will account for a significant percentage of your daily fat-gram allowance. Pretty soon you'll be selecting foods throughout the day and zeroing right in on your fat target without even consulting a chart or table. Millions have done it. Trust me.

But not all fat is the same. The difference is in the degree of saturation of the fat molecule. The more hydrogen atoms are attached to the fat molecule, the more saturated it is said to be. The more saturated a fat is, the more it tends to clog arteries. The saturated fats are solid or semi-solid at room temperature. The reason butter is harder to spread than margarine straight out of the refrigerator is that butter has more saturated fat.

Unsaturated fats fall into two categories: polyunsaturated and mono-unsaturated. The distinction comes, again, from the number of hydrogen atoms involved, or, conversely, how many spaces on the fat molecule are not occupied by a hydrogen atom. At first one might think, therefore, that polyunsaturated fats would be a far better choice than monounsaturated fats, since the former have more spaces unfilled by hydrogen atoms. For years, that was the consensus in the scientific and medical communities.

But there was one flaw in that reasoning. Many populations in the world consume a vast amount of monounsaturated fat in the form of olive oil, yet have very low rates of heart disease. To briefly summarize the many research projects that followed, we now know that monounsaturated fats can lower cholesterol levels as effectively as polyunsaturated fats when used to replace saturated fats in the diet. In fact, the mono-unsaturated fats may have a slight edge in view of the indication that they tend to reduce the bad LDL cholesterol selectively, leaving the good HDL untouched. Polyunsaturated fats tend to lower all types of cholesterol.

We'll discuss specific fats and oils in the section of this chapter that deals with shopping and selecting foods. Needless to say, you'll want to choose those with less saturated fats. But all foods contain a profile of saturated, polyunsaturated, and monounsaturated fats. That's true across the board, for butter as well as for corn oil. See Table 7 (page 334) for a comparison of fats and oils.

As much as we've heard about dietary cholesterol, and food manufacturers have rushed to satisfy consumer's demands by advertising "Cholesterol-Free" this and "No-Cholesterol" that, it turns out that saturated fat raises cholesterol levels in the blood more than dietary cholesterol itself. Indeed, much of the advertising is sheer nonsense, since cholesterol comes only from animal foods, never from plant foods. Thus *all* corn oil and *all* peanut butter is cholesterol-free.

Actually, by leaning toward foods of plant rather than animal origin, one can cut way back on saturated fats and can eliminate cholesterol entirely. There are only a few exceptions. Avocados, olives, and nuts are high in fat and must be consumed in moderation. Again, don't eliminate, but moderate. See Table 6 for specifics. And the so-called tropical oils—coconut oil, palm oil, and palm kernel oil—are high in saturated fats. Fortunately, as a result of consumer demands, manufacturers are removing the offending oils from their foods.

Unfortunately, they're replacing the tropical oils with hydrogenated oils. This has led to something of a controversy. By adding hydrogen atoms to corn oil, soybean oil, and so forth, manufacturers prolong the shelf life and consumer acceptance of their food products. But this makes those oils more saturated, and thus more likely to raise cholesterol levels in the blood and to clog arteries. While the hydrogenated or partially hydrogenated soybean oil in a food is a far cry better than the tropical oil or the lard it replaced, it's not as good as the pure soybean oil would be.

Some researchers aren't as concerned about this, however, pointing out that one must be more careful in observing what really happens to those fats during the hydrogenation process. First, some of the polyunsaturated fats may be converted to monounsaturated fats; as we've already seen, that's not at all bad. Second, not all saturated fats are as artery-clogging as others. The one most commonly formed saturated fat during hydrogenation, stearic acid, apparently has little or no effect on raising cholesterol levels in the blood, and, it would be expected, has less tendency to block arteries.

But another wrinkle has entered the hydrogenation dilemma. Some researchers are now concerned that such molecular manipulation changed the naturally occurring *cis* configuration of the molecule to the abnormal *trans* configuration. Apparently the trans fats are more artery-clogging than the cis types. You can expect to see and hear more about this in the coming months and years, as more research is done. In the meantime, bear in mind that the amount of trans fats fed in experimental diets being quoted is far higher than almost anyone could possibly expect to eat, even on a very high-fat diet.

The bottom line is to keep *all* fat intake as low as practical and possible. That's especially true for saturated fats.

But what about cholesterol? The American Heart Association calls for a maximum of 300 milligrams daily for the general public, no more than 100 milligrams per 1,000 calories eaten. But even the AHA concedes that's not good enough for someone who needs to lower his or her elevated cholesterol, especially those individuals who have established heart disease. For those of us in that situation, the ceiling should be 100 milligrams daily, certainly no more than 150 milligrams.

Actually that's not so hard to do. When you get rid of the saturated fat in animal foods, you automatically get rid of the cholesterol. By switching from whole milk to skim milk you go from more than 8 grams of fat to a mere fraction of a gram. At the same time, you drop from 34 milligrams of cholesterol to only 5 milligrams in an 8-ounce glass. Choose a cheese substitute over the regular cheddar, and the cholesterol is completely gone.

Take another look at Table 6 and notice the amount of cholesterol in the foods you're likely to eat. It's not all that difficult to limit yourself to 100 to 150 milligrams of cholesterol daily.

You'll be happy to learn that previous listings of cholesterol in shellfish were inaccurate. Clams, oysters, mussels, and scallops are actually very low in both fat and cholesterol. Crab and lobster are extremely low in fat, and have a fairly reasonable amount of cholesterol. Only shrimp are relatively high; but they're virtually devoid of fat. Eating a quarter pound of shrimp (obviously not deep-fried) will not exceed your cholesterol limit for the day.

The cholesterol-laden foods to avoid or completely eliminate are egg yolks and organ meats. Fortunately there are a number of very acceptable egg substitutes on the market. Remember, too, that egg whites have absolutely no cholesterol and virtually no fat. And very few of us will bemoan the loss of liver and kidneys and brains from the diet!

While discussing cholesterol, it might be worth noting that even though dietary cholesterol does not elevate cholesterol levels in the blood as much as saturated fat does, it might have problems of its own. Dr. Jeremiah Stamler of Northwestern University in Chicago has found that cholesterol has an artery-clogging tendency above and beyond raising levels in the blood. He currently believes that cholesterol intake constitutes a separate and independent risk of atherosclerosis. For those of us whose arteries are already blocked, that's a real consideration, and another reason to stick with the 100- to 150-milligram daily limit.

Since cholesterol is found only in animal foods, when we reduce the saturated fat by cutting back on those foods, we also limit our cholesterol intake. The foods that are particularly high in cholesterol, though relatively low in saturated fat, are egg yolks, shrimp, squid, crayfish, and organ meats.

I can just picture the look of doom and gloom on your face by this point. "Damn it, I won't be able to eat the kinds of foods that I love. Who wants to live like that?" I wish that you could see the way my family and I eat! That would completely change your attitude, and fast. We love meatloaf and mashed potatoes, pizzas, sloppy joes and hamburgers, omelets, and all sorts of things that are probably your favorites as well. But we take advantage of the tricks I've learned over the past few years, along with the new foods that have hit the market recently. Believe me, my way of eating represents zero deprivation.

After writing *The 8-Week Cholesterol Cure*, I received mail from across the country. Many admitted that they were amazed that they could reduce their cholesterol levels so effectively without feeling at all deprived. You can do it also. Maybe you'll even write me a letter yourself. Send it to me at P.O. Box 2039, Venice, CA 90294.

THE ROLE OF SOLUBLE FIBERS

Thus far we've concentrated on the kinds of foods we have to cut back on in terms of fats and cholesterol. But there's a whole category of foods that can actually lower our cholesterol levels while we enjoy them. They're the foods rich in soluble fiber.

It all started with a cereal that back in 1984 was virtually unknown. The only place I could find oat bran was in health food stores. It was worth looking for, since I'd read in some obscure medical journals that oat bran could lower cholesterol levels over and above the amount cut down by just eliminating fat.

Here's the way it works. Oat bran, and some other foods as well, are rich in soluble fiber. That distinguishes oat bran from wheat fiber, which contains primarily insoluble fiber. Both are a healthful part of the diet, but only oat bran can get the cholesterol out of the body.

Since the fiber is soluble, it forms a gel with water as it passes through the digestive tract. There it binds onto the bile acids that are used in the digestive process. Those bile acids are made from cholesterol, and when they are shunted out of the body in the stool, along with the fiber, the body must make more. It does so by drawing cholesterol out of the blood. Little by little, cholesterol levels fall.

Literally dozens of well-structured research studies have now been done across the country and around the world demonstrating this wonderful property of oat bran and other soluble fiber-rich foods. The results vary, with cholesterol reductions reported anywhere from 3 percent to 19 percent beyond that achieved by dietary restriction alone.

Yes, there has been some negative publicity along these lines. One study denied this effect. That study has since been criticized by outstanding researchers at a number of major research institutions. The nay-sayers fed oat bran or wheat cereal to 20 individuals, 16 of whom were women, most of whom were dietitians already eating a healthful diet, and all of whom had perfectly normal cholesterol levels to begin with. The average cholesterol level was 186; the average HDL cholesterol in the study group was 57. Those people didn't need any help at all. It was like giving aspirin to people who didn't have a headache, and then saying it didn't work.

The final proof of oat bran's efficacy was published in the April 10, 1991, issue of the *Journal of the American Medical Association*. Researchers compared oat bran, oatmeal, and farina in varying serving sizes in 156 adults with elevated cholesterol levels. Farina had no influence at all. A daily serving of two ounces of oat bran brought levels of LDL cholesterol down about 16 percent, and was significantly more effective than the same amount of oatmeal. That's because the oat bran contains far more of the cholesterol-lowering soluble fiber than oatmeal. It's unfortunate that the mass media did not give this carefully controlled research the same exposure given to the negative story a year earlier. But for those of us with a real interest in our cholesterol counts, the research confirmed what we've believed all along.

No, it won't do much good to eat potato chips with a bit of oat bran sprinkled over them. You need a reasonable amount of the cereal to see an effect. That comes out to two ounces, about a half cup, of oat bran daily, either as hot cereal or muffins. Quaker now also makes a ready-to-eat cold cereal that works just as well, ounce for ounce.

But oat bran is just the beginning. You can also get soluble fiber from dried beans and peas. A cup will provide the soluble fiber found in a half cup of oat bran. So each time you enjoy a bowl of split pea soup, or a garbanzo bean dip, or a side dish of black-eyed peas, you'll be working at lowering your cholesterol.

For more variety, try some rice bran. It's been shown to have the same cholesterol-lowering properties as oat bran. Try it in some baked goods. Or sprinkle some over frozen yogurt or one of the new nonfat ice creams. Two to three tablespoons of rice bran provide the soluble fiber for the day.

But what if you're tired of oat bran for breakfast, and you'd like a nice omelet made with an egg substitute and an English muffin with marmalade? There are two concentrated sources of soluble fiber that you can use to supplement such a meal.

Metamucil and a number of other laxative products are made with psyllium, a seed that's practically pure soluble fiber. Three teaspoons mixed with water supply all the soluble fiber you'd find in three oat bran muffins, a full day's requirement.

An alternative to psyllium is guar gum. You may have seen this on various food labels; it's used as a thickening agent in yogurt and puddings, for example. Like psyllium, guar gum is a very concentrated source of soluble fiber. Again, three teaspoons mixed with water, milk, or fruit juice will do the trick. Researchers at Stanford University have reported marvelous results with this amount of guar gum.

Here are two ways to incorporate it into your diet. Mix a six-ounce glass of orange juice, a teaspoon of honey, and a teaspoon of guar gum in your blender. The result, as I call it in *The 8-Week Cholesterol Cure Cookbook,* is an Orange Guarius. It's delicious. Or try mixing six ounces of skim milk with one teaspoon of guar gum, a ripe banana, and a teaspoon of cocoa powder. You'll have a wonderful, thick chocolate milk shake.

Soluble fiber continues to play an important role in my own program of cholesterol control. I've been using it in all its forms for the past several years, and my cholesterol level remains in the perfectly safe range. I think it should be a part of your program as well.

PRODUCTS WORTH PURSUING

Since writing *The 8-Week Cholesterol Cure,* companies regularly try to get me interested in their products so I can tell my readers about them in my *Diet-Heart Newsletter* (see page 337). Very few get mentioned, and seldom do I get excited about an entire product line. Happy to report, I am quite taken with the products of The NANCI Corporation of Tulsa, OK.

The star of their formulations is a special 100 percent soluble fiber. Unlike other fibers, this one mixes completely with water. As a result, it does not form a sludgy drink as is the case with psyllium-containing products such as Metamucil. A single-serving packet of their Fruity Fiber provides two grams of soluble fiber. It tastes like a refreshing beverage, much like Kool-Aid or Tang, not at all like something you'd consume just because it's "good for you."

This soluble fiber is also incorporated into the entire line of NANCI products. I'm particularly fond of a weight-loss preparation they call Lose-It. This is a meal-replacement shake, but totally superior to other products such as SlimFast which may contain up to 30 percent sugar. Instead, Lose-It can be mixed with fruit juice rather than just milk or water, and has just 50 calories per serving. My favorite is to mix it with a variety of fruit juices, especially cranberry. I use it as a convenient meal replacement when I'm on the run, a nice way to lose a pound or two when I've indulged a bit too much in some of those new nonfat desserts which still have plenty of calories, and as an additional source of soluble fiber.

Next on the list are two absolutely delicious cookies, oatmeal raisin and chocolate chip. Each two-ounce cookie provides 4.2 grams of soluble fiber and 1 gram of insoluble. And only 2.5 grams of fat! My son Ross went absolutely bonkers when he tasted them, and now eats them almost every day as his afterschool snack.

There's even a nutritious candy bar which packs a full six grams of fiber. It comes in caramel and peanut butter.

The NANCI products are formulated by the biochemist who developed what ultimately was marketed as the Science Diet for pets, which is now considered to be the gold standard for dogs and cats.

Those who have used the products routinely report wonderful results in terms of cholesterol lowering, weight control, and diabetes management. And preliminary research findings bear out the literally thousands of personal testimonials the company has received.

The question posed to researchers at the University of Texas Health Science Center in San Antonio was just how much effect NANCI's Lose-It could have on cholesterol levels. Two groups received two shakes daily. One had a total of 14 grams of the soluble fiber and the other got 7 grams daily. Both used the shakes as meal replacements. Neither group made any other changes in diet or exercise.

After six weeks, the group drinking two shakes containing 7 grams of fiber experienced a reduction in total cholesterol of 6.2 percent; their LDLs fell by 8.15 percent. Those drinking two shakes daily with a total of 14 grams of fiber had a 9.68 percent drop in total cholesterol and a 12.17 percent fall in LDLs.

I always travel with a supply of the products both in my suitcase and my attaché case. The shakes are wonderful when I'm on the run. And the cookies make great snacks on airplanes and in the hotel room in the evenings.

NANCI products are sold through independent distributorships across the nation. I'm absolutely sold on both the company and its products. For information on where you can buy the products (or perhaps even begin your own distributorship) call toll-free (800) 825-8848 and ask for Operator One. Or write to The NANCI Corporation at 7134 S. Yale, Suite One, Tulsa, OK 74136.

A HEALTHY SHOPPING TRIP

While I appear to be an exception to the rule, most of the grocery shopping is done by the woman rather than the man in the family. Since most heart attack patients are men, I'd like to urge my male readers to not skip over this section. Men need to get more involved with the food they eat. Moreover, a heart-healthy diet should be a family affair.

The best classroom for learning about food and making healthy choices is the supermarket aisle. All the information you need is typically right there on food labels for you to read. But most people just pick up items and toss them into their shopping carts without giving them much if any thought.

You wouldn't think of eating some unknown food offered to you by a stranger on the street, but you think nothing of buying and eating foods you know nothing about. The solution is quite painless. For the next three trips to the supermarket, give yourself an extra 20 minutes. That will give you enough time to read and compare labels on the foods on your shopping list. By the fourth shopping trip you'll find that you're repeating items, and you'll know just which ones to pick.

It's really important that both you and your spouse go shopping together those next three times. That way you can both learn and make decisions together. Some women may complain that the husband will get in the way, that the supermarket is no place for a man. It's difficult to break habits. But this is the start of a whole new way of looking at foods, and you both should be involved. If you still have children at home, you might want to involve them as well.

The worst thing you can do is prepare two or three meals each evening, so that while the heart patient can have healthy foods the rest of the family can eat "normally." Those "normal" foods aren't really that terrific for anyone, and all of us could benefit by cutting back on fat.

While shopping you'll find that there are two parts to each nutrition label, and that practically all packaged foods are labeled. First look at the breakdown of nutrients. You'll see protein, carbohydrates, and fats listed in terms of grams per serving. Since you now know just how many grams you have as your personal limit, you can decide whether this or that food will fit into your day's menu. Then look farther down the label and you'll see a declaration of the ingredients, in decreasing order by weight. Is the fat in the product from a healthy source such as soybean oil, or does it come from lard or tropical oils? With this information, you can make wise decisions. And once you've read that label, you needn't do so again.

Let's say you're walking down the aisle and you come to the luncheon meats. Pick up a package of regular ham and another of turkey ham, and you'll see that the turkey ham actually has more fat than the regular kind, which is actually quite low in fat. That's because turkey ham is made from the thigh meat rather than the low-fat breasts. Next you walk to the bread section to select some rolls with which to make sandwiches. You pick up two brands, and find that one is made with soybean oil while the other has animal fat. The next time you're shopping for luncheon meat and rolls you'll know exactly which ones to select. See how easy it gets?

Remember that cholesterol comes only from animal foods, so don't be fooled by advertising claims that boast "no cholesterol" for plant foods such as peanut butter or corn oil. What about those "no cholesterol" mayonnaises? Well, regular mayonnaise has only five milligrams of cholesterol per tablespoon, so removing it entirely is no big deal. Rather, read the labels for the fat content of mayonnaise. Look for Kraft Free mayo, completely free of fat.

Some products are very straightforward. You can see clearly that one 8-ounce glass of whole milk contains eight grams of fat while a glass of two-percent low-fat milk has 4.5 grams and skim milk contains virtually none. But look a bit more closely at how serving sizes and the number of servings are listed on other products.

A can of soup, for example, might have four grams of fat per serving. But the can is said to contain 2¾ servings, or 2⅓ servings. Needless to say, this complicates things and makes you do a bit of calculation. After a few experiences like that, however, you'll start rounding things off very quickly and accurately.

An increasing number of companies have begun to list not only the number of grams of fat per serving, but how that fat breaks down as polyunsaturated, monounsaturated, and saturated. Of course you'll want to choose those products that offer the least saturated fat.

A few companies also provide information about cholesterol, listing the number of milligrams per serving. This isn't mandatory, however, and it's usually the foods which have nothing to hide that state the facts. Remember, though, that you'll find cholesterol *only* in animal foods. The biggest single source of cholesterol in the diet is the egg yolk. Depending on size, the yolk will contain 210 to 250 milligrams. So watch for eggs listed as ingredients.

You have to become familiar with all the foods on your list, even those that seem innocuous at first. Take tortillas, for example. No problem with corn tortillas. But most flour tortillas are made with lard. Look for the ones produced with soybean oil instead; they'll be marked vegetarian.

There have been a number of conflicting reports on coffee. Fortunately, we now have data that give us the go-ahead for enjoying those steaming cups of java.

Researchers at the Harvard School of Public Health examined the relation of coffee consumption with the risk of heart attack or stroke, and the need for bypass surgery or angioplasty, in 45,589 men from 1986 through 1990. After a very thorough statistical analysis, adjusting for every possible variable, they concluded that coffee or caffeine consumption does *not* increase the risk of coronary heart disease or stroke. They published their data in the October 11, 1990 issue of the *New England Journal of Medicine*.

But what about arrhythmias? Doesn't caffeine increase the likelihood of irregular heartbeats? A study in the November 7, 1990 issue of the *Journal of the American Medical Association* provides reassurance along those lines as well.

Cardiologists at the Oregon Health Sciences University worked with 22 patients who were regular coffee drinkers and who had ventricular arrhythmias. First they took them off their anti-arrhythmia medications. Next they asked the patients to abstain from coffee for 24 hours. Then they gave them the caffeine equivalent of two to three cups of coffee. There were no additional arrhythmias, and the researchers concluded that caffeine has little effect on the "arrhythmia threshold."

Despite such assurances, however, recommendations from the American Heart Association's epidemiology meeting in March 1991 called for limiting coffee consumption to less than five cups a day. Others urge an even more prudent limit of two cups daily.

As for me, I'll stick with decaf because I drink a lot of coffee while at my typewriter and, combined with all the energizing exercise I do, that caffeine would give me jitters (though no arrhythmias). On the other hand, when I need a little pick-me-up at the end of a long day and when I still have a long evening to go, I do enjoy having a cup or two of the regular stuff.

The decision to drink alcohol or to avoid it must be made on an individual basis, and it's a good idea to discuss this with your physician if you have any doubts about your own situation. On the positive side of the ledger, alcohol tends to raise the levels of the good HDL cholesterol in the blood. Moreover, a number of studies have shown that those who drink alcohol in moderation are likely to live longer than those who totally abstain.

On the other side of the ledger, certain heart patients may well be better off without the booze. Alcohol raises blood pressure in those trying to control their hypertension. Depending on just how severe your hypertension is, your doctor might rule alcohol out altogether. In addition, recent research done in Framingham, Massachusetts has shown that some middle-aged men may increase their heart disease risk by drinking. It appears that any alcohol consumption, but especially three, four, or more drinks daily, leads to enlargement of the heart and resultant dysfunction. Women seem to be less affected than men.

Men in the study who already had enlarged hearts were placed in greatest danger by drinking alcohol. Again, those who drank the most had the most problems.

Other research has shown that heavy drinking can damage the heart muscle.

For those who do drink, and whose physicians see no reason that they should not do so, moderation must remain the key. This means no more than one or two drinks daily. That translates to two mixed drinks, two six-ounce glasses of wine, or two twelve ounce glasses of beer per day. The kind of liquor you drink doesn't matter; rather, it's the total amount of alcohol you consume.

I personally enjoy a cocktail before dinner. For me it's a way to put the work day behind me, and it gives me a chance to talk about this and that with my wife. On more relaxed occasions, we'll share some nice wine with dinner.

On the other hand, when I'm under a bit of stress, I cut out the alcohol entirely. Contrary to popular belief, booze is a depressant, and when under stress, that's the last thing I need. Moreover, alcohol interferes with a good night's sleep, which is what I sorely need when times are stressful.

As I started out saying in this discussion, the use of alcohol becomes a very personal decision. Talk about it with your doctor and if he or she gives the go-ahead, enjoy a drink or two, but always in moderation.

HEART-HEALTHY DINING OUT

One of the first things people think about when opting to eat a heart-healthy diet is dining out in restaurants. I think eating out is one of life's greatest pleasures, and you probably do too. So you'll be pleased to hear that you should have no problem at all; this is one time you can have your cake and eat it too. Just follow a few simple guidelines.

Advance Planning. Most of the people in the world eat a healthier diet than we do in the United States. That means that most ethnic restaurants offer a wide range of heart-healthy foods on their menus. You'll find you can eat to your heart's content at Chinese, Japanese, Korean, Thai, Italian, Mediterranean, and Middle Eastern restaurants. Actually, the only places I avoid these days are French restaurants that persist in using lots of cream and butter in all their sauces. Even at that, many French restaurants are now serving foods found on the French Riviera, those prepared with a much lighter touch.

Whenever possible, check out a restaurant's foods in advance. When you call for reservations, ask about menu selections. When you pass by a restaurant while shopping or visiting an area on business, drop in and check out the menu.

Many service organizations and charities sell coupon books that offer two-for-the-price-of-one dinners. This is a terrific way to save money and experience new restaurants. The book that my wife and I buy each year is *Entertainment,* which is published in 110 major cities. The book publishes the restaurants' menus, so we can make our choices in advance. To find out how you can get the *Entertainment* book for your area, you can write to Entertainment Publications, Inc. at 2125 Butterfield Road, Troy, MI 48084.

Have It Your Way! Remember that you're the boss at any restaurant. Ask the server all the questions you need to have answered. How is this sauce prepared? What are the ingredients in that pasta dish? Let the waiter or waitress know your needs: I don't eat butter or cream. Please bring some margarine for my bread. Let me have my salad dressing on the side. Ask the chef to sauté this dish in olive oil rather than butter. Please prepare my food with as little oil as possible.

It's a little-known fact that Chinese hosts honor their guests by lavishing much oil on their food. When dining out in a Chinese restaurant, then, ask the chef to go easy on the oil. The same goes for the MSG and soy sauce in order to hold down your sodium intake especially if you need to restrict it.

Most restaurants today offer large servings in order to justify higher prices. Don't feel shy about asking for a doggy bag so you don't eat the whole thing.

When traveling, don't leave your heart-healthy habits at home. See the Appendix for guidelines on taking those habits on the road. Hotels and their restaurants today cater to those who are more health-conscious.

Problems with Bingeing. If you're going to abandon your diet, it's most likely going to be in a restaurant. It's a special occasion. The sauce sounds terrific. The dessert cart creaks under its load of goodies. One thing leads to another, and before you know it you've consumed more fat than you'd want to eat in a week. That can be dangerous.

It's not just a matter of falling off the wagon and renewing your efforts the next day. A very high-fat meal can be outright dangerous for a person who has been limiting fat in the diet. Here's why.

A particularly high-fat meal produces a sluggish blood flow. The body responds by manufacturing more of a chemical called thromboxane which facilitates blood clotting. Chest pains following a fat-laden dinner are common. And sometimes that "just this once" treat can result in a heart attack. In fact, authorities have stated unequivocally that if one has decided to go back to a high-fat, high-cholesterol diet, it's best to do so a little at a time. I find it fascinating that the body has to "gear up" to handle that fat; it makes me feel that eating a lot of fat can't be very healthy in the first place, that to do so is unnatural.

EXERCISE AND CHOLESTEROL

Exercise has both direct and indirect effects on our cholesterol levels. First, it's a great way to deal with stress, which, as we know, can elevate those numbers. Next, a regular program of exercise helps control weight which, in turn, will help bring cholesterol counts down.

Not only will exercise bring levels of total cholesterol down, but it will also bring levels of the good HDL cholesterol up. Study after study has demonstrated that those who engage in regular physical activity have higher HDL counts than those who are more sedentary. Both aerobic and resistance exercise seem to have this beneficial effect.

BRINGING OUT THE BIG GUNS TO CONTROL CHOLESTEROL

For many, if not most, men and women, a program of diet, exercise, and stress control will bring cholesterol levels under control. But some of us need additional help.

The body makes its own cholesterol in the liver and, to a much lesser extent, in the intestine. But some of us make too much, and our bodies don't dispose of it adequately once it's made. Excess cholesterol builds up in the bloodstream and, well, you know the rest.

In fact, some people will find it impossible to lower cholesterol levels sufficiently with diet alone. A 1993 study done at the University of Minnesota showed that even after extensive counseling, which enabled them to greatly affect their diets, many individuals were able to reduce their elevated cholesterol levels by only 5 percent. Addition of a cholesterol-lowering drug, however, brought them all to desired levels.

A number of substances can help lower cholesterol levels. Please see chapter 16 for a full discussion of your options regarding medications.

Partial Ileal Bypass. One of the most drastic measures to lower cholesterol levels remains experimental at the time of this writing. Partial ileal bypass is a type of surgery of the intestine resulting in a shunting of food so that cholesterol cannot be absorbed by the body. This yields dramatic cholesterol reductions in the blood.

Over a ten-year period, 838 patients who had had a previous heart attack were divided into two groups at the University of Minnesota. One group received usual treatment and dietary recommendations; the other groups got the partial ileal bypass surgery. Researchers found that deaths due to heart disease were cut by 28 percent in the surgery group. The surgery group experienced 34 percent fewer heart attacks, and 63 percent fewer coronary bypass operations and angioplasties.

In the intervening years, according to Dr. Henry Buchwald, patients underwent angiograms to directly study their arteries. Each evaluation showed greater progression of the disease in the control group, while that with a greatly reduced cholesterol level demonstrated actual regression of heart disease.

Of course this is a very serious intervention. First there is the consideration of such major surgery itself; all surgery comes with its share of complications. Second, there are serious drawbacks. Patients could eat only small meals and had to eat repeatedly throughout the day. Vitamin deficiencies occurred, requiring supplement injections. And many experienced gastrointestinal distress including diarrhea. Much better to stick with far more pleasant ways to get and keep cholesterol levels down! However, the study does show the unequivocal benefits of cholesterol reduction.

LDL Pheresis. Here we have another experimental means of cholesterol reduction developed for those who have a genetically determined hyperproduction of cholesterol resulting in levels from 500 to 1000. Such individuals may not be able to control their levels even with drugs and the strictest diet.

The technique calls for blood to be "washed" in a manner similar to kidney dialysis. Patients must go to a laboratory each week to undergo the three-hour-long process, which can cost thousands of dollars annually. It is a very special treatment for very special patients.

Vegetarianism. Some might smile that I would include vegetarianism along with other "big guns" of cholesterol control. However, not everyone is willing to completely eliminate all animal products and most fats and oils from the diet for the rest of his or her life. But there's no doubt this can be a very effective means of cholesterol control.

Most individuals will find that they can effectively control their cholesterol counts without giving up animal foods entirely. Carefully selected dairy foods, poultry, and seafood are extremely low in fat and cholesterol. Moreover, some of the benefits ascribed to vegetarianism may be due more to what people do eat than to what they don't. That is to say that the vegetarian diet, by definition, is high in whole-grain cereals, fruits, vegetables, and dried beans and peas. A number of researchers who have investigated vegetarian diets have theorized that the nutrients in such foods may have a protective value over and above the lowering of dietary fat and cholesterol.

Dried beans and peas are rich sources of soluble fiber, known to directly lower cholesterol levels. Vegetarians rely on dried beans and peas as an excellent protein source in lieu of meat. Many fruits also provide significant amounts of soluble fiber.

And, as we'll see in the next section of this chapter, certain nutrients including vitamins C and E and beta-carotene may offer protection against heart disease. Fruits and vegetables are the principal sources of those nutrients in the diet. I've discussed Dr. Dean Ornish's research with reversing heart disease. His approach, involving a low-fat, near-vegetarian diet, exercise, and meditation, is spelled out in his book *Dr. Dean Ornish's Program for Reversing Heart Disease* (Random House, 1990). The book contains a nice section on vegetarian cookery, with some of the recipies supplied by Chef Wolfgang Puck, of L.A.'s famous Spago restaurant. It's a well thought-out book, and one you should consider adding to your heart-smart library.

If, like me, you prefer not to become a vegetarian, you still would be well advised to increase your daily intake of non-meat foods. A meatless meal once, twice, or even three times a week is a good idea. On those days, concentrate on pastas, egg substitutes, fruits and vegetables, dried beans and peas, and the low-fat and nonfat cheeses that have recently come onto the market.

ANTIOXIDANTS AND CHOLESTEROL

Yes, high levels of cholesterol in the blood increase the risk of heart disease. Yet some people manage to elude heart attacks even when their numbers are high. It could be that the way your body oxidizes cholesterol in the blood may point to susceptibility to heart disease.

At the University of Southern California in Los Angeles, Dr. Alex Sevanian said "your predisposition to atherosclerosis may depend much more on how much cholesterol oxide your body happens to produce than on the cholesterol levels in your blood." Ironically, the LDL carrier of cholesterol oxidizes more rapidly in the presence of polyunsaturated fats as found in corn and soybean oils. (That's another reason to start emphasizing monounsaturates rather than polyunsaturates in your diet.) So far, Dr. Sevanian's work has been on laboratory animals, but human studies are scheduled in a number of lipid research centers.

At a meeting of the American College of Cardiology in 1989, Dr. Thomas Carew of the University of California at San Diego said LDL, the bad cholesterol, may exert its deleterious influence only after it is oxidized and can then be taken up by scavenger cells known as macrophages. When the macrophages become laden with oxidized LDL, they imbed themselves in arterial walls, where they are transformed into foam cells, the first stage in the development of atherosclerosis.

What can one do about cholesterol oxidation? We have preliminary evidence that one can, indeed, limit this destructive process.

Dr. Carew, working with noted lipid researcher Dr. Daniel Steinberg in San Diego, found that the prescription drug probucol (Lorelco) limits cholesterol oxidation. Probucol has been prescribed for cholesterol reduction, but its use has been limited by the fact that it reduces the good HDL as well as LDL levels.

Working with another eminent lipid researcher, Dr. David Blankenhorn, of the University of Southern California, Dr. Sevanian has found that a non-drug approach may achieve the same results. He has shown that blood levels of cholesterol oxides can be reduced with vitamin E, which has long been known to be a potent antioxidant.

A report of Canadian researchers at the 1990 meeting of the American Heart Association showed the value of vitamin E in protecting patients from adverse effects of bypass surgery. A group of 14 patients received 300 mg of vitamin E daily, while another group of 14 got a placebo for two weeks prior to their operations. Those getting the vitamin E suffered less "metabolic dysfunction" during the procedure.

Scientists at the University of Toronto have been looking for ways to protect bypass patients from the decrease in heart function that occurs after they are taken off the heart-lung machine which keeps blood circulating and oxygenated during surgery. They have found that unstable molecules known as free radicals may be a major factor in the heart's inability to resume normal metabolic activity after the operation. In addition, surgery depletes the amount of vitamin E normally in the bloodstream.

Dr. Terrence Yau said that presurgical supplementation with vitamin E apparently improved the heart's ability to function, especially during the dangerous five-hour period immediately following the operation.

Two separate studies published in May 1993, in the *New England Journal of Medicine*, demonstrated the protective properties of vitamin E supplementation for both men and women. While no recommendations for the general population have been made, authorities note that there appear to be no adverse effects from taking 400 to 600 international units of vitamin E daily. The potential benefits appear to be enormous, with no apparent risks whatever. I believe that everyone who has had a cardiac event should consider taking vitamin E as well as other antioxidant supplements. I do.

Much of the initial research into the activities of free radicals has been done in Japan, and scientists there continue to investigate this important area. Now researchers report that free radical-induced oxidation of LDL cholesterol can be suppressed by supplementation with vitamins E and C. They conclude that vitamin C inhibits water-soluble radicals but could not scavenge fat-soluble radicals within LDL, while vitamin E scavenged fat-soluble radicals in order to break the chain reaction of LDL oxidation.

All the researchers involved in such studies point out the need for additional study, and state that they do not currently advocate self-supplementation. However, in private they admit that they themselves take anti-oxidants regularly. Moreover, the doses of supplements used is not excessive, and while the absolute evidence of benefit has not yet been delivered, the risk of taking reasonable doses of those vitamins is virtually absent.

And while we're on the topic of nutrient supplementation, add chromium to the list. When subjects were given a 200-microgram dose, their cholesterol levels fell by seven percent. The recommended "safe and adequate" intake for the trace mineral is 50 to 200 micrograms daily; it's found in oysters, brewer's yeast, and beer as well as in the organ meats which are on the no-no list for those of us cutting dietary cholesterol. A 1991 study showed that 90 percent of Americans consume less than 50 mcg. Daily intake of chromium should be no more than 200 mcg, however, since higher levels can lead to adverse reactions including skin rashes, mood changes, and anemia. Take a look at your vitamin/mineral supplement's formulation to see how much chromium is included. A dosage of between 50 and 200 mcg may do some good and won't do any harm.

Beta-carotene, the precursor of vitamin A, has also been shown to have advantages in heart disease. A study of beta-carotene was reported at the 1990 meeting of the American Heart Association in Dallas. Of 333 patients with documented coronary heart disease, those taking a beta-carotene tablet every other day suffered half as many cardiovascular events as those getting a placebo.

Charles H. Hennekens, M.D., of Brigham and Women's Hospital and Harvard Medical School, said the data provide the first evidence in humans of the potential efficacy of beta-carotene in protecting the arteries. His research, known at the Physicians' Health Study, is a national project involving about 22,000 male physicians aged 40 to 84.

The 333 individuals in the beta-carotene study are those physicians who had evidence of cardiovascular disease when they entered the project. In those taking the beta-carotene, there were half the number of strokes, heart attacks, sudden cardiac deaths, and bypass surgeries.

MOTIVATION AND COMMITMENT

Diet remains the basis of any cholesterol-cutting program. But it's up to you. Will you make the commitment to a real change in your diet?

All I ask is that you give it a real chance. A low-fat diet can be absolutely delicious, and there's no reason at all to feel deprived. If you saw the way my family and I eat you'd never know we were doing anything special; that's because the "all-American" foods we enjoy have been prepared with the fat taken out but with the fun and flavor left in. We all love dining out in restaurants. When there's something special to celebrate, I can feel just as festive in ordering a lobster or Alaskan king crab as in having the prime rib.

Perhaps at this point in your recovery you're saying to yourself that food is one of your life's pleasures, and you just don't want to give it up. Well, you don't have to give up all your favorites. You just have to make some simple modifications.

It's unfortunate that so many heart patients feel so sorry for themselves and that they use food as a consolation prize. It's even more unfortunate that they can't recognize their own self-destructive behaviors when bingeing on fats. Think about what you're really saying when you dig into that bacon-and-egg breakfast: "I'm not feeling well, and I'm not feeling good about myself, so I'm going to eat this food which is certain to make my condition worse rather than better." Yes, you might enjoy that meal. You'll have a certain amount of instant gratification. But consider the long term.

Feeling really good is the ultimate pleasure! You just don't know that yet, because you haven't given it a chance. I used to think that taking Alka Seltzer was a natural thing to do after a big meal. Bouts with indigestion were common. I'd lie in bed feeling lousy, never thinking that it was that huge meal dripping in butter and cream that was the culprit. You'll feel better in just days by deciding today to toss out the fatty foods and concentrate on a light approach to eating.

People ask me all the time if I don't miss certain foods that I've given up since my second bypass surgery in 1984. Sure, I'd really like to eat a bacon-and-eggs breakfast. Today I stick with egg substitute and Canadian bacon. There's just no substitute for sunnyside-up eggs and three or four strips of crisp bacon. But I've never given in to the temptation in all these years.

Why not? There's no breakfast in the world that could compare with another day of life and living. I wouldn't trade seeing a beautiful sunset for those sunnyside-up eggs. There's no hot fudge sundae that could tempt me to miss one of my daughter's birthday parties or my son's Little League baseball games. Every time I enjoy one of those special moments, I strengthen my resolve to stick with my diet.

Now, you might ask wouldn't it be all right to have a special treat just once in a while? Would that breakfast really do that much damage? Probably not. But here's the problem with having this or that "just once in a while." Today you have a piece of chocolate because you haven't had one in a month. Tomorrow you have a slab of prime rib because it's been so long since the last time. Then it's a lovely dessert. And a corned beef sandwich. And on and on and on. Add up all those "once in a whiles" and you have an "all the time" cheat.

Sometimes it's just a lot easier to make big changes rather than little ones. Compare this with the decision to quit smoking. One of the most masochistic things I ever did was to try to smoke just a few cigarettes a day after smoking two packs daily for years. I was in a constant state of withdrawal. Ask any former smoker and he or she will tell you the same thing. The same applies to exercise. Do it just now and then, and you'll never really get into it. But make the decision to do some physical exercise regularly and it becomes a part of your life.

Heart-healthy eating is, indeed, a part of my life. And I'm not alone. I've spoken with literally hundreds of men and women who've made the same changes in their own lives. Everyone who's given it a fair chance says that its amazing how little you miss certain foods. That's because you're concentrating on all those foods that are good for you. You can't order everything on the menu, so make your selections from the low-fat offerings.

Take the right mental approach to your decision to eat heart-healthy foods. Make it a hobby, trying to find new restaurants and new products in the supermarket. My family and I really got a big kick out of trying Entenmann's fat-free coffee cakes when they first came on the market. Then there was nonfat ice cream. And nonfat cheeses. The list keeps getting bigger and bigger.

When I made the decision that the entire family would benefit from a healthier diet, I discussed the matter with my son Ross, who was only seven years old at the time. I explained that there would be some foods and restaurants that would be off the "approved" list, but that it would get easier and easier as time went on. The reason, I said, was that more and more people were realizing the value of eating low-fat foods, and that the food industry would respond by providing more products that we could enjoy without the fat. That was in 1985, and my predictions have certainly come true. Moreover, we continue to see new and wonderful offerings all the time. No doubt about it, it's getting easier all the time.

But whether it's easy at certain times or difficult at others, the effort will be worthwhile. Every time you eat a bowl of oat bran cereal, every time you order the fish or chicken rather than the prime rib, every time you have frozen yogurt instead of ice cream, try to picture your coronary arteries. Visualize them getting cleaner and cleaner. "Feel" the blood coursing through your arteries without blockage.

Make an effort to think about all the wonderful, positive things in your life. Your children and grandchildren. Sports and hobbies. Nature and wildlife. Vacations and travel. Your career. Making love. Feeling love for all those around you. Then associate those good things in your life with your new dietary habits. Soon you wouldn't trade those moments for a hot fudge sundae any more than I would.

I promise that within days you'll feel better. And within eight weeks you'll experience significant improvements in your cholesterol levels and your attitudes. That's about the amount of time needed to show a change. When you go into the doctor's office for that next cholesterol check and he or she tells you with a broad smile that your efforts have paid off, you'll be on your way to a lifetime of healthier eating. Nothing succeeds like success.

So here's my challenge: Give it a try for at least eight weeks. Make a real effort to get the fat and cholesterol out of your diet. Don't cheat for that full eight-week period. You'll feel a whole lot better. You won't need those antacids. You'll start to see some weight loss. And then you'll see your results on the cholesterol test. I really doubt that after all that you'll ever want to go back to your old ways of eating.

Bon appétit!

CASE HISTORIES

When it comes to making some changes in your diet, only you can make the decision to make that commitment. Some men and women have a difficult time taking the first step. Take the case of Dr. John Smith. That's not his real name, and in a moment you'll see why I don't want to identify him. I met Dr. Smith at a Heart Association meeting in Dallas. After I interviewed him regarding his research, we chatted a while about our own lives. The subject of our cholesterol came up and it turned out his cholesterol level was dangerously high, sometimes nearly 300.

But Dr. Smith did little about it. Seems he was so busy with his research, his patient load, and trying to achieve tenure at the university that he had no time for his own health. Asked what he had for dinner, he replied that he and his family ordered pizza quite often. His wife also was a physician and neither had much inclination to prepare food.

OK, I said, how about ordering the pizza without cheese, and then spreading some low-fat or nonfat cheese substitute on when it arrived. A minute or two in the oven and the pizza would be ready to eat. Well, he replied, that would be a lot of effort. He'd have to stock the cheese, make a special request over the phone, and he didn't think he'd want to do that.

Hmmm, I thought, coming up with another suggestion. How about ordering the pizza with half the cheese, and getting all vegetable toppings? No, Dr. Smith said, rather sadly shaking his head, that, too, would be too difficult, since his wife and children refused to eat a lower-fat diet.

Getting a bit exasperated, I said he could get half the pizza with half the cheese. Uh, no, he said, then he would have to somehow decide which half was which, and, even then, it would take a special order. Besides, most of the time the kids ordered the pizza.

Needless to say, Dr. Smith can't find any time to do any exercise either. He was under enormous stress because of concerns over his tenure, but took no steps to alleviate that stress. And he was carrying about 20 pounds of extra weight around his waist. To make matters worse, Dr. Smith had a family history of heart disease. I wish him a lot of luck, but it's going to take more than that. It'll probably take a heart attack to get his attention. I hope he survives.

The next story is just as sad. I've heard it from at least two dozen women since writing *The 8-Week Cholesterol Cure*. Those women were trying to help their husbands get better after their heart attacks. That meant preparing more fish, more poultry, and more low-fat foods in general. But instead of thanks those women got complaints. "Why the hell don't we have steak anymore?" "I'm tired of cereal. I want some bacon and eggs." "Margarine just doesn't taste as good. Get some real butter." Many of the wives had tears in their eyes as they told their tales of woe.

Often clichés hold a lot of truth. You can lead a horse to water, but you can't make it drink. Same with those husbands. I often tell such women to get some Neiman Marcus fur catalogs and some cruise brochures and put them on the cocktail table. When asked by their husbands what those are all about, I tell the women to simply say they're figuring out what to do with the insurance money.

Too harsh? Actually that usually gets a laugh, since I deliver that advice with a smile on my face and tongue in cheek. But the fact remains that no one can lead another's life. You can't force someone to take the steps necessary for cardiac recovery or any other aspect of health.

But for every negative story, I can tell a dozen positive ones. Take the example of Sam Horwitz. Sam is a very successful businessman who must travel and attend dinners frequently. He finds no problem in requesting a fish alternative at banquets and is almost never turned down. He has his travel agent automatically order a low-cholesterol meal on all his flights. Sam knows which restaurants serve a wide variety of foods he and his wife can enjoy. And through such efforts he has lowered his cholesterol from the 250 range to well under 200. He's confident that he won't ever have another heart attack.

Sam is typical of young, dynamic men who have taken charge of their own destinies. They won't let that heart attack get in the way of living a full, rewarding life. And they know they have to take certain steps to provide the protection they want.

Keith Ingram, on the other hand, shows us how older individuals can also make remarkable recoveries. Even after having a bypass, performed by the eminent surgeon Dr. Michael DeBakey, Keith didn't do much to change his lifestyle. But then he was told that his disease had progressed to the degree that even another bypass was deemed inadvisable. "My doctor told me I wouldn't survive it," Keith said. At the age of 67 he couldn't enjoy his retirement, lived the life of a cardiac cripple because of angina pains, and made life a living hell for his wife Lucille.

Then Keith took charge. He changed his diet almost overnight, getting rid of most of the fat, and adding a lot of soluble fiber in the form of shakes made by The NANCI Corporation. Despite the angina, Keith forced himself to walk, a little more every day. To get his cholesterol down sufficiently from the horribly high point of 340, he took the prescription drug colestipol and took niacin daily. Knowing that he was doing something for himself, his attitude slowly changed for the better.

When I met him, Keith was 69, walking briskly three miles every day, with a normal blood pressure and a cholesterol reading under 200. His doctors are amazed. The angina pains are gone and he now lives his life to the fullest.

TAKE NOTE: NUMBERS ARE TRICKY AFTER HEART ATTACK OR SURGERY

Bonnie Farrell, R.N., who heads up the nursing staff at the Heart Institute of the Desert in Rancho Mirage, California, warns about trusting cholesterol tests taken shortly after heart attack or bypass. Both those cardiac events are known to lower cholesterol levels significantly, but only on a temporary basis.

A test taken about two months after the event should provide more accurate information. In the meantime, you should continue to stay on a low-fat, low-cholesterol diet.

Ms. Farrell also describes a frequent scenario in which the patient's cholesterol level is normal even after eating a regular diet in the hospital and consuming high-fat foods at home during the weeks following hospital discharge. Not only must one consider the cholesterol fluctuation mentioned above, but also the appetite decreases during those first weeks. Many patients lose weight, simply because they're not eating as much as before. Even though you might think that you're eating a lot of fat, the actual intake is likely to be lower. But when the appetite returns, fat intake—and cholesterol levels—are likely to rise unless you make some significant dietary modifications.

MODIFICATION, NOT DEPRIVATION

There's no reason not to enjoy all your favorite recipes. Just do a bit of modification and substitution. For openers, you can cut the fat content of virtually any recipe by half and not notice the difference. Next, make your changes one step at a time. Switch first from whole milk to two-percent low-fat and then on to one-percent and finally to nonfat skim. Then use the following list of substitutions to dramatically lower the fat content of all your recipes.

	INSTEAD OF	USE
DAIRY	Butter	Margarine, cooking oils
	Whipping/Heavy cream	Evaporated skim milk
	Sour cream	Nonfat yogurt
	Ice cream	Nonfat frozen yogurt, nonfat ice cream products
MEATS	Bacon	Canadian bacon
	Luncheon meats	Low-fat ham or turkey breast
	Ground beef (15–13% fat)	Round steak trimmed of all fat prior to grinding (5% fat)
	Veal cutlets	Sliced turkey breasts
	Duck, goose	Turkey, chicken
OTHER	Regular mayonnaise (11 grams fat/tbsp)	Reduced-fat mayonnaise (4–5 grams fat/tbsp)
	Regular salad dressings	Low-fat, nonfat dressings
	Potato, corn chips	Baked corn tortilla chips

TABLE 5A
Plasma Total Cholesterol (mg/dl) in Adult Males*

Age/Years	Average	5%	75%	90%	95%
0–19	155	115	170	185	200
20–24	165	125	185	205	220
25–29	180	135	200	225	245
30–34	190	140	215	240	255
35–39	200	145	225	250	270
40–44	205	150	230	250	270
45–69	215	160	235	260	275
70+	205	150	230	250	270

*Journal of the American Medical Association. 1983 Vol. 250, no. 12; pp. 1869–72.

TABLE 5B
Plasma Low-Density Lipoprotein Cholesterol (mg/dl) in Adult Males*

Age/Years	Average	5%	75%	90%	95%
5–19	95	65	105	120	130
20–24	105	65	120	140	145
25–29	115	70	140	155	165
30–34	125	80	145	165	185
35–39	135	80	155	175	190
40–44	135	85	155	175	185
45–69	145	90	165	190	205
70+	145	90	165	180	185

*Journal of the American Medical Association. 1983 Vol. 250, no. 12; pp. 1869–72.

TABLE 5C

Plasma High-Density Lipoprotein Cholesterol (mg/dl) in Adult Males*

Age/Years	Average	5%	10%	95%
5–14	55	35	40	75
15–19	45	30	35	65
20–24	45	30	30	65
25–29	45	30	30	65
30–34	45	30	30	65
35–39	45	30	30	60
40–44	45	25	30	65
45–69	50	30	30	70
70+	50	30	35	75

*Journal of the American Medical Association. 1983 Vol. 250, no. 12; pp. 1869–72.

TABLE 5D

Plasma Total Cholesterol (mg/dl) in Adult Females*

Age/Years	Average	5%	75%	90%	95%
0–19	160	120	175	190	200
20–24	170	125	190	215	230
25–34	175	130	195	220	235
35–39	185	140	205	230	245
40–44	195	145	215	235	255
45–49	205	150	225	250	270
50–54	220	165	240	265	285
55+	230	170	250	275	295

*Journal of the American Medical Association. 1983 Vol. 250, no. 12; pp. 1869–72.

TABLE 5E

Plasma Low-Density Lipoprotein Cholesterol (md/dl) in Adult Females*

Age/Years	Average	5%	75%	90%	95%
5–19	100	65	110	125	140
20–24	105	55	120	140	160
25–34	110	70	125	145	160
35–39	120	75	140	160	170
40–44	125	75	145	165	175
50–49	130	80	150	175	185
50–54	140	90	160	185	200
55+	150	95	170	195	215

*Journal of the American Medical Association. 1983 Vol. 250, no. 12; pp. 1869–72.

TABLE 5F

Plasma High-Density Lipoprotein Cholesterol (mg/dl) in Adult Females*

Age/Years	Average	5%	10%	95%
5–19	55	35	40	70
20–24	55	35	35	80
25–34	55	35	40	80
35–39	55	35	40	80
40–44	60	35	40	90
45–49	60	35	40	85
50–54	60	35	40	90
55+	60	35	40	95

*Journal of the American Medical Association. 1983 Vol. 250, no. 12; pp. 1869–72.

TABLE 5G
Plasma Triglycerides in Males*

Age/Years	Average	5%	90%	95%
0–9	55	30	85	100
10–14	65	30	100	125
15–19	80	35	120	150
20–24	100	45	165	200
25–29	115	45	200	250
30–34	130	50	215	265
35–39	145	55	250	320
40–54	150	55	250	320
55–64	140	60	235	290
65+	135	55	210	260

*Journal of the American Medical Association. 1983 Vol. 250, no. 12; pp. 1869–72.

TABLE 5H
Plasma Triglycerides in Females*

Age/Years	Average	5%	90%	95%
0–9	60	35	95	110
10–19	75	40	115	130
20–34	90	40	145	170
35–39	95	40	160	195
40–44	105	45	170	210
45–49	110	45	185	230
50–54	120	55	190	240
55–65	125	55	200	250
65+	130	60	205	240

*Journal of the American Medical Association. 1983 Vol. 250, no. 12; pp. 1869–72.

TABLE 5I
Plasma Cholesterol and Triglycerides in Children Before Puberty*

Levels in mg/dl	5%	50%	95%
Total cholesterol	125	155	200
LDL cholesterol	65	95	135
HDL cholesterol	38	55	75
VLDL cholesterol	5	10	20
Triglycerides	30	55	110

*Journal of the American Medical Association. 1983 Vol. 250, no. 12; pp. 1869–72.

TABLE 6
Calorie, Fat, Cholesterol, and Sodium Content of Foods

Food	Serving Size	Calories	Fat (grams)	Cholesterol (mgs)	Sodium (mgs)
Candy					
Carnation Breakfast Bar	1 bar	210	11.0	1	140–220
Milk chocolate bar or 6–7 Kisses	1 oz.	150	9.2	5	7
Milk chocolate with almonds	1 oz.	155	9.3	4	22
Cheese					
American	1 oz.	105	8.4	27	318
Blue	1 oz.	103	8.5	21	390
Brick	1 oz.	103	8.5	25	157
Brie	1 oz.	94	7.8	28	176
Camembert	1 oz.	84	6.9	20	236
Cheddar	1 oz.	112	9.1	30	197
Colby	1 oz.	110	9.0	27	169
Cottage (1% fat)	½ cup	82	1.6	5	460
Cottage (2% fat)	½ cup	100	2.2	9	460
Cottage (4% fat)	½ cup	120	4.7	12	460

Table 6 (continued)

Food	Serving Size	Calories	Fat (grams)	Cholesterol (mgs)	Sodium (mgs)
Cheese					
Cream cheese	2 tbsp.	99	9.9	34	84
Edam	1 oz.	87	5.7	25	270
Feta	1 oz.	74	6.0	25	312
Gouda	1 oz.	100	7.7	32	229
Gruyère	1 oz.	115	8.9	31	94
Monterey Jack	1 oz.	105	8.5	30	150
Mozzarella	1 oz.	79	6.1	22	104
Mozzarella (part skim)	1 oz.	78	4.8	15	148
Muenster	1 oz.	104	8.5	27	178
Neufchâtel	1 oz.	73	6.6	21	112
Parmesan (grated)	1 tbsp.	23	1.5	4	93
Parmesan (hard)	1 oz.	111	7.3	19	454
Provolone	1 oz.	98	7.3	19	245
Ricotta (13% fat)	½ cup	216	16.1	63	104
Ricotta (8% fat)	½ cup	171	9.8	40	155
Romano	1 oz.	110	7.6	29	340
Roquefort	1 oz.	105	8.7	26	513
Swiss (pasteurized processed)	1 oz.	95	7.1	26	388
Cheezola	1 oz.	89	6.4	1	448
Countdown	1 oz.	39	0.3	1	434
Lite Line	1 oz.	50	2.0	10	410
Light n' Lively	1 oz.	70	4.0	15	350+
Cheeze Whiz spread	1 oz.	80	6.0	15	490
Lo-Chol	1 oz.	105	9.0	4	130
Formagg	1 oz.	70	5.0	0	140
Kraft-Free	1 oz.	45	0.0	0	420
Combination Foods					
Beefaroni	7 oz.	229	7.9	50	1044
Beef pot pie	1 pie	443	25.4	41	1008

Table 6 (continued)

Food	Serving Size	Calories	Fat (grams)	Cholesterol (mgs)	Sodium (mgs)
Combination Foods					
Beef stew	1 cup	186	7.3	33	966
Chicken & noodles	6 oz.	151	4.9	20	816
Dennison's Chili con Carne	16-oz. can	320	17.0	30	10
Egg roll	3½ oz.	210+	6.7+	12+	530+
Morton Salisbury Steak Dinner	1 oz.	373	15.6	47	1213
Franco-American Macaroni and Cheese	1 cup	180	8.0	26	900
ARMOUR CLASSIC LITE DINNERS					
Beef Pepper Steak	1	270	9.0	55	900
Chicken Burgundy	1	230	4.0	75	920
Chicken Oriental	1	240	4.0	75	730
Fillet of Cod Divan	1	280	7.0	80	990
Chicken Breast Marsala	1	270	7.0	NA	NA
Seafood, Natural Herbs	1	240	5.0	25	1440
Sliced Beef with Broccoli	1	280	7.0	70	2140
Turf n Surf	1	260	8.0	105	690
Turkey Parmesan	1	260	7.0	75	960
Veal Pepper Steak	1	280	8.0	90	480

Table 6 (continued)

Food	Serving Size	Calories	Fat (grams)	Cholesterol (mgs)	Sodium (mgs)
Combination Foods					
LEAN CUISINE (Stouffer's)					
Cheese Cannelloni	1	270	10.0	45	950
Chicken & Vegetables with Vermicelli	1	260	7.0	40	1250
Chicken Cacciatore with Vermicelli	1	280	10.0	40	1040
Chicken Chow Mein	1	250	5.0	25	1160
Fillet of Fish Florentine	1	240	9.0	100	800
Glazed Chicken	1	270	8.0	55	840
Linguini/Clam	1	260	7.0	40	860
Meatball Stew	1	250	9.0	65	1165
Oriental Beef	1	260	8.0	35	1270
Oriental Scallops	1	220	3.0	20	1200
Spaghetti	1	280	7.0	20	1400
Stuffed Cabbage	1	210	9.0	40	830
Zucchini Lasagna	1	260	7.0	20	1050
KRAFT					
Macaroni & Cheese	¾ cup	290	13.0	5	530
Spiral Mac. & Cheese	¾ cup	330	17.0	10	560
Egg Noodles & Cheese	¾ cup	340	17.0	50	630
Egg Noodles & Chicken	¾ cup	240	9.0	35	880
Spaghetti Dinner	1 cup	310	8.0	5	730
Spaghetti Dinner Meat Sauce	1 cup	370	14.0	15	720

Table 6 (continued)

Food	Serving Size	Calories	Fat (grams)	Cholesterol (mgs)	Sodium (mgs)
Combination Foods					
Velveeta Shells & Cheese	¾ cup	260	10.0	25	720
Condiments					
Mayonnaise	1 tbsp.	100	11.0	5	80
Tartar sauce	1 tbsp.	95	10.0	10	141
White sauce	2 tbsp.	54	4.1	4	125
Kraft-Free	1 tbsp.	12	0.0	0	190
Imitation mayo.	1 tbsp.	60	4.0	10	100
Miracle Whip	1 tbsp.	70	7.0	5	85
Kraft sandwich spread	1 tbsp.	50	5.0	5	75
Dairy Foods					
Whole milk	1 cup	150	8.1	34	120
Low-fat milk	1 cup	122	4.7	20	122
Skim milk	1 cup	89	0.4	5	128
Nonfat dry	1 cup	81	0.2	4	124
Canned evaporated skim	1 oz.	23	trace	1	35
Buttermilk (skim)	1 cup	88	0.2	10	318
Goat milk	1 cup	163	9.8	27	83
Yogurt (nonfat)	1 cup	127	0.4	4	174
Yogurt (low-fat)	1 cup	143	3.4	14	159
Yogurt (whole-milk)	1 cup	141	7.7	30	107
Half & half	1 tbsp.	20	1.7	6	6
Light cream	1 tbsp.	29	2.9	10	6
Medium cream	1 tbsp.	37	3.8	13	6
Light whipped cream	1 tbsp.	44	4.6	17	5

Table 6 (continued)

Food	Serving Size	Calories	Fat (grams)	Cholesterol (mgs)	Sodium (mgs)
Dairy Foods					
Heavy whipped cream	1 tbsp.	52	5.6	20	6
Sour cream	1 tbsp.	26	2.5	5	6
Aerosol whipped-cream topping	¼ cup	25	2.0	10	10
Desserts					
Cinnamon roll	1 ave.	174	5.0	39	214
Brownie	1 ave.	146	9.4	25	75
Angel-food cake	2 oz.	161	0.1	0	170
Carrot cake	3½ oz.	356	20.4	30	246
Devil's-food cake	3 oz.	323	15.0	37	357
Gingerbread	2 oz.	175	4.3	0.6	190
Marble cake	3 oz.	288	7.6	40	225
Choco.-chip cookies	1 ave.	52	2.3	6	44
Ladyfingers	1 large	50	1.1	50	10
McDonald's cookies	1 box	292	10.5	9	328
Oatmeal cookies	1 ave.	63	2.2	7	23
Peanut-butter cookies	1 ave.	57	2.3	7	21
Hostess Devil's Food Cupcakes	1	185	6.0	5	282
Hostess Ding Dongs	1	187	10.5	10	121
Hostess Ho Hos	1	118	6.0	14	63
Hostess Suzy Qs	1	256	10.9	10	301
Hostess Twinkies	1	152	6.2	20	203
Custard mixes	½ cup	143	4.6	19–24	125+

Table 6 (continued)

Food	Serving Size	Calories	Fat (grams)	Cholesterol (mgs)	Sodium (mgs)
Desserts					
Doughnuts	1 ave.	125+	6–12	8–100+	75+
Ice Cream:					
16% fat	1 cup	349	23.8	84	108
10% fat	1 cup	257	14.1	53	116
sandwich	1	238	8.5	34	100+
Eskimo Pie	1	270	19.1	35	100+
Ice milk	1 cup	222	4.6	13	163
Frozen yogurt	1 cup	244	3.0	10	121
Tofu dessert	1 cup	130	10.8	0	95
Sherbet	1 cup	268	4.0	7	92
Pies:					
Hostess Apple	3½ oz.	331	18.1	35	320
Hostess Cherry	3½ oz.	352	17.1	10	180
Sara Lee Bavarian Cream	3½ oz.	352	25.1	23	80
Morton Coconut Custard	3½ oz.	290	15.0	60	150
Lemon meringue	3½ oz.	227	7.5	93	282
Morton Peach	3½ oz.	260	12.0	10	230
Morton Pumpkin	3½ oz.	210	8.0	40	270
Puddings:					
Canned tapioca	3½ oz.	129	3.1	53	185
Vanilla (whole-milk)	½ cup	175	4.1	16	251
Vanilla (skim-milk)	½ cup	147	0.3	3	258
Dips					
Kraft Premium (various types)	1 oz.	50	4.0	10–20	150+

Table 6 (continued)

Food	Serving Size	Calories	Fat (grams)	Cholesterol (mgs)	Sodium (mgs)
Dips					
	1 oz.	50	4.0	10–20	150+
Guacamole	2 tbsp.	50	4.0	0	210
Buttermilk	2 tbsp.	70	6.0	0	240
French onion	2 tbsp.	60	4.0	0	260
Green onion	2 tbsp.	60	4.0	0	170
Bacon-horseradish	2 tbsp.	60	5.0	0	200
Clam	2 tbsp.	60	5.0	0	250
Garlic	2 tbsp.	60	4.0	0	160
Egg & Substitutes					
Whole egg	1 med.	78	5.5	250	59
Egg yolk	1 med.	59	5.2	250	12
Egg white	1 med.	16	trace	0	47
Eggnog	1 cup	352	19.0	149	138
Egg Beaters	¼ cup	25	0	0	80
Eggstra	¼ cup	30	0.8	23	56
Eggtime	¼ cup	40	1.0	0	120
Lucern	¼ cup	50	2.0	trace	NA
Second Nature	¼ cup	35	1.6	0	79
Scramblers	¼ cup	60	3.0	0	150
Fast Foods					
McDonald's:					
Big Mac	1	541	31.4	75	963
Egg McMuffin	1	352	20.0	191	911
Fish fillet	1	402	22.7	43	707
French fries	1 serv.	211	10.6	14	112
Hamburger	1	257	9.4	26	525
Hamburger with cheese	1	306	13.3	41	724
Apple pie	1	295	18.3	14	408
Quarter Pounder	1	418	20.5	69	278
Quarter Pounder with cheese	1	518	28.6	95	1206

Table 6 (continued)

Food	Serving Size	Calories	Fat (grams)	Cholesterol (mgs)	Sodium (mgs)
Fast Foods					
Vanilla shake	1	324	7.8	29	250
Kentucky Fried Chicken:					
Original recipe chicken	3½ oz.	290	17.8	133	535
Extra-crispy chicken	3½ oz.	323	20.8	116	446
Cole slaw	1 serv.	110	5.9	4	237
Mashed potatoes w/ gravy	1 serv.	74	2.0	3	353
Dinner roll	1	52	1.1	trace	83
Fats & Oils					
Bacon fat	1 tbsp.	126	14.0	11	150+
Beef suet	1 tbsp.	216	23.3	21	18
Chicken fat	1 tbsp.	126	14.0	9	0
Lard	1 tbsp.	126	14.0	13	0
Vegetable oil	1 tbsp.	120	13.5	0	0
Butter	1 tbsp.	108	12.2	36	124
Margarine	1 tbsp.	108	12.0	0	Variable
Butter Buds	1 oz.	12	0	0	NA
Fish & Shellfish					
Caviar (sturgeon)	1 tsp.	26	1.5	25	220
Clams (canned)	½ cup	52	0.7	80	36
Clams (raw)	3½ oz.	82	1.9	50	36
Cod (raw)	3½ oz.	78	0.3	50	70
Crab (king)	3½ oz.	93	1.9	60	Variable
Fish sticks (frozen)	3½ oz.	176	8.9	70	180
Flatfish	3½ oz.	79	0.8	61	78
Haddock	3½ oz.	141	6.6	60	71
Halibut	3½ oz.	214	8.8	60	168
Herring	3½ oz.	176	11.3	85	74
Lobster	3½ oz.	91	1.9	80	210

Table 6 (continued)

Food	Serving Size	Calories	Fat (grams)	Cholesterol (mgs)	Sodium (mgs)
Fish & Shellfish					
Mackerel	3½ oz.	191	12.2	95	148
Oysters	3½ oz.	66	1.8	50	73
Salmon	3½ oz.	182	7.4	47	50
Salmon (canned chinook)	3½ oz.	210	14.0	60	300+
Sardines (canned in oil)	3½ oz.	311	24.4	120	510
Scallops	3½ oz.	81	0.2	35	255
Shrimp	3½ oz.	91	0.8	150	140
Trout (brook)	3½ oz.	101	2.1	55	50
Trout (rainbow)	3½ oz.	195	11.4	55	50
Tuna (raw)	3½ oz.	133	3.0	60	37
Tuna (canned in oil)	3½ oz.	197	8.2	63	800+
Tuna (canned in water)	3½ oz.	127	0.8	63	41
Grain Products					
Breads:					
Cracked-wheat	1 slice	66	0.6	0	132
English muffin	1 slice	133	1.0	0	203
French	1 slice	75	0.5	0	140
Pita (pocket)	1 slice	145	1.0	0	86
Pumpernickel	1 slice	79	0.4	0	182
Raisin	1 slice	66	0.7	0	91
Rye	1 slice	61	0.3	0	139
White	1 slice	68	0.8	0	127
Whole-wheat	1 slice	61	0.8	0	132
Crackers:					
Matzo	1	118	0.3	0	10
Melba toast	3	60	2.0	0.6	2
Saltines	4	48	1.3	1.0	123
Egg noodles	1 cup	200	2.4	50	3

Table 6 (continued)

Food	Serving Size	Calories	Fat (grams)	Cholesterol (mgs)	Sodium (mgs)
Grain Products					
Pancake mix	1 ave.	367	5.0	33	1192
Stuffing mix	½ cup	198	8.0	45	515
Meats					
Beef: Composite cooked, well-trimmed	3 oz.	192	9.4	73	57
Eye round steak	3 oz.	158	6.0	59	52
Top round steak	3 oz.	166	5.9	72	52
Tip roast	3 oz.	167	7.0	69	55
Bottom round	3 oz.	201	9.3	81	44
Sirloin steak	3 oz.	185	8.3	75	56
Top sirloin	3 oz.	182	8.7	65	57
Rib steak	3 oz.	200	10.9	68	58
Rib roast	3 oz.	217	12.9	68	62
Blade pot roast	3 oz.	241	14.3	90	60
Arm pot roast	3 oz.	205	9.3	85	56
Brisket	3 oz.	230	14.3	77	66
Tenderloin	3 oz.	183	8.9	72	54
Ground beef (27% fat)	3 oz.	251	16.9	86	71
Ground beef (18% fat)	3 oz.	233	14.4	86	69
Lamb: Composite, cooked, trimmed	3 oz.	176	8.1	78	71
Lamb shank	3 oz.	156	6.0	81	54
Lamb loin chop	3 oz.	188	8.9	82	71
Lamb blade chop	3 oz.	195	10.9	82	80
Lamb rib roast	3 oz.	211	12.9	78	67
Pork: Composite, cooked, trimmed	3 oz.	198	11.1	79	50

Table 6 (continued)

Food	Serving Size	Calories	Fat (grams)	Cholesterol (mgs)	Sodium (mgs)
Meats					
Leg roast	3 oz.	187	9.4	80	55
Top loin chop	3 oz.	219	12.7	80	57
Top loin roast	3 oz.	208	11.7	67	39
Shoulder blade	3 oz.	250	15.0	99	64
Spareribs	3 oz.	338	25.8	103	79
Center loin chop	3 oz.	196	8.9	83	66
Tenderloin	3 oz.	141	4.1	79	57
Sirloin roast	3 oz.	221	11.1	94	50
Center rib chop	3 oz.	219	12.7	80	57
Center rib roast	3 oz.	208	11.7	67	39
Bacon	1 slice	40	3.0	5	120
Ham (3% fat)	3 oz.	120	6.0	45	240
Chicken:					
Light, no skin	3 oz.	153	4.2	66	54
Dark, no skin	3 oz.	156	5.4	78	72
Dark, & white, with skin	3 oz.	210	12.6	75	66
Chicken gizzard	1 cup	215	4.8	283	83
Chicken liver	1 cup	200	5.0	800	68
Turkey:					
Light, no skin	3 oz.	153	4.2	66	54
Dark, no skin	3 oz.	156	5.4	78	72
Light & dark, with skin	3 oz.	210	12.6	75	66
Bologna, franks	1 oz.	71	5.4	37	336
Ham	1 oz.	40	1.5	28	280
Pastrami	1 oz.	34	1.6	29	525
Salami	1 oz.	50	3.5	26	454

Table 6 (continued)

Food	Serving Size	Calories	Fat (grams)	Cholesterol (mgs)	Sodium (mgs)
Meats					
Veal:					
Lean only (leg, loin, cutlet)	3 oz.	120	2.7	84	48
Lean & fat (most cuts)	3 oz.	183	9.0	84	39
Lean & fat (rib, breast)	3 oz.	267	23.1	87	42
Duck:					
Flesh only	3 oz.	141	6.9	62	63
Flesh & skin	3 oz.	276	24.3	60	63
Goose:					
Flesh only	3 oz.	135	6.0	63	72
Organ meats:					
Beef kidney	3½ oz.	252	12.0	375	253
Beef liver	3½ oz.	140	4.7	300	73
Chicken liver	3½ oz.	165	4.4	746	61
Beef tongue	3½ oz.	244	16.7	140	61
Beef heart	3½ oz.	179	5.7	274	104
Brains	3½ oz.	106	7.3	2100	106
Sweetbreads	3½ oz.	90	6.6	132	99
Luncheon meats:					
OSCAR MAYER					
Bologna	1 oz.	88	8.1	15+	292
Canadian bacon	1 oz.	45	2.0	13	384
Chopped ham	1 oz.	64	4.8	14	387
Ham & cheese loaf	1 oz.	70	5.6		372
Headcheese	1 oz.	55	4.1	28	
Honey loaf	1 oz.	39	1.7	8	377
Liverwurst	1 oz.	139	9.1	35	81
Olive loaf	1 oz.	64	4.5	10	416
Salami (dry)	1 oz.	112	9.8	22	540

Table 6 (continued)

Food	Serving Size	Calories	Fat (grams)	Cholesterol (mgs)	Sodium (mgs)
Meats					
Spam					
(Hormel)	1 oz.	87	7.4	15	336
Hot dog	1.6 oz.	142	13.5	23	464
Ham	3½ oz.	120	5.0	50	1527
Salad Dressings					
Blue cheese	1 tbsp.	71	7.3	4–10	153
Green					
goddess	1 tbsp.	68	7.0	1	150
Russian	1 tbsp.	74	7.6	7–10	130
Thousand					
Island	1 tbsp.	70	7.0	9	98
French	1 tbsp.	66	6.2	0	219
Italian	1 tbsp.	83	9.0	0	314

TABLE 7
Comparison of Dietary Fats and Oils

Type	Saturated Fatty Acids (% of total)*	Monounsaturated Fatty Acids (% of total)*	Polyunsaturated Fatty Acids (% of total)*
Canola oil	6	62	32
Walnut oil	9	23	64
Safflower oil	10	13	77
Sunflower oil	11	20	69
Corn oil	13	25	62
Olive oil	14	77	9
Soybean oil	15	24	61
Peanut oil	18	49	33
Margarine (tub)	18	47	31
Cottonseed oil	27	19	54
Tuna fat	27	26	21
Chicken fat	30	45	11
Margarine (stick)	31	47	22
Shortening (can)	31	51	14
Lard	40	45	11

Table 7 (continued)

Type	Saturated Fatty Acids (% of total)*	Monounsaturated Fatty Acids (% of total)*	Polyunsaturated Fatty Acids (% of total)*
Mutton fat	47	41	8
Palm oil	49	37	9
Beef fat	50	42	4
Butterfat	62	29	4
Palm kernel oil	81	11	2
Coconut oil	86	6	2

*Percentage are averaged and thus may not total exactly 100 percent.

SOME NOTABLE FOOD PRODUCTS

The easier it is to enjoy delicious, though low-fat or nonfat, foods, the easier it will be to make dietary modifications that you can live with. The food industry has responded to an increasing public demand for heart-healthy foods, and new ones enter the market each week. I report these new products regularly in my *Diet-Heart Newsletter* (see page 337). Here are some notable products that make my life a lot more enjoyable, and which I think you should add to your own shopping list.

When I first started to get serious about my diet, I virtually eliminated red meat. Now I don't have to, thanks to Dakota Lean Meats. A three-ounce serving of USDA choice New York steak packs nearly seven grams of fat, and that's after trimming all the visible fat. And most of us want to eat more than just three ounces. Well, a three-ounce Dakota Lean New York steak has just a little over one gram of fat. That means you can enjoy a hefty seven-ounce steak, for instance, with barely more than three grams of fat.

Dakota Lean beef has less fat than chicken breast and most fish. That means you can enjoy it as often as you wish. How do they do it? It's a matter of cross-breeding of cattle along with a special feeding program. And to make things even better, this beef is 100 percent free of hormones and antibiotics.

But how does it taste? In a word, delicious! Prepare your beef over the charcoal or under the broiler. It cooks faster than ordinary beef, and tastes best when rare. Don't overcook.

You can have Dakota Lean steaks, roasts, and ground beef delivered to your door by second-day delivery. To place an order or to get more information you can call toll-free (800) 727-5326 or write to Dakota Lean Meats, 136 West Tripp, Winner, SD 57580.

Talking about meat, how about some sausage? Commercially prepared sausages, even those claiming to be low-fat, are laden with fat and cholesterol. But now there's a way to enjoy breakfast sausage, pepperoni, bologna, salami, and jerky and stay heart-healthy.

Here's the way it works. Just mix a package of Spice 'n' Slice herbs and seasonings and special curing ingredients with two pounds of ground low-fat meat. You might use low-fat beef or ground turkey breast. Then shape into logs and pop into the oven for about an hour to make salami, pepperoni, or bologna. Or combine meat with the jerky mix, roll thin, and allow to dry in a low-heat oven. Especially on weekends, we look forward to having one of two flavors of breakfast sausage. Just mix the packet of seasonings with low-fat meat, form into patties, and sizzle on a nonstick pan.

To place an order or get additional information, call (602) 861-4094 or write to Spice 'n' Slice at P.O. Box 26051, Phoenix, AZ 85068.

And what about cheese? That's one of the worst sources of saturated fat, cholesterol, and sodium in the diet, yet one of the foods most of us hate to give up. Now you can enjoy the flavor of cheese without the guilt.

Finally, of all the different egg substitutes available, I think the best one is Second Nature. It looks and tastes closest to fresh, beaten eggs. You can find it in the egg case or sometimes in the dairy case in most supermarkets. To introduce the readers of my books to Second Nature egg substitute, the company is offering a free recipe brochure and discount coupons to anyone who calls toll-free (800) 441-3321.

Using these and other products makes life a lot more enjoyable. After all, eating is one of the joys of life. The trick to following a heart-healthy diet is to get rid of the fat and keep the fun and flavor!

THE DIET-HEART NEWSLETTER

To keep you on top of current happenings in the ever-expanding area of diet and heart disease, I've developed the *Diet-Heart Newsletter*. This quarterly publication summarizes current articles in the medical literature, presenting ideas that are not often available to the public.

You'll receive insights from medical meetings and seminars, and you'll get newly developed recipes and dietary suggestions about new products. There's also a regular question–answer forum in which you can participate.

For a sample of the *Diet-Heart Newsletter* and subscription information, send a stamped, self-addressed business-size (large) envelope to:

The Diet-Heart Newsletter
P.O. Box 2039
Venice, CA 90294

CHAPTER 14

Dealing with Diabetes

D iabetes places one at increased risk of heart attack and undermines efforts to prevent a second event. But the good news is that you can take charge of the situation and bring diabetes under control.

Diabetes is a metabolic disorder in which patients do not properly metabolize sugar in the blood. As levels of blood sugar, known as glucose, rise, especially over a prolonged period of years, the sugar becomes toxic to a number of systems of the body including the cardiovascular system.

There are two types of diabetes to consider. The type I, insulin-dependent form of diabetes normally occurs before the age of 30. It was previously termed juvenile diabetes. Type II, non-insulin-dependent diabetes, has its onset later in life and afflicts women more often than men, especially those who are overweight and sedentary. Both kinds have adverse effects on the cardiovascular system.

Patients with diabetes are likely to experience a heart attack earlier in life, and the disease may be more severe. Often diabetic patients are also hypertensive, each condition magnifying the ill effects of the other, and both intensified by obesity. Poor diabetes control, with elevated sugar levels in the blood, tends to contribute to rises in cholesterol and triglyceride counts.

INCREASED ODDS OF "SILENT" HEART ATTACK

One of the results of poor diabetes control and rampant blood sugar levels is the development of neuropathy or nerve damage. Damaged nerves prevent proper transmission of sensations including those of heat, cold, touch, and pain. The patient may not be aware of the pain that results from the heart not getting sufficient oxygen. Without this warning signal, one may not be conscious of angina or even heart attack. This is known as "silent ischemia" or "silent heart attack."

If a heart attack occurs, it might be passed off as indigestion or other minor discomfort since there wouldn't be the crushing chest pain or radiating shoulder/arm pain normally experienced. The results of not seeking immediate medical attention can be fatal. In less severe attacks, the evidence isn't discovered until the patient has a routine ECG or treadmill test. If a number of attacks occur in this way, the function of the heart muscle can be affected, resulting in congestive heart failure.

DAMAGE TO ARTERIOLES

When sugar levels in the blood remain high, damage can occur in the tiniest of the blood vessels transporting oxygen to tissues. These tiny arteries or arterioles become scarred and clogged with cholesterol-containing plaque. The damage in such cases is widespread throughout the body, with virtually all tissues receiving less than adequate supplies of blood and oxygen. This chronic oxygen deficit to the heart muscle can lead to gradual, insidious damage to the heart which may not be detected until the heart's function is severely impaired.

HEART RATE AND BLOOD PRESSURE IMPAIRED

Diabetes adversely affects the cardiovascular system indirectly by impeding blood pressure control and restricting heart rate. That happens when nerve damage leads to improper regulation of blood pressure and pulse rates, preventing the nerves from controlling those functions when the body requires them to speed up or slow down.

Normally the least effort results in some change in blood pressure and heart rate. Even getting up from a chair is enough to set the heart beating a bit faster in normal individuals. But without such fine-tuning, blood has a tendency to pool, blood pressure is abnormally low, and the individual has a tendency to faint.

KNOWLEDGE IS KING

If you have either type I or type II diabetes, it's absolutely essential that you thoroughly understand your disease. The ill effects are gradual but certain, and without proper attention the result will be tragic.

Only you can manage your disease. Yes, your doctor can prescribe insulin for type I or oral medications for type II diabetes. But ultimately you must be the one in control on a day-to-day basis.

Entire books and extensive pamphlets have been written about diabetes. Take the time to really learn about your condition. Then discuss your management with your doctor.

The good news is that diabetes can be well controlled. In both type I and type II, diet and exercise play major roles and are absolutely essential as integral parts of treatment.

THE DIABETIC DIET

As is true for the general population, diabetic patients benefit greatly from a low-fat, low-cholesterol diet. An additional consideration, however, is restriction of sugars and other simple carbohydrates. The best dietary approach is that provided in the exchange lists provided by the American Diabetic Association. This is particularly essential for the type I patient who must keep his or her diet/exercise/insulin equation properly maintained in a tight range.

For the type II patient, weight control is the principal goal. And, of course, the best diet for controlling calories is one which restricts fat, since fat is the most concentrated source of calories. Read chapter 13 thoroughly, and follow the suggestions you'll find there.

THE DIABETIC EXERCISE PROGRAM

Exercise is indispensable for both the type I and type II diabetes patient. Those recovering from heart disease will, quite literally, be able to kill two birds with one stone in terms of controlling both their heart disease and diabetes.

Especially if you're getting started on an exercise program, a periodic examination by your doctor to monitor your progress will allow you to achieve the best results.

Regular exercise helps you to lower blood sugar levels, since the muscles use glucose to provide energy. Even after the exercise session, your muscles will continue to take in glucose from the blood for hours. Your metabolic rate will increase, allowing you to burn more calories, and thus facilitate weight loss and weight control. And you'll potentially see an increase in the protective levels of HDL cholesterol.

STACKING THE ODDS IN YOUR FAVOR

Diabetes places a major obstacle in front of your efforts to make a speedy and complete recovery. The disease magnifies other risk factors, increasing the potential for recurrence. Fighting heart disease with uncontrolled diabetes is like fighting with one arm tied behind your back.

Stack the odds in your favor by doing all you possibly can to work with your doctors to bring your diabetes under strict control if you have type I, and completing eliminating the symptoms if you have type II.

THE SEVENTH STEP:

Beating the
Blood Pressure Blues

CHAPTER 15

The Invisible Nemesis

How's your blood pressure today? Unless you had it checked, you can't be sure. That's because there are no symptoms of high blood pressure, also known as hypertension. But we do know that it's one of the Big Three risk factors in heart disease along with cigarette smoking and elevated cholesterol levels, and it's the Number One risk factor for strokes. We also know that we can completely control blood pressure in almost every case.

You're not alone. It's estimated that nearly 60 million men and women in the United States have an elevated pressure. To a large extent the condition is another part of your genetic heritage, and your blood pressure has probably been slowly but surely increasing since you were much younger, perhaps even back to your childhood.

On its most basic level, blood pressure is quite easy to understand. It refers to the pressure required to pump blood from the heart through the arteries to all parts of the body. Through a complex system of checks and balances, blood pressure is regulated and adjusted. During exercise pressure goes up, and at rest it comes back down. Different pressures may be needed in different parts of the body at different times.

Blood pressure is something we just don't think much about since we can't feel it. Even when one is completely calm and relaxed, blood pressure may be elevated. Over a period of time, hypertension leads to a thickening or hardening of the arteries, which are also weakened in the process.

There are two important blood pressure measurements. The first is the *systolic* pressure, the pressure of the blood pushing against the artery wall as the heart beats. The second is the *diastolic* pressure, a measurement between beats when the heart rests. A reading of 120/80 is stated as "120 over 80" with the systolic being 120 and the diastolic 80. That reading, by the way, is completely normal, and the patient would be termed *normotensive*.

For years there was controversy as to what would be considered high blood pressure. Then in 1972 the National High Blood Pressure Education Program was launched by the National Heart, Lung, and Blood Institute in conjunction with the nation's major medical organizations. This program has initiated efforts to educate both patients and physicians as to the seriousness of hypertension and methods of controlling it. Today there is virtual consensus as to the classification of blood pressure in adults 18 years or older.

The risk of cardiovascular problems related to blood pressure increases with greater levels of both systolic and diastolic pressure. Diastolic pressure is normally of greatest concern, but systolic pressure is also considered. You'll note in the following breakdown that the term "mild hypertension" is used. That's somewhat deceptive and should not be construed to mean that such an elevation is of no consequence. *All* elevations of blood pressure should be treated and controlled.

You've had your blood pressure measured many times, but you may not know exactly how the measurement is made. The apparatus used is called a *sphygmomanometer* ("sfig-mo-ma-na-meh-ter"). It consists of a cloth or rubber cuff to wrap around the arm, a rubber air bulb to pump air into the cuff, and a manometer, which measures pressure in millimeters of mercury in a glass tube similar to a thermometer. As air enters the cuff, mercury rises in the manometer. The cuff temporarily cuts off blood flow in the forearm.

As air is gradually let out of the cuff, blood begins to flow again and the mercury in the glass tube drops. The doctor or nurse (or other trained person) listens to the blood flow through a stethoscope placed on the artery just below the cuff. One first hears a thudding or tapping sound as the blood spurts out. It occurs when the air pressure in the cuff is a bit lower than the pressure in the artery. The reading on the glass tube at the time of that first sound is your systolic pressure.

Mercury continues to fall as more air is released from the cuff. When the tapping sound stops, blood is smoothly flowing between heartbeats. The moment the sound stops a reading is taken from the manometer tube. This is your diastolic pressure.

Your blood pressure varies from day to day, situation to situation, and even minute to minute. That's why to get an accurate assessment the doctor will take two, three, or even more readings. He may also take both sitting and standing pressures. And to be absolutely certain of your condition, at least two examinations on different days are needed.

See Table 9 (page 348) for a classification of blood pressure readings.

WHO GETS HYPERTENSION?

As mentioned earlier, nearly 60 million men and women in the United States have hypertension. That makes it this country's most common chronic illness. No one is totally immune, though some are more likely than others to develop hypertension.

In nine out of ten cases, no particular cause can be determined. The condition for such patients is termed *primary hypertension*. If elevated blood pressure results from another cause, such as kidney disease and disorders of the blood vessels, the ailment is called *secondary hypertension*. Occasionally the underlying cause of secondary hypertension can be eliminated by surgery or medical treatment. But for primary hypertension there is no cure. On the other hand, we can very effectively control it such that the condition poses no health risks.

Certain factors may predispose individuals to develop hypertension. Those with a family history are more likely to develop it than those without this genetic background. At least 50 percent of those with high blood pressure have one or more parents with the condition.

While hypertension can develop early in life, sometimes even in childhood, most patients see their blood pressure rise between the ages of 35 and 50. By the age of 64, more than half the population has an elevated pressure.

Normally we think of hypertension as a man's problem, but that's true only until age 50. After that, women catch up and by age 60 more women than men have high blood pressure. For both men and women, this is a major risk factor in heart disease, though death caused by complications from hypertension such as stroke is more frequent in men.

Race plays an important role. Regardless of age, blacks have twice the incidence of hypertension. In fact, blacks develop the condition much younger than do whites, and for them it is the leading cause of death. Apparently both genetics and environment are involved. Black dietary preferences have been implicated, and blacks have been shown to retain sodium more readily than do whites. For blacks, salt and sodium restriction is mandatory in almost all cases.

Nearly four out of ten overweight persons have hypertension. Conversely, those who lose weight show a significant decrease in blood pressure. As we'll see, that becomes a necessary part of hypertension treatment.

About 70 percent of patients with high blood pressure are in the "mild hypertension" category. Twenty percent fall into the moderate classification, and about ten percent have severe hypertension.

Your doctor may have told you that you have *labile hypertension*. This means that your blood pressure is sometimes but not always high, and it might reflect a stressful situation. Some patients, about 10 to 25 percent, progress from labile hypertension to mild hypertension.

Other patients, including me on occasion, will have what's known as *white coat hypertension*. This means our blood pressure goes up in the doctor's office during examinations, but would otherwise be normal. In my case, I often react to doctor's examination in the same way as I would

TABLE 9
Blood Pressure Classification in Adults Over 18

DIASTOLIC BLOOD PRESSURE	(measured in millimeters of mercury)
Normal blood pressure	less than 85
High normal pressure	85–89
Mild hypertension	90–104
Moderate hypertension	105–114
Severe hypertension	more than 115
SYSTOLIC BLOOD PRESSURE	(when diastolic pressure is less than 90)
Normal blood pressure	less than 140
Borderline hypertension	140–159
Systolic hypertension	more than 160

to a test in school or an athletic competition. After a few minutes of conversation and relaxation the pressure drops to normal.

There is a rare type of high blood pressure that requires intensive treatment to prevent severe damage to the body's organs and even death. This is called *accelerated* or *malignant hypertension*. In such cases, which have nothing to do with cancer, diastolic pressure goes to 130 and beyond, with systolic pressure above 200. This severe form of hypertension quickly gets worse and calls for emergency measures to bring it under control.

Regardless of your blood pressure measurement, your doctor will keep close watch on it, testing during every visit. We can't do much about risk factors affecting our cardiovascular health such as genetics, age, or sex. But hypertension is something we can alter. Since 1972, when doctors started to get serious about blood pressure, the mortality rate due to strokes has dropped 50 percent. That's impressive. And there's no reason you shouldn't succeed in controlling your own blood pressure and thus eliminating a major heart disease risk factor.

Again, there are no symptoms. Yes, stress can result in an increase in blood pressure, but only temporarily. The only way you can tell how you're doing is by close monitoring. You might even want to invest in home equipment. You'll find a wide variety available, including some very easy to use devices which show your measurement in a digital readout. Talk with your doctor about whether this would be a good idea for you, and, if so, which type would be best for your needs.

There is no cure for primary hypertension. But methods of control can be so effective that the condition need not be a concern. The important thing is to make the commitment to that control.

The treatment you and your doctor decide upon for your blood pressure control will depend on the severity of hypertension and your willingness to make some lifestyle modifications. In some cases, prescription drugs will be absolutely necessary, at least at the beginning to quickly reduce your health risks. If you, like most patients, have a mild hypertension, lifestyle modifications alone may be enough for control.

It's wrong to think that just swallowing a few pills is an effective method of control. First, lifestyle changes will make the drugs more effective. Second, you can get by with fewer drugs, and possibly none at all, with some modifications. That's important, since antihypertensive drugs may involve some side effects, and few patients want to take more medicine than they absolutely have to.

WEIGHT REDUCTION

A large number of studies, both in this country and around the world, have shown that obesity and hypertension are closely linked. The more weight one gains, the higher the blood pressure goes. Conversely, by losing that extra weight one can achieve a significant reduction in pressure. Try to get as close to your ideal body weight as possible. Yes, it's hard to do at first, but it's really worth the effort.

A recent study at the University of Mississippi has demonstrated that weight loss can be as effective as drugs in controlling mild hypertension. The 800 patients involved had diastolic pressures of 90 to 100. Some received a weight-reduction diet while others were given antihypertensive drugs. After six months, weight loss exceeding 10 pounds equalled the benefits of the medication, with patients exhibiting a 12.1 drop in diastolic blood pressure. According to Dr. Herbert Langford, the threshold of benefit appears to be 10 pounds of weight loss. Of course the more the better, down to ideal body weight.

Dr. Langford also found that weight loss boosted the effectiveness of drugs given to patients. Those losing more than 10 pounds while on medications saw a fall of 18.6 in diastolic pressure.

Interestingly, the benefit of weight loss was found even in those patients who did not significantly restrict their alcohol or sodium consumption. This demonstrates that weight loss alone can be responsible for impressive hypertension control.

What's the best way to achieve weight loss? Reducing the total fat intake, which is also the best way to control cholesterol, is the most effective path to *permanent* weight control. Fat represents the richest source of calories in the diet. Simply put, if you don't eat fat, you won't be fat.

An excellent way to both limit fat intake and cut total calories for the day is through a sound program of meal replacement. The NANCI Corporation mentioned on page 297 makes a product called Lose-It which can facilitate weight loss and weight control. Try using it to replace lunch and for a midafternoon snack, in conjunction with a low-fat diet. I know from personal experience and observation that Lose-It really works.

Weight reduction provides a number of benefits beyond hypertension control. You'll see an automatic reduction in cholesterol levels. Diabetes is more easily controlled, and in many cases the need for medication is greatly lessened or even eliminated. And, very importantly, you'll feel a lot better about yourself. Since self-esteem is such a vital part of recovery from heart disease, that element cannot be overemphasized.

ALCOHOL RESTRICTION

Most patients with mild to moderate hypertension can continue to drink moderately. But excessive amounts of alcohol can result in elevated blood pressure. Heavy drinking also lessens inhibitions and may lead to behaviors including overeating that impede blood pressure control.

If you enjoy a drink now and then, do so in moderation. Don't drink more than the equivalent of 1 ounce of ethanol, pure alcohol, daily. That comes out to 2 ounces of 100-proof whiskey or other distilled spirits, 8 ounces of standard table wine, or 24 ounces of beer.

Alcohol also provides a lot of empty calories. A 12-ounce bottle of beer packs about 150 calories; a 4-ounce glass of wine has about 80 calories. And 2 ounces of gin, whiskey, or scotch contain about 170 calories. That really adds up over the course of the week, and makes weight control much more difficult.

Life is often a matter of give and take. If you enjoy that glass of wine with dinner, or that bottle of beer during the football game on TV, just remember that you are consuming calories. Compensate for that intake by cutting back on other nonessential calories.

Of course, your own program of hypertension control may call for even more stringent alcohol restriction. By all means discuss this with your doctor. He may suggest abstinence for a while. Then you might be able to add back a drink now and then and see whether you can maintain control.

EXERCISE

Exercise is so important an element in a heart-healthy lifestyle that you'll see it come up again and again in this book. We discuss regular physical activity in chapter 11. One of the dramatic benefits of exercise is blood pressure control. Numerous studies have shown that patients can often control mild hypertension with exercise and diet alone, with no need for drugs. This remains a bit controversial for some doctors, who feel more comfortable when prescribing drugs that they can adjust and control. The fact remains, however, that drugs can often be avoided. If you're like most patients, you will want to keep the number of medications you take to a minimum.

What to do if your doctor is adamant about your taking drugs to control mild hypertension? You may decide to go along with him for the time being, while actively pursuing your own program of diet and exercise as spelled out in this book. Assuming that these non-drug approaches are effective for you, your doctor will soon see that there is no need for the drugs.

If you have a moderate or severe form of hypertension, the diet and exercise regimen may not completely replace the need for medications, but certainly the amount of drugs will be lessened. Perhaps instead of needing two pills three times a day, you'll only need to take one.

By all means it's necessary to have a good relationship with your doctor so you can work out the formula that's best for you. If you don't think such a relationship is possible with your current doctor, you might think about a change. Take a look at some suggestions along these lines in chapter 9.

AVOIDING TOBACCO

Just in case you need one more reason to quit smoking, controlling your blood pressure should give you the final incentive. Smokers have a higher frequency of accelerated or malignant hypertension, the highly dangerous form of high blood pressure.

As with exercise, quitting those cigarettes may allow you to use less medication. Studies have shown that the more one smokes, the more antihypertensive drugs one needs. One particular drug tested along these lines has side effects including impotence and fatigue; the more one needs to take to control blood pressure, the greater those adverse reactions. Here's a case in which you just might have to choose between making love and smoking a cigarette. There's no doubt as to which one I prefer. How about you?

SODIUM RESTRICTION

For many years we have heard the unequivocal advice that all Americans should significantly reduce their salt consumption. This was based on the fact that a percentage of us develop a type of high blood pressure that is aggravated by a salty diet. For some patients, the need to cut back on salt is very real, and most of us could be more moderate with the salt shaker.

But the total picture on salt and sodium consumption is not so clear. Not everyone needs to greatly restrict salt intake. On the other hand, most Americans consume far too much. View this entire discussion as a call for moderation.

The International Intersalt study is the most comprehensive population study yet undertaken to get some answers. Researchers looked at blood pressures and sodium intake in people in 32 countries. The results revealed little link between sodium intake and blood pressure in people around the world.

Yes, in populations where sodium intake is extremely low—at a level at which most of us would find the diet virtually inedible—blood pressure is low. That was true in 4 out of 52 centers studied. But in the other 48 centers where there was wide variation in sodium intake there was little if any difference in blood pressure. These findings suggest that unless sodium intake is very severely limited, most people will not see any improvement. Any drop in blood pressure will be clinically insignificant.

A study published in the *Archives of Internal Medicine* (January 1990) also failed to show a strong sodium–hypertension link. For three years, 841 men and women were observed for the blood pressure-lowering effects of diet. Some restricted sodium alone, a second group cut back on calories, a third group reduced both sodium and calories, while a fourth group was put on a low-sodium, high-potassium diet. The group with the greatest drop in blood pressure was that which reduced calories. Those cutting back on sodium showed little benefit.

It may even be possible that a low-salt diet may hurt more than help. Dr. Brent Egan reported his findings at the American Heart Association meeting in New Orleans in 1989. He and other researchers at the Medical College of Wisconsin in Milwaukee found that a low-salt diet will not reduce blood pressure in 50 percent of people with higher-than-normal blood pressure and in 80 percent of those with normal blood pressure. In fact, for some people, salt restriction actually may result in higher blood pressure.

Dr. Egan takes a very practical approach with his own patients. He has them monitor their blood pressure for a week before starting a low-salt diet in order to establish a baseline. Then they keep track of their pressure after cutting down on salt. If there is no reduction in blood pressure after one to two months, he tells them to discontinue salt restriction.

Dr. Carter Newton, a cardiologist at the University of California at Los Angeles who practices in Santa Monica, believes this is the best approach, but points out that it takes cooperation and time. He suggests that patients might have to "push" their MDs to do this with them.

Certainly some people are salt-sensitive. It is estimated that 25 to 60 percent of people with high blood pressure, or about 10 to 15 percent of the general population, is sodium sensitive. Only those individuals are likely to benefit from stringent sodium restriction. Eventually we'll have a test for such sensitivity, but right now the only way to tell is by trial and error.

Moreover, it appears now that not all sodium can be clumped in the same "villain" category as salt. While you may be sensitive to salt and may need to cut back on intake, you may not respond at all to other sodium compounds in the diet such as MSG (monosodium glutamate). Again, trial and error is the only completely effective way to tell just what you can and cannot consume without adversely affecting your pressure.

Advocates of salt and sodium restriction for everybody across the board say that such an approach will mean that some individuals will benefit, and no one will be harmed since no one needs the salt or sodium in the diet anyway. At first glance this makes sense, but upon closer examination, there are two major flaws in such thinking.

First, why give something up when you don't have to? Second, salt makes food taste better. For those of us trying to keep the fat content of our diets down, overly restricted salt intake might torpedo our efforts.

As in most things, moderation should be the watchword in salt and sodium intake. The National Research Council indicates that a "safe and adequate" daily sodium intake is about 1,100 to 3,300 milligrams daily for adults. To put that into perspective, one teaspoon of salt contains about 2,000 milligrams of sodium. That's how much we need to maintain good health under normal circumstances. How much do Americans actually consume? The frequently quoted range is from 2,300 to 6,900 milligrams daily. Many Americans, and many foreign populations, consume much more than that. There's a big difference between salting all food until it's virtually white and sprinkling on a few grains here and there.

Actually, researchers have demonstrated that the best way to cut back on salt is to reduce or eliminate it in cooking. That way you can enjoy a sprinkle at the table. When they measured the amount consumed in that way, the total intake was way down.

Actually, most of the salt and sodium in the American diet gets there by way of processed foods and foods in fast-food restaurants. Those are the same foods which are highest in saturated fats and cholesterol. So if you cut down on them in your efforts to lower your cholesterol level, you'll automatically reduce your salt and sodium intake.

THE ROLE OF OTHER MINERALS

While we've heard a lot about cutting down on sodium, the research on other minerals hasn't received as much publicity. Reduced potassium intake may be associated with high blood pressure. By increasing your potassium intake, you might be able to decrease your hypertension. That means consuming more foods such as bananas, oranges, and potatoes. Talk about this with your doctor. And ask whether the drugs he may have prescribed for you will, in and of themselves, affect potassium levels in your blood.

The other mineral in the blood pressure equation is calcium. When Dr. David McCarron of Oregon Health Sciences University in Portland first suggested that calcium deficiencies in the diet might be correlated with hypertension, many were skeptical. Today additional studies appear to corroborate his initial beliefs.

One cardiovascular benefit derived from calcium is a lessening of high blood pressure. Another study demonstrated a 23 percent decrease in hypertension in women getting an 800-milligram calcium supplement.

Dr. McCarron does not advocate unlimited sodium intake to be negated by calcium supplements or extra glasses of milk. Rather, he says, there appears to be a threshold at which if one has a very low dietary calcium intake there is more likely to be an incidence of hypertension. Rather than limiting sodium in such patients, the better approach may be to increase calcium.

How much calcium do you need? The recommendation here is the same as for all healthy adults, 800 milligrams per day. That's about what you'd get from two eight-ounce glasses of milk and an ounce of cheese or a cup of yogurt. Of course you'll want to make those the low-fat or nonfat types. Other foods including salmon and sardines with bones intact, leafy green vegetables, and corn tortillas are also calcium sources. For those not getting enough in the diet, calcium supplements should be considered.

While magnesium has been mentioned as another mineral to be considered in hypertension control, data do not appear to bear out the hypothesis. In one study at Wayne State University, patients with mild hypertension received 480 milligrams of magnesium for three months. At Harvard, subjects got 360 milligrams for two months. At the conclusion of the studies, blood pressure was no lower for those getting the magnesium than for those getting a placebo.

FISH AND FISH OILS

According to some people, fish oil capsules appear to be the cure for whatever ails you. Unfortunately, fact does not match fancy. Despite the publicity, those capsules have little if any direct benefit for the heart patient. They don't lower cholesterol levels, and they may actually increase the amount of the "bad" LDL cholesterol in the blood. Oil capsules do not reduce blood pressure, though they can lower triglycerides. Moreover, the potential disadvantages far outweigh the advantages for most patients.

Instead of popping fish oil capsules, try to increase the amount of fish in your diet. That provides two benefits. You'll get the oils which may offer some protection from heart disease, and you'll replace fatty meats with much leaner fish.

STRESS REDUCTION AND RELAXATION

Some people are able to control their blood pressure completely by non-drug methods. As noted earlier, diet and exercise can play important roles. Another factor in the equation is the ability to control stress and to relax. You can't lose with this winning combination. In addition to the blood pressure control achieved, you'll simply feel better.

The relaxation response can elicit a fall of four to five systolic points and two to three points of diastolic pressure. That's good, but it's not clinically significant. Certainly one feels better when using the relaxation response, and I try to work it into my own life regularly.

But for really effective hypertension benefits, we need something more potent. One such method appears to be biofeedback. Dr. Keith Sedlacek discusses this fully in his book *The Sedlacek Technique: Finding the Calm Within You* (1989). In research at St. Luke's Hospital in New York, he worked with hypertensive patients who practiced biofeedback techniques for as little as 10 weeks. They averaged a reduction of 14 points systolic and 12 points diastolic.

The patients in Dr. Sedlacek's study suffered from hypertension for more than two years, and 27 out of 30 were on medication. Pressures fell from an average of 144/95 to 130/83. Many patients were able to significantly reduce their need for antihypertensive drugs.

Biofeedback may or may not be the answer for you. It does take a degree of effort and commitment, and skills get better as one practices on a regular basis. It's not quite as simple as doing a breathing exercise or utilizing the relaxation response. For the most thorough and intensive biofeedback experience you may wish to consider working with a professional counselor. He or she can train and coach you in techniques whereby you control your body's response to the environment. All practitioners utilize some manner of "feeding back" information as to how well you're responding.

In the most elaborate setups, patients are literally "wired" to detect their body temperature, heart rate, breathing, and palm sweatiness. It is, in effect, the apparatus used in lie detection. On a lesser, much simpler, level one may use an ordinary fever thermometer held in the grip of the hand to monitor temperature changes. Some utilize specially designed strips or rings which remind one of the mood ring fad of some years ago but which are more accurate today.

The first step is to relax the body and mind. The procedure typically is deep breathing and/or variations on the relaxation technique. Once the person is fairly relaxed and receptive to further calming, he or she will concentrate on increasing the body's temperature. He or she breathes in and out regularly and in a controlled manner. The concentration on the body's temperature and breathing, as well as on heart rate in some cases, enables one to remove oneself from surrounding stresses and pressures of life. To aid the concentration, one looks at the thermometer, ring, strip, or other device now and then to gauge progress.

As I've said, practice makes perfect. At each session, one attempts greater and greater control over the heat-generating capability and the speed at which improvement in calming is "fed back." Does it work? Indeed it does for many thousands who have given it a real trial.

DRAW A PICTURE

Biofeedback works so well because one becomes focused on the process itself. For some, prayer can be equally effective, again because of the total immersion involved. A method of relaxation will not be as effective if it allows the mind to wander.

Think back to the last time you saw a child with his or her crayons coloring in a book. Picture those little fingers holding the crayon, trying to stay within the lines. The eyes are intent, and perhaps the tip of the tongue protrudes in deep concentration. That child is thinking of nothing else at that moment. Wouldn't it be great to share in that complete sense of calm?

Well, you can. I've suggested this before, but it's worth repeating. Go out and buy a box of crayons and a nice little coloring book. Don't laugh. It's fun! In fact, it's even more fun if you invite a little child, perhaps your grandchild, to join you. Or borrow a neighbor's little one. That child can act as your "calming counselor" and guide you in the world of coloring.

Does this sound ridiculous to you? I'm here to tell the world that despite my extensive college training, my degrees, my world travel, it's nice to settle back into childhood once in a while. I surprise my kids now and then by pulling out the coloring book and crayons and spending 30 minutes or so with them. We all enjoy it, and I've noticed a very similar warming of the hands during the process, signalling a calming effect which helps control blood pressure.

You may even want to go beyond the crayon stage and "graduate" to more sophisticated painting or drawing. You can find no-cost or low-cost instruction at most community centers, senior centers, and YMCAs. Bring out your creative side and you'll find a marvelous new way to relax.

Too complicated for you, but you'd like something a bit more "adult" than crayons? How about one of those paint-by-numbers kits? Yes, they still make them, and you can find some kits that will help you produce a really beautiful painting you'll actually want to frame and hang on a wall. Most important, you'll achieve a level of calming far deeper than you can get by watching TV or reading a book.

GET A PET

There's a little friend out there waiting for you, one who'll never argue with you, will love you unconditionally, and will always be there for you to confide in and love. A pet can be good for what ails you, especially in terms of helping to control blood pressure.

Pets can provide a sense of self-esteem and a feeling of being needed and wanted. Most dogs and cats live at least 10 years; that's longer than many marriages survive today! Pets reduce stress and tension as they provide companionship and affection.

Dr. Aaron Katcher, a University of Pennsylvania psychiatrist, contends that pets supply a kind of mental medicine that lowers stress levels and blood pressure, making people feel more secure. His research indicates that hypertensive patients with pets live longer and live happier.

As we age, family and friends often don't need us as they used to, leaving us to feel abandoned and useless at times. A pet can help fill this void. Unequivocal data prove that loneliness causes an increase in sickness and death.

We also know that active people live longer and pets often make demands on us that keep us active. Dogs need their walks, giving us that nudge to go out for some exercise ourselves. You're likely to walk farther with a dog than alone, since it's less boring and lonely.

A number of studies indicate that when people talk, blood pressure rises. That's especially true when talking quickly and pointedly. But it's quite the opposite when we talk to our pets. At least four studies I've read show that blood pressure actually falls when one talks with a dog or cat. Talk *with* you ask? Yes, we get feedback from our pets, in the form of a purr or a wag of the tail.

When we address pets we talk more quietly and slowly, much as we would with a small child. And since so many pet owners are convinced that their pets understand them, the experience becomes remarkably calming.

Owning a pet can help us live longer. Dr. Katcher has found that pet owners have a real survival edge. Only 3 out of 53 pet owners died within one year of admission for coronary heart disease while 11 out of 39 non-pet owners died during the same period. Amazingly, that remarkable difference in survival rates was independent of physiological status. That is to say, no matter how sick the patient was, he or she was likely to fare better by owning and loving a pet.

Just about anyone can find the wonderful benefits of pet ownership. A study at San Diego State University demonstrated that petting a dog lowered blood pressure even more than resting or reading a book. The subjects studied who had the best attitudes toward their pets tended to have lower blood pressures across the board.

DRUG TREATMENT

The benefits of all the non-drug methods of controlling blood pressure we've discussed cannot be disputed. All contribute to substantial improvement and should be included in your complete program of recovery. But some patients, despite their best efforts and intentions, are unable to bring their blood pressures to a safe level without the aid of prescription drugs.

Your first reaction may be quite negative, since antihypertensive drugs have received a lot of bad publicity owing to adverse reactions such as fatigue, irritability, and, most notorious, impotence. Rest assured that tremendous progress has been made since the early days of treating high blood pressure with drugs.

No doubt the most important factor is having a good doctor–patient relationship so you can work out the best possible drug treatment as part of a complete blood pressure control program. While one patient may do very well with a given drug, another will respond negatively. Some simply give up, refusing to take medications at all. That's the wrong approach. Instead, you'll have to find a drug or drugs tailored to your specific needs.

At the risk of being redundant, it's vital to remember that there are no symptoms of hypertension. Just because you feel fine doesn't mean that you can stop taking your medications. In fact, that's the single biggest problem facing doctors and their patients. It's vital, literally in many cases a matter of life and death, to remain on the drugs your doctor has prescribed.

By all means you'll want to do everything in your power to keep the drugs needed to a minimum. You can do that by controlling your weight, getting plenty of exercise, quitting the cigarettes, curbing stress, and limiting your alcohol and salt intake. But the drugs may give you the edge in keeping hypertension at bay.

You'll find a complete listing of antihypertensive drugs used in medical treatment today in chapter 16. But I'd like to provide a brief overview of just how the drugs work and the various categories your doctor may prescribe for you.

First, you might ask, is taking antihypertensive drugs really worthwhile? Since you don't feel any different, can you expect real benefits? The answer is an unequivocal yes.

Drug therapy to reduce blood pressure definitely decreases cardiovascular morbidity and mortality in those with diastolic blood pressures of more than 104. Studies of patients with mild hypertension, from 90 to 104, have shown that antihypertensive drugs protect against stroke, congestive heart failure, increases in hypertension severity, and all-cause mortality. And a 30- to 50-percent reduction in both fatal and nonfatal strokes has been demonstrated in those taking medications. Needless to say, if one can prove the benefits of drugs so clearly in even mild cases of hypertension, the health advantages for patients with moderate and severe hypertension are even greater.

Be patient. Expect a period of trial and error as you and your doctor work together to find the winning combination of drug and non-drug therapy. Don't be discouraged. Ask all the questions you want, make sure you understand the dosages and the schedules your doctor wants you to try. Find out if there are certain side effects or adverse reactions that you should be aware of. Let your doctor know if you're taking any other drugs, since one drug may interact with another. Find out whether taking the drug while driving a car, working on hazardous equipment, or drinking alcohol is OK. In other words, become an active participant in your treatment.

Doctors most often initiate antihypertensive drug therapy with diuretics. These "water pills" lower your blood pressure by eliminating excess sodium and fluid the body would otherwise retain. By cutting down on the amount of fluid in the bloodstream, pressure in the arteries decreases.

At least for the first few days you'll find yourself needing to urinate frequently. That's because there's been a buildup of fluid in your tissues. This will lessen over time. To avoid the need to wake up with a "bathroom call" in the middle of the night, don't take your diuretic after about six in the evening.

For the most part, diuretics don't pose significant problems, but the right dosage schedule is important. In the summer, for example, you may find that you lose more fluid than desired. This could lead to feeling light-headed or faint.

Because diuretics sometimes wash away potassium, you may be asked to eat more potassium-rich foods such as bananas, oranges, and potatoes. Your doctor may even prescribe a potassium supplement. Again, each patient is different, and it's important to keep your doctor informed on your progress and any difficulties you're experiencing.

One distinct disadvantage of the diuretics is that they tend to elevate cholesterol levels in the blood. You'll want to have your cholesterol count measured regularly to make sure this does not get out of control.

Diuretics are often prescribed in combination with other drugs. That's because they help those other drugs work more effectively, and thus they keep the necessary dosage to a minimum.

Drugs in the category of sympatholytics act on the sympathetic nervous system. They lower blood pressure by reducing the amount of blood the heart pumps and decreasing the heart rate so your heart doesn't work so hard. Other drugs in this classification work by relaxing the blood vessels indirectly by blocking nervous system signals that cause them to contract.

Drugs known as vasodilators relax blood vessels directly, causing a widening of the lumen and allowing blood to flow more easily. They have a particular advantage for patients whose arteries are blocked by cholesterol buildup.

ACE inhibitors are the newest drugs in the antihypertension arsenal. ACE stands for angiotensin converting enzyme. By reducing the production of angiotensin, a chemical produced in the kidney which controls blood pressure, one can regulate hypertension.

Here's another incentive for you to work as hard as possible to get that blood pressure down: for patients with mild hypertension who have controlled their blood pressure for at least one year, doctors are now advising a stepwise reduction in drugs. This will be particularly effective if you've made some of those lifestyle modifications we've discussed. Conversely, if you don't keep up the good work with those non-drug approaches, you may find that you'll have to return to medications.

The progress made in controlling hypertension during the past 20 years has been nothing short of spectacular. Blood pressure reduction has resulted in a substantial reduction in the incidence of and deaths from strokes. While it has had much less effect on coronary heart disease when viewed alone, together with cholesterol reduction and other lifestyle modifications, controlling hypertension can significantly improve your chances for cutting your risks. This is definitely a risk factor that you can take charge of in a very positive way. It's a major step forward in your complete recovery from heart disease.

THE EIGHTH STEP:

Mastering Medications

CHAPTER 16
The Cardiac Pharmacy

I t's almost certain that your doctor has prescribed special medications for you as a heart patient. Some will be taken on a temporary basis, while you might need to take others for the rest of your life. And it's just as certain that you're more than a bit confused about those pills, capsules, tablets, and whatnot.

Cardiac medications comprise a major segment of the entire pharmaceutical industry. There are hundreds of choices for your doctor to make in prescribing just the right drugs to put you on the road to recovery. What do the drugs do? How do they work? Why do you need this particular dosage? What about potential side effects? Will the medications interact with other drugs? How about with foods? Is it really important to take each and every dose? And if you miss a dose, should you take two the next time?

I took these and other questions to a man with the answers, a man who could help me sort through the vast amount of information available on each and every drug. Hiro Nishi, Pharm.D., is Senior Pharmacist at Daniel Freeman Memorial Hospital in Inglewood, California. When I told him what I wanted for my readers, his first reaction was, "Bob, you could write a whole book on that! It could be huge!"

The problem, indeed, was to limit the amount of information in this chapter. I want to simplify your life, not make it more complicated. So Dr. Nishi and I worked together to provide general guidelines on cardiac medications and specific information on the drugs you're taking. He designed the charts at the end of the chapter so that you can easily find the information you need about your own medications in a moment.

First let me say that no one likes the idea of taking medicine. Just the notion of swallowing this pill or that nostrum makes one feel like a sick person. I understand that feeling entirely, even though my own father was a pharmacist. But there are two things you must keep in mind at all times.

One is that those medications are vital to your recovery and long-term wellness. Many have been introduced only during recent years and are directly responsible for the improved outlook for the heart patient. And the other thing is that by following the steps outlined in this book, you can gradually but dramatically cut back the amount of medication you must take.

So, if you really hate taking those heart medications, the best thing you can do is follow your doctor's prescription to the letter and do everything in your power to convert yourself into a former heart patient.

But just keeping track of your medications can be difficult, especially with so many other things on your mind. To help you with that aspect I'd like to share a trick I learned at the Heart Institute of the Desert in Rancho Mirage, California. The nurses there help patients make their own, individualized medication charts. You can do the same for yourself.

Find a piece of stiff cardboard about the size of a sheet of typing paper. At the top write your name and "heart medications." Tape one of each of the tablets, capsules, and pills you've been prescribed to the cardboard and write the following information alongside each one with the help of your doctor or nurse.

Drug (brand name) _____

(generic name) _____

Take _____

Purpose _____

_____

Precautions _____

Doctor's Comments _____

_____

As an example, you might write that the brand name of your drug is Inderal; its generic name is propranolol. Your doctor might tell you to take the tablet twice daily, once in the morning and once in the evening. The purpose of the drug is to help control blood pressure, to ease arrhythmias, and to slow down the rate of the heart so it won't have to work so hard. Precautions might include a warning not to stop taking the medication abruptly. Your doctor's comments may remind you that this drug might lead to drowsiness. Finally, you may wish to add something you've learned in this chapter to keep it close at hand.

By glancing at your heart medication chart now and then you'll be able to easily keep track of your prescriptions. But, if you're like most patients, you're likely to be taking other medications as well. Another doctor may have prescribed tablets for arthritis, diabetes, or other chronic, long-term conditions. Be certain to tell your cardiologist, and later your personal physician, about *all* the vitamins and medications you take, including those you can buy without a prescription.

On the other side of your heart medication chart, make a daily medication dosage plan. List the drugs you are to take in the morning, those to be taken with lunch, those for the evening, and at whatever special times your doctor might advise. On that dosage plan, include all the medications for the day, including both your heart prescriptions, those for other conditions, and those you buy across the counter.

Each time you have a doctor's appointment, be certain to take your chart in with you. You may have questions about a certain drug. Or your physician may wish to make an alteration in the type or dosage of a particular pill.

Now, certainly you're not going to carry this chart along with you wherever you go throughout the day. But the chart will help you keep them organized in your mind, and, after a while, you'll probably rely on it less and less.

Dr. Nishi offers the following 10 guidelines for all medications. Following these rules will help facilitate your recovery by providing your medications' full benefit, with the least chance of complications.

1. Take medications specifically as directed. This will provide maximum effectiveness with a minimum of side effects.
2. Understand what your medications should do for you. This is the best way to avoid possible adverse reactions.

3. Plan medication taking around your regular routine so that it will become part of your lifestyle.

4. Leave reminders in conspicuous places, such as bathroom, mirror, television set, refrigerator, etc.

5. Keep *all* medications in their original containers labeled with specific directions *even when traveling.* (If you need another bottle to keep, say, at the office, ask the pharmacist to divide the prescription into two identically labeled bottles.)

6. If you consider taking *any* over-the-counter medication, consult your doctor first. Some medications may alter the effectiveness of your prescribed medications.

7. *Never* take anyone else's medications, even if they have the same medical condition that you have. And *never* let anyone take your medications.

8. If you have questions about your medications, talk with your doctor and pharmacist. The more you understand, the more comfortable you'll feel.

9. Be careful not to run out of your medication. Obtain refills *before* you run out. Plan for weekends and holidays.

10. *Never take more* than prescribed, even if you skip a dose. And *never stop* taking your medications without consulting your doctor first.

FOOD AND DRUG INTERACTIONS

Every drug has been developed to achieve a specific goal. But just as an opponent can block a shot in sports, other drugs and certain foods can interact with your cardiac medications. I'll provide a few examples in just a moment, but it would be impractical if not impossible to list every potential combination. That underlines the importance of telling your cardiologist about *all* the other drugs you take regularly or even once in a while. Also make it a point to talk with both your doctor and your pharmacist about potential drug and food interactions.

Cholestyramine and colestipol, drugs given to reduce cholesterol, may interfere with the absorption of other drugs. That's why it's best to take those other drugs four to six hours after the cholesterol drugs.

Two other cholesterol-fighting drugs, clofibrate and gemfibrozil, enhance the action of "blood-thinning" agents that prevent excessive clotting. Your doctor may cut the dosage of the anti-clotting drug to balance the medications.

Niacin, in all its forms, can increase the body's production of uric acid and decrease the body's ability to metabolize glucose. These characteristics could be important for gout patients and diabetes patients, respectively.

Just think of all the drugs in the pharmacy, and consider the combinations. It's mind-boggling! So do remember to talk about those interactions.

And don't forget to discuss foods. Your doctor might temporarily prescribe an antidepressant during your initial recovery. If those medications are in the class known as MAO inhibitors, they can interact with a kitchen full of foods including herring, cheese, sausages, wine, and soy sauce. Taken together, the combination of those foods and drugs can lead to headache, fever, and blood pressure increases.

Beta-blockers work best when taken with food, maximizing their effectiveness. The effectiveness of other antihypertensives and vasodilators, on the other hand, can be impeded by salty foods. And those blood-thinners can work *too* well when taken with boiled or fried onions!

Digitalis preparations are among the oldest cardiac medications. But high-fiber foods may decrease the drugs' effectiveness. Obviously, since you'll want to increase the amount of fiber-rich foods in your diet in order to control cholesterol levels, this dilemma calls for a doctor–patient discussion.

ASPIRIN AND OTHER ANTIPLATELET AGENTS

One of the most frequent immediate causes of a heart attack is the formation of a blood clot which blocks the flow of blood in an already-occluded coronary artery. It's logical, then, to think that preventing excessive clotting could reduce the incidence of heart attacks and strokes. And certainly we've all heard about the wisdom of taking an aspirin a day, or every other day, to ward off the potential of a heart attack, especially for those who have already had an event.

The proof of efficacy came from a study in which 22,000 doctors took either one 350 mg aspirin tablet or a placebo every other day. Those taking the aspirin rather than the placebo had nearly 50 percent fewer heart attacks. In fact, the study was cut short because the benefits of the aspirin regimen were so obvious. That project began in 1982 and was to run until 1990; but when the data were monitored in 1988, preliminary results showed "extreme beneficial effects on nonfatal and fatal myocardial infarction." The researchers decided those findings had to be shared with the world immediately.

Virtually all physicians and researchers agree on the benefits of aspirin in terms of preventing another heart attack. We now have evidence of effectiveness for both men and women. The only question is whether to take it daily or every other day. That will be your doctor's decision, based on your individual medical history and specific considerations. In no case, however, should you decide that if one is good, two must be better. Indeed, that could be harmful.

Especially if you have had bypass surgery, your doctor may have prescribed the drug Persantine (dipyridamole). Like aspirin, this medication is an antiplatelet agent used to prevent clotting. That's particularly important after the surgery to keep the grafted vessels open and flowing. Your doctor may decide to discontinue the Persantine after a period of time.

Take Persantine an hour before meals unless your doctor prescribes otherwise. Other medications may increase or decrease the effects of Persantine. For this reason, don't take anything at all without talking with your doctor first. That's particularly true for preparations containing additional amounts of aspirin.

The third drug in this category is Anturane (sulfinpyrazone). Its purpose and special considerations are similar to those of aspirin and Persantine.

ANTICOAGULANTS

This category of drugs is also designed to prevent clotting. These medications are commonly referred to as "blood thinners." The generic name is warfarin, with brand names Coumadin and Panwarfin. Warfarin, like aspirin and Persantine, lengthens clotting time. It does so by affecting clotting factors in the blood, while aspirin and Persantine act by affecting the function of blood platelets.

Warfarin is often given to patients with certain types of artificial heart valves to reduce the possibility of small clots forming on the valves.

The amount you take will be determined by the results of a "pro-time" blood test. Your doctor will prescribe a standard daily dose or may give you a specific dosage schedule to follow. Take your medication at the same time each day, and do not stop taking it without consulting your physician. You may be taking warfarin for some time, perhaps indefinitely.

If bleeding from a cut continues for several minutes, contact your doctor. Talk with him about signs of unusual bleeding as well, including black stool, pink or red urine, nose bleeds, or bruising with severe swelling.

Do not take aspirin or preparations containing aspirin while taking warfarin. If you have a headache, one of the non-aspirin pain relievers such as Tylenol may be taken instead.

Do not drink excessive amounts of alcohol. More than one or two drinks, or drinking even that amount regularly, can alter the effect of your anticoagulant. Major changes in diet, such as eating unusually large amounts of fish or leafy green vegetables, can alter your response to the drug. Try to keep your diet regular, without binges or splurges.

While these precautions and warnings may sound severe to you now, remember that anticoagulants have been prescribed for many years for thousands of patients. They have major benefits your doctor wants you to get. In a short period of time you and your doctor will work out just the right dosage, and taking this medication will become second nature to you.

NITROGLYCERIN AND NITRATES

I have a deep and abiding respect for nitrates, since I believe these drugs kept me alive during my heart attack in 1978. I experienced that heart attack the night before my scheduled angiogram, and fortunately my cardiologist had put me on a high dosage of nitrates, which are designed to keep the arteries open. Without the effects of those drugs, my attack might very well have been worse.

The nitrates are used mainly for acute relief and prevention of angina pectoris. They work by relaxing the smooth muscle tissue of the blood vessels, resulting in dilation of both veins and arteries. This, in turn, yields increased blood flow and decreased oxygen consumption by the heart. Another effect may be a reduction in both systolic and diastolic blood pressure.

There are a number of ways to deliver nitrates, for either long-term or short-term benefits. Nitroglycerin, which I'll discuss in more detail in a moment, provides a quick burst of vasodilation, but the vessel-opening effect doesn't last long. The long-term nitrates don't have as dramatic an effect, but they keep the vessels open over a longer period of time. Your doctor may prescribe one or more of the nitrates, to be taken as tablets (swallow, don't chew), ointment, skin patches, or sprays.

Contraindications include severe anemia, head trauma, cerebral hemorrhage, and hypersensitivity to nitrates. The drugs can result in postural hypotension, that is, dizziness which occurs when you change position suddenly, such as standing up from a seated position. Since alcohol makes this tendency worse, it's best to avoid or limit drinking. Large nitrate dosage can produce headaches. Talk with your doctor if headache develops; often patients become more tolerant to nitrates.

If you experience angina pectoris, your doctor will very likely prescribe nitroglycerin, either alone or in addition to other nitrates. It enables the heart muscle to get more blood which, in turn, provides more oxygen and relieves the pain.

Unless instructed otherwise, place a nitroglycerin tablet under your tongue at the start of chest pain. You may experience a dull headache, one of the ways you know that the nitroglycerin has gotten into your bloodstream. If your chest pain doesn't go away within five minutes, take another tablet. If pain still persists, after another five minutes take a third tablet. And if that doesn't work, contact your physician. For severe or worsening pain, seek immediate medical attention.

Dr. Nishi offers these tips regarding nitroglycerin usage:

1. Do not drink water with this pill, and don't swallow it. Let it dissolve under your tongue.
2. It's best to sit down or lie down when taking nitroglycerin, as it may cause a temporary drop in blood pressure and resulting dizziness.

3. Don't be concerned about normal side effects including headache, dizziness, a warm flushed feeling, and a burning sensation under the tongue.

4. This medication can easily lose its potency. Don't store in a hot or even very warm place, and keep it out of the sun. Keep nitroglycerin in its original, brown glass container. Studies have shown that even the heat generated by keeping the container in a shirt pocket next to the skin is enough to destroy nitroglycerin's potency.

5. Replace opened bottles of nitroglycerin at least every six months. Properly stored, unopened bottles should be good until the expiration date on the label.

6. If you *don't* get the dull headache that typically occurs when taking nitroglycerin, assume that the pills have lost their potency.

7. Keep bottle top tightly closed.

As with all other medications, discuss nitroglycerin with your doctor or pharmacist. Dr. Nishi recalls a patient who claimed he had no questions, and fully understood all his medications. Then the pharmacist spotted the patient's nitroglycerin on a windowsill in direct sunlight. After mentioning that, a 15- to 20-minute discussion and Q&A session followed.

BETA-BLOCKERS

Here's another case where a drug has been scientifically demonstrated to decrease the likelihood of a subsequent heart attack following an initial event. Nine out of ten studies have shown that beta-blocking drugs, which interfere with nervous stimulation of cells in the heart called beta-adrenergicreceptors, increase heart attack patients' chances of survival. The beta-blockers literally slow down the beat of the heart. Since it doesn't work as hard at the slower rate, the heart muscle needs less oxygen. And since oxygen-deficit to the heart muscle is the heart patient's biggest concern, the beta-blockers help to prevent angina attacks as well as heart attacks.

It's interesting to note that some doctors and medical students have been known to "pop" a beta-blocker tablet just before delivering a presentation. Why? The medication prevents the rapidly beating, pounding heart that many people experience when they have to do any public speaking. You may find this to be a very pleasant "side effect" of the drug.

Despite the generally good publicity in the medical literature, beta-blockers have received their share of criticism. First, studies have shown that the drugs can lower the levels of the protective HDL cholesterol, thus balancing out the beneficial effects. Second, since beta-blockers slow down heartbeat, will they interfere with the goals of exercise in the recovery process? Fortunately, studies have demonstrated that even those taking the drugs continue to achieve the benefits accruing to physical exercise. On the other hand, it may be possible to duplicate the benefits of the beta-blockers merely by doing sufficient exercise regularly to slow the heart rate at rest. Again, we have research data to prove that this can be achieved by patients who do strenuous exercise on a regular basis. In those studies, exercise and drugs had a similar effect on resting heart rate.

But the biggest controversy regards the length of time beta-blockers should be prescribed. The protection against subsequent heart attack has been proved for only the critical six months to a year after the initial event. After that, critics maintain, there's just no reason to continue the drug.

On the other hand, beta-blockers also have an antihypertensive effect. That alone may be reason enough for your doctor to want you to stay on the medication beyond the first year. Talk with him about it. And, of course, if you demonstrate that your exercise program is paying off with improved resting heart rates, decreased blood pressure, and fewer problems with angina pectoris, it's likely that your doctor will go along with gradually cutting down the dosage and perhaps even eliminating it altogether.

But here's a strong note of caution: Do not stop taking beta-blockers abruptly or without your physician's consent. There have been instances of patients stopping their dosage suddenly and suffering a heart attack as a result.

CALCIUM-CHANNEL BLOCKERS

Calcium-channel blockers, also known as calcium antagonists, seem to work by preventing or slowing the flow of calcium into muscle cells. Calcium activates contraction of muscle, so if it is blocked, cardiac and arterial muscle will not contract as much. This is an obvious benefit for the patient, as a strong contraction in the coronary artery may be enough to totally occlude the flow of blood, especially when the artery is already compromised by the buildup of cholesterol-laden plaque. The actions of calcium-channel blockers make them useful in managing angina, hypertension, and arrhythmias.

Research reports in the medical literature have shown the following benefits derived from calcium blockers: They improve coronary flow, suppress arrhythmias, diminish cell damage in the heart muscle during times of oxygen deficit, reduce platelet aggregation, and reduce excessive growth of the left ventricle caused by excessive work resulting from the need to beat rapidly to provide oxygen. As with beta-blockers, there has been some evidence that prescribing calcium blockers can reduce the incidence of subsequent heart attack. However, the data are not as clear, and some controversy remains. Again, this will be your doctor's decision as to which medication to prescribe.

ACE INHIBITORS

This classification of drugs includes three brands which are listed in the charts at the end of this chapter. These drugs are prescribed for patients with hypertension and heart failure. They work by inhibiting the production of an enzyme (angiotensin-converting enzyme) involved in the increase of blood pressure. Without as much of the enzyme released into the bloodstream, less angiotensin II is produced. The latter is a hormone which triggers blood pressure to go up.

ACE inhibitors help to keep blood vessels open rather than constricted, thus limiting the demands placed on the heart to beat to supply oxygen. For those patients whose left ventricles have been damaged, and thus have to work particularly hard to provide needed oxygen, this is a particular benefit. By slowing down the workload of the ventricles, the excessive thickening of the heart wall is retarded, thus diminishing the progress of heart failure.

Should a cough or cold occur when taking the ACE inhibitors, you should *not* take a cough medication that contains pseudoephedrine or phenylpropanolamine (read the labels), since they may cause rises in blood pressure due to vasoconstriction. Discuss this important consideration with your doctor if you develop a cough. Cough medicine can also interfere with the action of the ACE inhibitors.

Women may experience an itching in the external genitals area after starting to take ACE inhibitors. While this is a rare occurrence, it's worth mentioning since otherwise the patient might not associate the two.

DIGITALIS/DIGOXIN/CARDIAC GLYCOSIDES

In the years before modern medicine, "witch doctors" in England gave their clients a preparation made from the leaves of the foxglove plant to aid their failing hearts. Doctors of the day scorned the practice, but today we know that foxglove is the natural source of the drug digitalis, long a mainstay in the treatment of heart disease.

Digitalis belongs in the class of drugs known as cardiac glycosides. Today potent synthetics known as digoxin and digitoxin predominate.

Digitalis increases venous tone, increases renal blood flow, slows heart rate, and increases the contracting force of the heart muscle. The result of all its actions is increased efficiency for the heart's work.

Digoxin and digitoxin are given orally, as tablets or capsules. Prescribing just the right amount is both an art and science, and your doctor will work with you to zero in on the precisely correct dosage. It's important that you follow his prescription to the letter, taking neither more nor less than directed. An extra dose may lead to cardiac disturbances, while stopping the drug may lead to heart failure. Dr. Nishi recalls one cardiac rehab patient who did well, was discharged, and then was readmitted to the hospital after several days because he had taken extra doses of his digoxin.

We've talked before about food and drug interactions. In the case of digoxin, there is an interaction between the drug and exercise. Everyday exercise, even walking, can cause up to a one-third drop in digoxin levels. The converse is also true. Active people who stop exercising suddenly, for example during the flu, can experience a one-third rise in levels.

This, too, shows the need for working closely with your doctor. Talk about your exercise program; include normal exercise plans as well as occasional bursts of activity. Your physician will conduct digoxin-level testing to make certain that you're taking just the right amount.

ANTIARRHYTHMIC AGENTS

The healthy heart is a finely tuned instrument, beating in a very predictable manner throughout life. It is so predictable, in fact, that your cardiologist can determine a great deal about its health simply by looking at the paper tracing produced during an electrocardiogram (ECG) as the pumping action renders easily recognized waves and blips. But this rhythm can become abnormal in a number of ways.

Just as there are a vast array of arrhythmias, there are a large number of drugs from which your doctor may choose. Some of the medications are specifically designed to treat arrhythmias, while others control heartbeat as one of their functions. The beta-blockers, for example, not only slow the rate of the heartbeat, but control its rhythm as well. It may be necessary for you and your doctor to experiment with more than just one of those potential drugs before finding the ideal treatment. Your doctor may choose not to prescribe any antiarrhythmic agent at all, even though you are uncomfortable with the arrhythmias you experience. That's because studies have shown serious problems with certain drugs, and there has been question as to the value of medications to treat arrhythmias that are not life-threatening. Again, its a matter of teamwork, and it's important for you to follow the prescription to the letter rather than deciding on your own that you need more today or less tomorrow.

ANTIHYPERTENSIVE AGENTS

To treat, or not to treat, that is the question. Some doctors believe that all patients with high blood pressure should be treated, even if their conditions are mild. Others disagree, pointing to the potential effects of diet and exercise alone, and citing data which show no particular therapeutic advantage to taking the drugs.

There's no question, however, that hypertension is one of the major risk factors in heart disease and should be controlled in order to prevent future cardiac events. This is especially true for women, who do far worse following heart attack or bypass if their blood pressures are even slightly elevated. Blacks, too, are at increased risk when hypertension enters the equation.

Mild hypertension can be defined as a blood pressure of 140–160 systolic over 90–100 diastolic. This range describes 80 percent of the hypertensive population.

Norman Kaplan, M.D., is chief of the hypertension division at the University of Texas Health Science Center in Dallas. He voices the concern of many in the medical community about the benefits of treating mild hypertension with drugs.

"The data on the treatment of mild hypertension and protection against coronary heart disease are simply nonexistent," he explained at a meeting of the American Heart Association. "In four of the nine studies conducted to compare hypertension treatment with nontreatment, the benefits were seen on the wrong side, that is the nontreatment side of the study. There has simply been no significant decrease in coronary mortality among the treated population of mild hypertensives. Lowering blood pressure to the lowest possible level simply may not be in the best interests of our patients."

One of the most common ways to treat hypertension is with diuretic drugs. But diuretics may cause a rise in cholesterol levels. Moreover, diabetic patients may suffer owing to decreased glucose tolerance.

Moreover, even if one has been taking hypertension medications, is it necessary to remain on the drugs for life? Once it was believed that such therapy would need to be continued forever. Now some experts are saying that many patients can safely quit their medications or at least cut way back on the dosage.

But that's possible *only* when the patient takes an active role in the management of blood pressure. And that means weight control, proper diet including salt and sodium restriction if sensitive to sodium, and regular physical exercise.

As you can probably tell, I believe in the least possible medication, relying as much as practical on diet and exercise. But there certainly are patients for whom drugs will be necessary even when doing their very best with non-drug methods. For those with very high blood pressure which does not entirely respond to diet and exercise, there are a wide variety of drugs the physician can choose to bring the condition under control.

Remember that regardless of the means used to achieve the end, control of hypertension is essential to prevent future cardiac events. Discuss these matters with your physician. Talk about the different drugs listed in the chart at the end of this chapter and listen to why one or another might be the choice for you. Then follow your doctor's prescription exactly. Don't forget that after a while you may be able to cut that dosage down through your program of weight control, diet, and exercise. But do *not* alter your medication dosage without your physician's prior permission.

POTASSIUM REPLACEMENT PRODUCTS

One of the expected adverse reactions of taking diuretics to control hypertension is loss of potassium from the blood through the urine. Potassium is essential in protecting the heart's muscular wall, and must be replaced.

Natural sources of potassium in the diet include oranges, bananas, potatoes, melons, and dried fruits. See Table 10 (page 382) for a listing of foods and their potassium contents. Moreover, salt substitutes pack a lot of potassium, as shown in Table 11.

Your doctor may also feel that you need a supplemental source of potassium. This is one nutrient that you can't purchase without a prescription. There are many brands on the market, as tablets, liquids, capsules, and effervescent tablets.

Unfortunately, all potassium replacement products can cause stomach upset. That's why it's best to take them with a meal. Many patients

TABLE 10
Food Sources of Potassium

Food	Amount	Potassium (mg)
Honeydew melon	¼ melon	940
Potato (baked)	1 medium	844
Dried figs	5 whole	666
Prunes	10 medium	626
Dates	10 whole	541
Tomato puree	½ cup	525
Dried apricots	10 halves	482
Banana	1 medium	451
Winter squash	½ cup	445
Raisins	⅓ cup	375
Lima beans	½ cup	370
Cantaloupe	¼ melon	341
Orange (navel)	1 medium	250
Strawberries	1 cup	247

object to the taste, and you may have to taste-test a few brands to see which is most palatable.

Potassium replacements are not as benign as other nutritional supplements. That's why they're not sold without a prescription. If you experience severe nausea and/or vomiting, severe stomach pain, black stools, or weakness or tingling in the hands or feet, be certain to report to your doctor.

Talk with your doctor about combining the potassium replacements prescribed with potassium-rich foods and salt substitutes. That way you'll need less of the prescription product.

While the nutrients in foods are listed in milligrams (mg), the potas-

TABLE 11
Potassium Content of Salt Substitutes

Salt Substitute (one tsp)	Potassium (mg/mEq)
Morton Lite Salt	1500/38
Morton Salt Substitute	2800/72
No Salt	2500/64
No Salt (Seasoned)	1330/34

sium content of prescription potassium replacement products is measured in milliequivalents (mEq). Each milliequivalent is equal to 39 milligrams.

You'll need to do a bit of arithmetic to see how much food you'd need to match a given prescription product. Let's say that an orally taken liquid has 10 mEq per tablespoonful. That is the same as 390 mg. You can get that much from a ½-cup serving of lima beans.

Added to food, salt substitutes can provide a significant amount of potassium and can be used instead of some of the prescribed potassium replacement. A note of caution: excessive use while also taking a potassium replacement could lead to a condition termed hyperkalemia in which abnormally high levels of potassium are concentrated in the blood. This is a particular concern if you're taking the potassium-sparing diuretics. Talk with your doctor or pharmacist about this.

MEDICATIONS FOR CONTROLLING CHOLESTEROL AND TRIGLYCERIDES

Like hypertension, high cholesterol levels pose one of the major risks for heart disease. Left uncontrolled and elevated, cholesterol continues to clog the arteries and the disease progresses. But, as with hypertension, you can do much to control cholesterol without drugs.

The first line of defense, once again, is a prudent program of diet and exercise. We've talked about the details before. You've seen the data proving that heart disease can be stopped dead in its tracks and maybe even reversed with the right kind of program.

But some of us simply can't do the job alone. Our bloodstreams contain increased amounts of cholesterol and triglycerides even though we cut back on the foods which raise those levels. Fortunately, there are a number of agents at our disposal to lower our levels into a safe zone.

Let me summarize what I've said earlier, however, as to what a truly safe range is for the person who has already had a heart attack or bypass surgery. It's just not good enough to settle for a cholesterol level under 200. That might slow the process down a bit, but it won't stop it and it absolutely won't make it go in the opposite direction.

To do that takes more effort. Heart patients must shoot for cholesterol levels well under 180, preferably even lower, ideally down in the

140–160 range. In terms of the subfractions of cholesterol, the "bad" LDL cholesterol should be down around 100 or so, not just below 140 (which is the target for the general population). For men, the "good" HDL should be no lower than 45 and for women the number is 50. And while triglycerides have not been shown to be as much a risk as cholesterol, it's best to keep those numbers under 200, preferably down around 150 to be on the safe side.

Don't be fooled by your cholesterol levels shortly after your heart attack or bypass. Levels tend to drop dramatically for a while. Many patients think they don't have a problem when they get their test results. But the levels return to pre-heart attack or pre-bypass points two to three months later.

Once you've established what your cholesterol levels really are, for total, LDL, and HDL as well as for triglycerides (those all are collectively termed lipids), then try your level best to get those counts down as low as possible with your diet and exercise program. Take a closer look at chapter 13, and perhaps you'd like to read *The 8-Week Cholesterol Cure* for more detail.

After giving the diet–exercise a fair trial and finding that your lipids are still elevated, your doctor very well may want to put you on one of the agents known to reduce cholesterol. There's a fairly wide choice available.

NIACIN/NICOTINIC ACID

Technically niacin is a vitamin, a necessary nutrient in everyone's diet. But in very high doses, many times the required daily allowance (RDA) for the nutrient value, niacin can be a very effective cholesterol fighter. Niacin is available in pharmacies and health food stores, and is also known as nicotinic acid. Note that *only* niacin, and not the niacinamide form of the vitamin, works to lower cholesterol levels. And although you can purchase niacin without a prescription, at the high doses needed for effectiveness you require medical supervision. Never take niacin without your doctor's permission.

Niacin decreases the liver's manufacture of VLDL, a precursor of LDL, thus limiting the production of LDL. At the same time, it raises levels of HDL and lowers triglycerides. It performs that combination of benefits better than any other substance available, with or without a prescription. As such, the National Cholesterol Education Program has listed it as a first-choice agent in cholesterol control.

Only niacin has been shown effective in lowering another risk-predicting lipid in the blood known as lipoprotein(a), abbreviated as Lp(a). Neither diet nor prescription cholesterol-lowering drugs can lower Lp(a).

Unfortunately, not everyone can take niacin. First there are a number of contraindications including past or present liver dysfunction, diabetes, gout, severe arrhythmias, and ulcers. Second, some side effects may occur which would prevent patients from taking the large doses needed. Gastric upset may be overcome by taking niacin with meals. And the flushing which typically follows niacin's entering the bloodstream can be limited by preceding the dose with a half tablet of aspirin about 20 to 30 minutes before. Moreover, sustained-release tablets have been developed which reduce or even eliminate the flushing for most patients.

The brand of niacin I personally have taken for many years with excellent results is called Endur-acin. This formulation is a sustained-release preparation which has been studied in detail by Dr. Joseph Keenan at the University of Minnesota. He reported his work in the *Archives of Internal Medicine* in 1991.

A total of 158 patients, both men and women, completed the study. They began with a diet providing 30 percent of calories as fat and limiting cholesterol to no more than 300 milligrams daily. And they were given varying dosages of Endur-acin or placebos. Subjects receiving 1500 milligrams (1½ grams) of Endur-acin had a 19 percent fall in LDL cholesterol and a 10 percent rise in HDL. This resulted in a very dramatic improvement of the cholesterol risk ratio. Smaller dosages were not as effective, and doses of 2000 mg (2 grams) produced no greater benefit.

Patients taking standard rather than slow-release niacin typically need more than 1500 mg to achieve the desired effect. In a well-publicized study showing reversal of blockage in the arteries, Dr. David Blankenhorn at the University of Southern California gave patients an average of 4.3 grams of niacin along with the prescription drug colestipol. Some doctors have given patients as much as eight or nine grams daily. It will be up to your own physician to determine if you're a good candidate for niacin therapy and, if so, what kind and how much you should use. (Endur-acin is available only by mail order. For order information write to Endurance Products Company at P.O. Box 230489, Tigard, OR 97281-0489, or call 503-684-8506.)

If you'd like your doctor to learn about the benefits of Endur-acin, have him send a request on his letterhead to the Endurance Products Company. They will send your doctor a reprint of Dr. Keenan's article.

Let me repeat: do not take niacin without medical permission and supervision. Niacin works at the site of the liver where cholesterol is manufactured, and it places an additional burden on that organ as it is metabolized. Some studies have shown that slow-release niacin is harder on the liver than standard niacin. It would appear that while smaller doses of sustained-release niacin can achieve the cholesterol-lowering effects of larger doses of standard niacin, one can also expect the potential liver toxicity of larger doses. Reports have shown that those who switch from standard niacin to an equal dosage of slow-release niacin may have problems. Your doctor will need to study your liver function by way of a simple blood test to determine whether your body is properly handling the niacin. Moreover, your doctor will decide which form of niacin is best for you, and at what dosage.

If you or your physician would like additional information about niacin, I've devoted an entire chapter to it in *The 8-Week Cholesterol Cure*.

BILE SEQUESTRANT DRUGS

The two brands of medications in this category (Questran [cholestyramine] and Colestid [colestipol]) work by binding onto the bile acids your body produces in the digestive tract and shunting them out along with your bowel movement. They are also called the resin drugs. The National Cholesterol Education Program has also listed these medications as first-choice agents for treating those for whom dietary efforts at lowering cholesterol levels have failed.

Most typically the drugs are prescribed as a powder or in granules which are mixed with water or juices and gulped down two or three times daily. A "candy" bar form is also available. Unfortunately, the taste is not pleasant, and patient compliance may be low as a result. And there may be some gastrointestinal upset.

The resin drugs may also bind onto other medications you may be taking, thus rendering them useless or at least causing them to be absorbed less efficiently. Thus you should take the two drugs with as much time in between as possible.

The combination of niacin with resin drugs has been tested a number of times and has been shown to be particularly effective.

FIBRIC ACID DERIVATIVES

While two drugs are in this category, only one is normally prescribed. Lopid (gemfibrozil) works very well at reducing triglyceride levels, though its cholesterol-controlling capabilities are not as good as those of other drugs. On the other hand, Lopid has been shown to increase the level of HDL cholesterol. The Helsinki Heart Study in Finland showed a significantly lower incidence of heart attacks in men taking this drug, and the benefits have been largely ascribed to the HDL effect.

The typical dosage is 600 mg taken twice daily. There are few side effects, and patients tolerate the drug well with good compliance.

The other drug in this classification is Atromid-S (clofibrate). It has fallen out of use with most doctors because of a report of an increase in mortality from taking the drug during a World Health Organization study.

PROBUCOL

This drug is the only one in the category. Probucol is the generic name, and the brand name is Lorelco. Once used more widely owing to its effectiveness in reducing cholesterol and its low incidence of side effects or adverse reactions, probucol has dropped by the wayside because it significantly lowers levels of the protective HDL. As I discussed in the chapter on cholesterol, probucol has been shown to decrease cholesterol oxidation. As a result of that study, the drug has received some recent attention.

HMG-CoA REDUCTASE INHIBITORS

I won't trouble you with the full spelling of this one. Suffice it to say that drugs in this category decrease synthesis of cholesterol by the liver by partially inhibiting an enzyme necessary for its production.

The first drug to receive FDA approval in this category was lovastatin (Mevacor, Merck). More than one million patients now take the drug in daily doses of 20 mg, 40 mg, or more depending on the severity of cholesterol elevation.

The major advantage of Mevacor is that, in most cases, only one or two tablets per day will do the job very effectively. The drug is easy to take and patients report few if any side effects at the lower dosages. However, since Mevacor, like niacin, works in the liver, it could possibly do some damage there. Thus your doctor will have to do regular liver function tests to make sure you're tolerating the drug well. The most serious side effect has been an inflammation of muscles; fortunately, that adverse reaction is quite rare.

Dosage typically begins with one tablet, taken with the evening meal. That's because most of the body's cholesterol gets made in the evening and night hours. If one 20-mg tablet doesn't get the cholesterol level low enough, the dosage may be increased to two tablets, and perhaps up to a maximum of 80 mg daily.

As this is a very new medication, we don't have a long-term track record for it. However, millions of prescriptions have already been written, and the drug appears to be safe and effective at least at low dosages typically prescribed.

One of the major limitations of Mevacor is its high price. This medication can, depending on dosage, cost $2000 a year or even more.

A second and third drug in this category were approved by the FDA in 1991. Pravastatin (Pravachol) and simvastatin (Zocor) are prescribed to be taken once a day at bedtime. The effects are similar to those achieved with Mevacor. Side effects are also similar, and regular liver function testing is necessary.

Both Mevacor and Pravachol have been shown to be particularly effective when prescribed in combination with bile sequestrant drugs, either cholestyramine or colestipol. And both require the patient to follow a low-fat, low-cholesterol diet in addition to taking medication.

Antiplatelet Agents

Medication	Brand Name	Type/Purpose	Special Instructions	Expected Side Effects	Side Effects to Report to M.D.
DIPYRIDAMOLE	Persantine	Inhibits the clotting of platelets	Take 1 hour before meals	Transient dizziness	Flushing, skin rash
ASPIRIN	ASA, Bayer, Ecotrin, Bufferin, Empirin, Alka Seltzer, cold remedies	Same as above	May cause upset stomach; take with food or after meals		Unusual bleeding (black or bloody stools), stomach pain, bronchospasm, skin rash
SULFINPYRAZONE	Anturane	Same as above	May cause upset stomach; take with food, milk, or antacids Avoid aspirin-containing products Drink plenty of water		Same as above

Potassium Replacement Products

Medication	Brand Name	Type/Purpose	Special Instructions	Expected Side Effects	Side Effects to Report to M.D.
POTASSIUM CHLORIDE (KCL) POTASSIUM GLUCONATE POTASSIUM BICARONATE/ CITRATE	K-Dur, Klotrix, K-tab, Slow-K, Ten-K, K-Lor, Micro-K, Kato, Kaochlor, Kay Ciel, Kolyum, K-lyte/Cl, Kaon, K-lyte, Klor-Con, etc.	Potassium supplement	May cause upset stomach; take after meals or w/ food w/ a full glass of water Liquids, powders, effervescent tabs: mix and dissolve in water/beverage	Stomach discomfort	Severe nausea/ vomiting, stomach pain, black stools, weakness, tingling of hands or feet
NITROGLYCERIN	Nitrostat	Angina—acute attack or prevention (sublingual tablets)	Sit, dissolve under the tongue, may repeat every 5 minutes × 3. Protect bottle from light/heat	Headache, dizziness, flushing	Call MD if pain not relieved after 3 doses Blurred vision, dry mouth, persistent headaches
	Nitrolingual	Angina—acute attack or prevention (sublingual spray)	Sit, spray under tongue; may repeat every 5 min. Do not inhale spray	Same as above	Same as above
	Nitrogard	Angina (buccal, controlled-release tablets)	Place tablet between lip and gum above incisors, or between cheek and gum	Same as above	Blurred vision, dry mouth, persistent headaches

	Nitro-Bid, Nitro-span, Nitroglyn	Angina (Oral, sustained-release capsules)	Take on empty stomach w/ water. Swallow whole, do not chew	Same as above	Blurred vision, dry mouth, persistent headaches
	Transderm-Nitro, Nitro-Dur, Nitro-disc, Deponit	Angina (transdermal patches)	Apply to clean, hair-free site; use different site daily	Same as above. Warmth and/or redness at the site	Blurred vision, dry mouth, persistent headaches
	Nitrol, Nitro-Bid, Nitrostat	Angina (topical ointment)	Apply, using applicator papers. Rotate sites. Avoid getting on fingers	Same as above	Blurred vision, dry mouth, persistent headaches
AMYL NITRITE	Amyl Nitrite Vaporole, Aspirols, (inhalant)	Angina—acute attack	Crush capsule and wave under nose; 1 to 6 whiffs from 1 capsule are usually sufficient	Headache, dizziness, flushing	Call MD if pain not relieved (may repeat in 3 to 5 minutes)
ISOSORBIDE DINITRATE	Isordil, Sorbitrate (chewable and sublingual)	Angina—acute attack and prevention	Usually taken every 2 to 3 hrs	Same as above	Call MD if pain not relieved. Blurred vision, dry mouth, persistent headaches
	Isordil, Sorbitrate (oral tablets)	Angina	Take on empty stomach with water	Same as above	Same as above

continued

Potassium Replacement Products *(continued)*

Medication	Brand Name	Type/Purpose	Special Instructions	Expected Side Effects	Side Effects to Report to M.D.
ERYTHRITAL-TETRANI-TRATE	Cardilate (sublingual and oral tablets)	Angina	Oral tablets—take on empty stomach with water	Same as above	Same as above
PENTA-ERYTHRITAL-TETRANI-TRATE	Peritrate, P.E.T.N. (oral tablets, sustained-release tablets and capsules)	Angina	Tablets: take ½ hr before or 1 hr after meals Sustained-release: take on empty stomach	Same as above	Same as above

392

Beta-Blockers

Medication	Brand Name	Type/Purpose	Special Instructions	Expected Side Effects	Side Effects to Report to M.D.
ACEBUTOLOL	Sectral	Arrhythmias Hypertension	Do not stop medications abruptly, except on advice of MD	Fatigue, transient drowsiness and dizziness	Dizziness, symptoms, of congestive heart failure, confusion, slow pulse rate, bronchospasm, skin rash
ATENOLOL	Ternormin	Angina, M.I. Hypertension	Same as above	Same as above	Same as above
BETAXOLOL	Kerlone	Hypertension	Same as above	Same as above	Same as above
CARTEOLOL	Cartrol	Hypertension	Save as above	Same as above	Same as above
LABETALOL	Trandate, Normodyne	Hypertension	Same as above	Same as above	Same as above
METOPROLOL*	Lopressor	Angina, M.I. Hypertension	Same as above	Same as above	Same as above
NADOLOL	Corgard	Angina Hypertension	Same as above	Same as above	Same as above
PENBUTOLOL	Levatol	Arterial hypertension	Same as above	Same as above	Same as above
PINDOLOL	Visken	Hypertension	Same as above	Same as above	Same as above

*Food enhances the absorption of Metoprolol and Propranolol

continued

Beta-Blockers *(continued)*

Medication	Brand Name	Type/Purpose	Special Instructions	Expected Side Effects	Side Effects to Report to M.D.
PROPRANOLOL*	Inderal (tablets, liquid) Inderal LA (sus- tained-release capsules)	Angina, M.I. Hypertension Arrhythmias IHSS and others	Same as above	Same as above	Same as above
TIMOLOL	Blocadren	Hypertension M.I.	Same as above	Same as above	Same as above

*Food enhances the absorption of Metoprolol and Propranolol

Calcium-Channel Blockers

Medication	Brand Name	Type/Purpose	Special Instructions	Expected Side Effects	Side Effects to Report to M.D.
NIFEDIPINE	Procardia, Adalat Procardia XL	Angina Hypertension	XL: swallow whole, do not crush or chew. Empty tablet may appear in the stool	Flushing, headache, dizziness	Shortness of breath, irregular heartbeat, swelling of hands or feet, pronounced dizziness
DILTIAZEM	Cardizem Cardizem SR	Angina Hypertension	Take before meals	Headache, dizziness	Same as above
VERAPAMIL	Calan, Isoptin Calan SR, Isoptin SR Verelan	Angina, arrhythmias Hypertension	Take with meals	Constipation, dizziness	Same as above
NICARDIPINE	Cardene	Angina Hypertension		Flushing, headache, dizziness	Same as above
ISADIPINE	DynaCirc	Hypertension		Headache, flushing	Same as above
BEPRIDIL	Vascor	Angina	May be taken with meals if nausea experienced	Upset stomach, drowsiness	Same as above

Angiotensin Converting Enzymes (ACE) Inhibitors

Medication	Brand Name	Type/Purpose	Special Instructions	Expected Side Effects	Side Effects to Report to M.D.
CAPTOPRIL	Capoten	Hypertension Heart failure	Take 1 hour before meals Avoid cough/cold/allergy meds except on recommendation of MD Do not stop med w/o MD knowledge	Initial dizziness, taste alteration	Rash, fever, cough, sore throat, mouth sores, irregular heartbeat, chest pain, swelling of extremities
ENALAPRIL	Vasotec	Hypertension Heart failure	Avoid cough/cold/allergy meds except on recommendation of MD Do not stop med w/o MD knowledge	Same as above	Same as above
LISINOPRIL	Prinivil Zestril	Hypertension	Same as above	Same as above	Same as above

Oral Antiarrhythmic Agents

Medication Name & Group	Brand Name	Type/Purpose	Special Instructions	Expected Side Effects	Side Effects to Report to M.D.
I. MORIZICINE	Ethmozine	Helps regulate heart rhythm		Transient, dizziness, headache	Nausea/vomiting, heart rhythm or pulse changes, dizziness
IA. QUINIDINE	Quinora Cin-Quin Quinidex Quinaglute Cardioquin	Same as above	Take with food	Upset stomach, diarrhea	Ringing in ears, dizziness, headache, visual disturbances
IA. PROCAIN-AMIDE	Pronestyl Procan-SR	Same as above	Do not break or chew sustained-release (SR) products	Upset stomach	Nausea/vomiting, soreness of the mouth/gums, joint pain, rash
IA. DISOPYRAM-IDE	Norpace Nospace CR	Same as above	Check w/ MD before taking cold or allergy meds	Dry mouth, constipation	Shortness of breath, swelling, blurred vision, persistent urinary hesitancy, constipation
IB. PHENYTOIN	Dilantin	Same as above	Take with food	Drowsiness	Nausea/vomiting, skin rash, sore gums, dizziness

continued

Oral Antiarrhythmic Agents *(continued)*

Medication Name & Group	Brand Name	Type/Purpose	Special Instructions	Expected Side Effects	Side Effects to Report to M.D.
IB. TOCAINIDE	Tonocard	Same as above	Take with food	Drowsiness	Nausea/vomiting, sore throat, shortness of breath, palpitations, easy bruising
IB. MEXILITENE	Mexitil	Same as above	Take with food	Drowsiness	Nausea/vomiting, shortness of breath, irregular heartbeats, palpitations
IC. FLECAINIDE	Tambocor	Helps regulate heart rhythm	Take exactly as prescribed	Drowsiness	Dizziness, visual disturbances, shortness of breath, heart rhythm or pulse changes
IC. INDECAINIDE	Decabid	Same as above	Swallow whole, do not crush or chew	Same as above	Same as above

IC. PROPAFENONE	Rythmol	Same as above	Take with meals	Drowsiness, metallic taste	Same as above
II. PROPRANOLOL	Inderal Inderal LA	Same as above	Do not stop medication abruptly except on advice of MD	Fatigue, transient drowsiness & dizziness	Dizziness, symptoms of congestive heart failure, confusion, slow pulse rate, skin rash
II. ACEBUTOLOL	Sectral	Same as above	Same as above	Same as above	Same as above
III. AMIODARONE	Cordarone	Same as above	Take exactly as prescribed Take with meals Avoid prolonged exposure to sun	Upset stomach	Nausea/vomiting, shortness of breath, irregular heartbeat, dizziness, skin rash
IV. VERAPAMIL	Calan Isoptin	Same as above	Take with meals	Constipation, dizziness	Shortness of breath, irregular heartbeat, swelling of extremities, pronounced dizziness

Oral Antihypertensive Agents

Medication	Brand Name	Type/Purpose	Special Instructions	Expected Side Effects	Side Effects to Report to M.D.
CHLOROTHIA-ZIDE HYDROCHLO-ROTHIAZIDE	Diuril Hydrodiuril, Esidrix, Oretic	Thiazides and related diuretics (Lower high blood pressure, rid body of excess water)	May cause upset stomach; take with food or milk Take daily dose in the morning	Frequent/increased urination Postural hypotension may occur; get up slowly	Muscle weakness, cramps, nausea, vomiting, diarrhea, dizziness
METHYCLO-THIAZIDE METOLAZONE	Enduron Zaroxolyn, Diulo, Microx				
CHLORTHALI-DONE INDAPAMIDE	Hygroton Lozol				
FUROSEMIDE ETHACRYNIC ACID BUMETANIDE	Lasix Edecrin Bumex	Loop diuretics	Same as above	Same as above	Same as above
SPIRONOLAC-TONE	Aldactone	Potassium-sparing diuretics	Same as above Avoid excessive potassium-rich food	Same as above	Stomach cramping, diarrhea, lethargy, headache, skin rash, menstrual abnormalities, voice changes

AMILORIDE	Midamor		Same as above	Same as above	Weakness, fatigue, muscle cramps
TRIAMTERENE	Dyrenium		Same as above Avoid prolonged sun exposure	Same as above	Weakness, headache, nausea, vomiting, sore throat, fever
DIURETIC COMBINATIONS	Dyazide Aldactazide Maxide Moduretic	Thiazide plus potassium-sparing diuretic	Same as above	Same as above	Same as above
METHYLDOPA	Aldomet	Antiadrenegic/ centrally acting		Postural hypotension, drowsiness	Prolonged tiredness, fever, dizziness
CLONIDINE	Catapres			Same as above, drowsiness, dry mouth	Persistent drowsiness, fatigue, constipation, hypotension
GUANABENZ	Wytensin		Protect meds from light	Drowsiness	Persistent sedation, dry mouth, dizziness, weakness, headache
GUANFACINE	Tenex		Should be taken at bedtime	Same as above	Same as above

continued

Oral Antihypertensive Agents (continued)

Medication	Brand Name	Type/Purpose	Special Instructions	Expected Side Effects	Side Effects to Report to M.D.
RESERPINE	Serpasil	Antiadrenergic/peripherally acting	May cause upset stomach; take with food/milk	Same as above	Persistent neusea and vomiting, dizziness, mood/sleep changes
GUANETHIDINE	Isemelin		Watch for postural hypotension	Same as above	Frequent dizziness or fainting, severe diarrhea
GUANADREL	Hylorel		Watch for postural hypotension	Same as above	Frequent dizziness or fainting
PRAZOSIN TERAZOSIN DOXAZOSIN	Minipress Hytrin Cardura		Watch for postural hypotension especially with the first dose	Same as above	Frequent dizziness, headache, weakness
HYDRALAZINE	Apresoline	Vasodilators	Take with meals	Headache, nausea	Tiredness, fever, muscle/joint pain
MINOXIDIL	Loniten			Hair growth, drowsiness	Increased heart rate, swelling of extremities, angina

Cardiac Glycosides (Digitalis)

Medication	Brand Name	Type/Purpose	Special Instructions	Expected Side Effects	Side Effects to Report to M.D.
DIGOXIN	Lanoxin (tablets, capsules, elixir, injections)	Increases the heart's ability to pump more effectively; control arrhythmias	Take after meals. Do not stop or increase or decrease the amount you are taking w/o your MD's knowledge.		Nausea/vomiting, unusual tiredness, changes in pulse, blurred vision, skin rash
DIGITOXIN	Crystodigin	Same as above	Same as above		Same as above

Anticoagulants

Medication	Brand Name	Type/Purpose	Special Instructions	Expected Side Effects	Side Effects to Report to M.D.
WARFARIN	Coumadin Panwarfin	Blood thinner	Take exactly as prescribed; do not take any other meds w/o your MD's knowledge. Avoid alcohol, aspirin, and drastic dietary changes. Take dosage at same time each day		Unusual bleeding or bruising, red or dark brown urine (blood), black or bloody stools

Cholesterol-Lowering Agents

Medication	Brand Name	Type/Purpose	Special Instructions	Expected Side Effects	Side Effects to Report to M.D.
CHOLESTYRA-MINE	Questran Cholybar (chewable)	Bile acid-binding resins	Mix in noncarbonated liquid Include fiber in diet or stool softener Take before meals Avoid concurrent administration of meds	Constipation, abdominal pain, heartburn, nausea, belching, bloating	Persistent gastrointestinal (GI) effects
COLESTIPOL	Colestid				
NICOTINIC ACID/ NIACIN	Niac Nicobid Endur-Acin Nico-400 Nicolar Slo-Niacin	Also lowers triglycerides Raises HDL	Take with meals Aspirin 325 mg. taken 30 minutes prior to dose may help if flushing persistent (check w/MD)	Face and upper body flushing Itching, tingling GI upset Dizziness	Pronounced and persistent cutaneous effects Nausea, vomiting

		Also lowers tri-glycerides	Take with meal(s)	GI upset, muscle weakness/pain, insomnia, rash, liver enzyme elevations	Persistent GI effects
LOVASTATIN PRAVASTATIN SIMVASTATIN	Mevacor Pravachol Zocor	Also lowers tri-glycerides	Take with meal(s)	GI upset, muscle weakness/pain, insomnia, rash, liver enzyme elevations	Persistent GI effects
GEMFIBROZIL	Lopid	Lowers triglycer-ides and LDL Raises HDL cho-lesterol	Take 30 minutes before meals	GI upset, fatigue, rash, liver enyzme eleva-tions, dizziness	Persistent GI effects
PROBUCOL	Lorelco		Take with meals	GI upset Prolong Q-T inter-val Dizziness	Persistent GI effects

A third drug in this category, simvastatin, is expected to receive FDA approval. It appears to be very similar to lovastatin, and will offer the advantage of once-a-day dosing.

ONE FINAL THOUGHT ON CHOLESTEROL CONTROL

You may be tempted to rely on cholesterol-controlling drugs and forget about the importance of diet. In fact, many doctors just prescribe drugs without even giving diet a trial. That's absolutely wrong, for two reasons.

First, you want to take the least medication possible. No drug will work as well without dietary modification as it will with a well-planned low-fat diet. Obviously, since you want to prevent another cardiac event you want your cholesterol level in the healthiest range, between 150 and 180.

Second, by just taking the drugs, you'll never know how much benefit you can derive from diet and exercise. In a perverse sort of way, taking drugs without dieting is like hitting your head with a hammer while taking aspirin for the headache!

AND A FINAL THOUGHT ON DRUGS IN GENERAL

As I said at the outset of this chapter, no one likes the idea of taking medications, especially when one might have to do so for the rest of one's life. But that's one mental barrier you're just going to have to get over. The drugs your doctor prescribes very likely will prolong or even save your life.

Millions of dollars have been spent on research and development to bring these medicines to the cardiac pharmacy, and even more millions went into testing and retesting them at medical centers in this country and around the world. It's been money well spent, in my opinion, and you'd be foolish to discount it by refusing to cooperate by taking the prescriptions exactly as your doctor advises.

Remember, too, that the more you do to improve your own health status by way of weight control, diet, exercise, stress management, and a life of moderation, the more likely it is that your drug requirements will drop considerably over time. In the meantime, your fullest possible compliance in your medications will be a major step in your recovery and in your becoming a former heart patient.

CHAPTER 17

Taking the Heart-Healthy Program on the Road

It's one thing to do your exercise and stick with your heart-healthy diet at home, but what about when you travel? It may take a bit of extra effort and commitment, but you definitely can take the program on the road with you.

Do all recovering heart patients stay with it? Research from the University of Houston indicates that individuals with heavy demands on their time tend to slip in terms of exercise. When eating alone, as on a business trip, they're likely to eat foods higher in fat than they would if at home or even if eating with others.

No doubt about it, we're living in a mobile society, and that puts a strain on your commitment. Most of us spend a lot of time on the road, traveling on business or for pleasure.

As with all other aspects of your recovery, you've got to view this one with a positive, upbeat attitude. Don't view it with doom and gloom like Nathan Pritikin did in his books when he called restaurants "the enemy camp" to be avoided at all costs. Even a respected heart researcher like Dr. William Castelli of the Framingham Heart Study has sounded pessimistic about the prospects when he told a group of physicians that "if you have to eat out in America, you are as good as dead."

Well, I'd like to take major exception with those two negative opinions. I've traveled extensively following the publication of *The 8-Week Cholesterol Cure,* at times spending as much as 70 percent of the month on the road, at other times traveling nonstop, city-to-city for a month or more at a time.

I've flown on virtually every airline in the sky, stayed at every major hotel chain and dozens of little independent motels, visited large cities and small towns, and eaten in countless restaurants. I can speak with some authority, then, when I say that it's not only possible, but actually easy, to take one's heart-healthy program on the road.

The travel industry recognizes a giant trend toward the desire to make healthy choices in exercise and dining. They're responding beautifully, more strongly than locally based restaurants and food companies. That's no doubt because the traveler tends to be more educated, more affluent, and more in tune with the compelling necessity to take care of himself and herself.

Robert Lang, vice president for food quality standards for Marriott, reflects the desire to best serve the international chain's clientele. He says Marriott's customers are speaking up, and Marriott is listening. They're sending chefs to training sessions and continuing education programs. The hotel restaurants and room-service menus offer substitutions such as olive oil, margarine, and Egg Beaters. At some locations one can order a sauté done with Pam.

If you have special dietary requirements, Mr. Lang says, let the hotel know. In fact, he actually encourages you to complain in those facilities which haven't totally made the changes the chain is striving for. Speaking up will let the management know that they need to get on the stick if they want to keep your business. "Be outspoken and be proud of your healthful eating habits," he says.

In Canada, 1,500 regular hotel customers did just that. When interviewed about what they wanted in foods, they spoke up about healthy alternatives to heavy, rich dishes. As a result, 32 Holiday Inn hotels across the country now offer menu items developed in cooperation with the Canadian Heart Foundation. They call such items as filet of salmon, chicken Shanghai, and spinach salad with sesame seed dressing "Heart Smart."

Taking a cruise is usually synonymous with indulging in lavish meals that aren't intended to be heart-healthy. Sure, you can ask for the fish to be broiled and to be served without sauce. But then you see and smell all those wonderful dishes arriving at tables around you, and willpower starts to melt. But Commodore Cruise Lines offers the perfect solution with foods from their Lite Cuisine Menu for all meals. Every single listing comes complete with calorie, fat, cholesterol, and sodium information. Imagine barley soup, veal chops, and lemon soufflé for dinner, with a total fat count of a mere 10 grams. Every meal is delicious and imaginative.

I mention these things to let you know that you're not in the minority. Rather, you're riding the crest of a trend that's sweeping across the country if not most of the western world. Start taking the attitude that the first thing to pack when traveling are your healthy program and practices. Don't leave home without them!

A good start is to get acquainted with an accommodating travel agent. If you don't already know this, it costs no more to arrange your travel arrangements with an agent than to do so yourself. In fact, very often an agent can do the bookings for far less.

GIVING YOUR PROGRAM WINGS

I'm not at all sure that "getting there is half the fun." In fact, air travel, in my opinion, lost all its glamour years ago. Today it's a grind, a typically disenchanting necessity. But advance planning can make all the difference.

Let's face it, airline food has never been one of flying's major attractions. The fare is fair at best, and just plain terrible at worst. Like hospital food, airline meals have been the basis of countless jokes and stories. And to make it worse, the food that doesn't taste very good is also likely to be laden with fat and cholesterol. Why cheat with food that doesn't make your taste buds tingle?

Instead, make advance arrangements for healthy alternatives. You can do so yourself by calling the airline 24 hours in advance. Or you can simply leave a standing order with your travel agent to do so on your behalf.

Every airline has a different list of choices, and some are a lot better than others. Very often, however, you'll be the envy of your fellow passengers when your special meal arrives. The reason for the superiority of those special plates is that they have to be made to order, rather than in assembly-line fashion. Fresher food is better food.

Most airlines don't broadly advertise about those special meals. They cost a lot more than those normally served. Why not take advantage of the situation?

To get a heart-healthy tray brought to your seat you can order a low-cholesterol/low-fat meal, a vegetarian platter, a fruit plate, or a cold seafood assortment. The latter is particularly good on American Airlines, including lobster and shrimp.

What might you expect to get? Breakfast might be hot or cold cereal, a muffin, maybe some yogurt, a little fruit salad, and skim milk and juice. Many airlines have been leaning to cold plates and sandwiches for lunch rather than hot meals. Most customers, myself included, prefer it that way. Dinner will include either chicken or fish, with salad, vegetables, pasta or potato, and most often fruit for dessert. You'll get margarine instead of butter and skim or low-fat milk with all meals served.

If you're really picky, or if you travel so much that you run into the same offerings over and over, your travel agent can even inquire as to the menus for the flights you might be interested in, comparing two or three airlines. A nice egg-substitute omelet with fresh fruit and squeezed orange juice might be the incentive for you to fly one airline over another.

Then again, you might not want to eat the airline's food at all. This is a great time to "brown bag" it with foods brought from home or picked up in the airport terminal. Many's the time I've had the guy sitting next to me drooling when I pull out a turkey breast sandwich on sourdough bread dressed with lettuce, tomato, and a bit of avocado.

And every frequent flyer can expect delays and more delays. It's become an anticipated part of travel these days. So I make certain that there are some "emergency foods" in my attaché case for all my flights. I might bring a couple of oat bran muffins, pieces of fresh fruit, dried fruits, and one of those low-fat, high-fiber bars or cookies you can pick up in health food shops or buy from the NANCI Corporation (page 297). There have been times when, after the captain has announced a delay, I've wished I had a shopping bag full so I could sell some of my goodies to the envious people around me. Be prepared!

Sitting on a plane for more than an hour can lead to blood pooling in the lower legs and ankles, as well as a general feeling of sluggishness. I make it a point to get an aisle seat on all flights so that I can get up frequently and walk a few lengths of the cabin without disturbing my fellow passengers.

On long flights, especially, it's a good idea to have a routine of stretches that you can do in your chair. Don't worry about others staring; they'll probably follow your example. Here are a few to keep you from stiffening up.

- Shoulder shrugs. Sitting upright, simply rest your hands on your thighs and shrug your shoulders up, hold, release, and repeat six or seven times.
- Arm raises. Just reach straight up with both arms, stretching out the shoulders and upper body.
- Elbow shrugs. Lean slightly forward in your seat, bend your arms at 90° angles, and shrug your elbows behind your back as though trying to touch your shoulder blades.
- Head rolls. Swivel your head three times in one direction and three times in the other, starting with your chin on your chest, rolling your ear to your shoulder, and around.
- Tummy tucking. Sitting straight, tighten your abdominal muscles, hold for a count of 10, release, and repeat.
- Leg lifts. Still sitting, raise your feet off the floor an inch or two, hold for a count of 10, release and repeat.
- Foot stretches. Point one foot at a time straight out as though on point like a ballet dancer, hold for a count of 10, release and repeat. Now reverse the process by bringing your toes upward toward your knee, hold, release and repeat.

Doing these stretches will make you feel a lot more relaxed when you land. I make it a point to do them when the captain is making his approach and the seat and table are in their upright and locked positions. There's an additional benefit in that such activities make one aware of the body and one's continuing efforts to take good care of it.

While we all like to find nonstop flights, layovers are a necessary evil much of the time. Don't waste your time by sitting in one of those uncomfortable chairs and grousing about the inconvenience. Rather, take a long walk through the airport's terminals. In many of the major cities that can be a long walk! Step briskly, as though you're late for a flight, and you'll find your heart rate going up nicely. Without exaggeration, you can easily get your whole day's exercise allotment of 30 minutes or so right there in the airport.

Still have some time on your hands? Again, don't waste it. Instead, do some deep breathing exercises, meditation, biofeedback, or whatever relaxation technique you've been using at home. It'll help make the time fly, and you'll be far more relaxed when you reach your destination.

Now and then you'll get one of those "connections made in hell" flights with three or more hours between flights. Or there might be a time when you originally thought you'd have only a one-hour layover but thanks to a "slight mechanical repair" or a "weather condition" in the next flight's originating city, you find yourself with a four-hour delay.

Yes, you can yell and scream and raise your cholesterol level and blood pressure by getting all stressed out. Or you can get in some relaxing, therapeutic exercise at a nearby hotel facility. You can ask about availability and short-term rates by calling from the free phones frequently found in the baggage area. Then take the shuttle to and from.

Here are just a few hotels that will allow travelers to use their health clubs for a reasonable fee:

EAST
   Marriott Hotel La Guardia (New York)
   Grand Hyatt Washington (D.C.)
   Ramada Renaissance (Atlanta)

MIDWEST
   St. Louis Marriott (St. Louis)
   Sheraton Hopkins Airport Hotel (Cleveland)
   Westin Hotel O'Hare (Chicago)

WEST
   Hilton & Towers Los Angeles Airport (Los Angeles)
   Westin Hotel San Francisco Airport (San Francisco)
   Stapleton Plaza Hotel (Denver)
   Hyatt Regency DFW (Dallas/Fort Worth)

TABLE 12
Airlines' Toll-Free Phone Numbers

Air Canada	800 422–6362
Alaska Airlines	426–0333
America West	247–5692
American Airlines	433–7300
Continental	525–0280
Delta	221–1212
Northwest	225–2525
Southwest	531–5601
TWA	221–2000
United	241–6522
USAir	428–4322

TABLE 13
Hotels' Toll-Free Phone Numbers

Doubletree Hotels	800 528–0444
Embassy Suites	362–2779
Hilton Hotels	445–8667
Holiday Inns	465–4329
Hyatt	228–9000
Loews	223–0888
Marriott	228–9290
Meridien	543–4300
Radisson	333–3333
Ramada Inns	272–6232
Sheraton	325–3536
Stouffer	325–5000

MAKING HOTELS BETTER THAN HOME

Like Marriott, most of the big hotel chains have made major accommodations for those of us trying to stay heart-healthy. In a very real way, I find it *easier* to follow my program while away than while at home. After all, I'm the guest, and I get to have it my way.

It all starts with good planning. Find out what kind of exercise facilities the hotel has. Ask in detail, learning whether they have treadmills, exercycles, a lap pool, and so forth. Don't accept vague answers. Great that they have that lap pool, but is it open at this time of year? Is it heated?

If you don't get all the answers you need, ask to speak with the concierge if they have one. He or she is specially trained to provide such assistance. Perhaps there's a health club near the hotel with reciprocal arrangements.

Pack your bag appropriately, including walking/running shoes, workout clothing, and swim gear. Take enough for your entire stay.

Even if you stay at a hotel with absolutely no exercise equipment or access to any, you can still get a workout. Find out where you can go for a 30-minute run or walk. It's a great way to see the sights.

What if it's raining or the temperature is below zero? Still no excuse. Put on your walking shoes and head to the stairwell. Walking those stairs can be a really strenuous workout; in fact, keep close tabs on your heart rate, counting the beats regularly so you don't overdo it.

Back in your room, get in your stretching exercises. This is a good time to know how to jump rope, since a rope takes so little room in your suitcase.

OK, let's say the stairwell is locked, it's raining outside, you can't skip rope, there's no exercise equipment or pool, and you want some exercise. Don't despair. Take out a couple of hefty phone books and use them to step up and down, one foot at a time. Here's the routine: right foot up, left foot up, left foot down, right foot down, left foot up, right foot up, right foot down, left foot down, and so forth. That's the way doctors used to get the heart rate going when doing an exercise test in the days prior to treadmill testing. It really works.

You can also use those phone books as weights to do some resistance training in your room. Think of them as barbells.

Especially if I haven't had a chance to do so prior to a flight, I really like getting a workout in as soon as I get into my hotel. It gets the kinks out, relaxes me, gets me into a mood and appetite for dinner, and somehow seems to adjust my internal clock to that city's time.

EATING ON THE ROAD

One of the first things I do when I check into a hotel is take a look at the menus in the restaurants for lunches and dinners. Happily, the major chains offer a number of low-fat choices to accommodate their health-conscious clientele. If I spot something I'd really like, but it's made with butter and cream sauce, I ask whether it could be made without those offending ingredients. That way when I go into the restaurant later during my stay I won't be surprised or disappointed.

I've learned that when ordering food I have to be very specific. Once I asked if an entree was prepared with butter or olive oil. I was assured that it was sautéed in olive oil. But when the dish came, it was swimming in butter. Rather irate, I called over the waiter who haughtily informed me that it was "sautéed in olive oil, but *finished* with butter!" Now I just say that I want no butter or cream in any of my food.

Breakfasts are getting easier all the time. Most hotel restaurants offer egg substitutes which I can enjoy scrambled or in omelets. Hyatt makes a wonderful frittata, a light sort of omelet with just a glaze of low-fat cheese. Moreover, you can order egg-white omelets just about anywhere; they're quite good, and no one is surprised by the order.

For breakfast side dishes, try Canadian bacon or ham. Ask for hash brown potatoes to be prepared "dry" and for your toast or muffin to be presented without butter. Margarine is usually available.

But most of the time I bring some breakfast food to my room to enjoy while watching the morning news. I pack some oat bran cereal, bananas, and a few snack items. That way all I need is some skim milk and juice, which I can get for "take-out" at the coffee shop along with a cup of decaf. This saves time and money, since the lines are long in the morning as all those businessmen want to be fed at the same time, and the prices are ridiculously high.

Those snack items I pack come in really handy, especially in the evening when I return to my room after a long day's work. It's at those times when one can be easily tempted to indulge in a candy bar or chips or cookies from the mini-bars often placed in the room. Instead, I have my fruit and nonfat or NANCI cookies to munch on. Planning ahead really pays off.

BITING THE BULLET

OK, I'll admit that I've painted a rosy picture thus far. There definitely are times when the hotel restaurants have absolutely nothing to offer along the lines of dishes that are delicious as well as nutritious, with interesting sauces and side dishes. You have two choices.

One, ask the concierge where some ethnic restaurants are located fairly close to the hotel. Opt for Italian or Oriental food that night. You can always find some healthy pasta or stir-fry dishes in such spots, anywhere in the world.

Two, you can bite the bullet that night. By that I mean that once in a while it's necessary to order spartan food in the face of artery-clogging temptations. Yes, it's tough to forego the sauces and have a piece of fish simply broiled, and to give up on dessert and wait till you get to your room to have a piece of fruit. Yes, it's not easy to eat that baked potato .plain, or that piece of bread without a spread if they have no margarine. But it can be done once in a while. You'll be proud of yourself in the morning.

BANQUETS AND BINGEING

Banquets pose a special problem for businessmen, whether traveling or at home. Seldom are such meals planned with health in mind. But you don't have to give in. First of all, banquet food isn't the greatest anyway, so it's not as though you're really giving up something wonderful. Second, it's easier than ever to request an alternative. Certainly that's best accomplished by ordering a substitute meal in advance, but even on short notice the kitchen can come up with something that will tide you over.

If you're going to have a splurge, by all means do so now and then. As part of a routinely low-fat diet, a now-and-then binge won't significantly affect your cholesterol level. But wouldn't you rather enjoy that splurge in a fine restaurant with your spouse? I put banquet food in the same category as airline cuisine, and treat it the same.

Don't be ashamed or embarrassed to ask for a special meal. Be proud of your commitment. You'll probably impress those you do business with as being a person whose standards are high and firm.

As a last resort, you can always eat prior to going to the banquet. Have a sandwich and some soup in the coffee shop. Then you won't be hungry, and you can simply nibble at the banquet. No one will even notice. I do it often.

ENJOYING A HEART-HEALTHY VACATION

It's really a paradox to go on a vacation and abandon your good habits. The idea of a vacation is to renew oneself, to refresh and strengthen the mind and body. It's a mistake to throw your principles to the winds when vacationing. Happily, you don't have to do so at all. Plan a healthy holiday!

Once again, a good travel agent comes in handy at such times. There are spas, resorts, dude ranches, fishing camps, cruises, and tours which feature healthy activities and foods. Don't ever forget that by eating and living a heart-healthy lifestyle, you're on the cutting edge. In today's society that means that more and more people are doing the very same thing. And in turn the vacation industry has responded with some very healthy choices.

Why not start planning for your next vacation well in advance? Call your travel agent and ask her to start collecting information about healthy destinations. Put together a file on such places and enjoy letting your imagination go, thinking about cruising the Caribbean or walking along a sandy beach. Looking forward to future pleasures is one of life's greatest joys.

Planning to travel abroad? Obviously you can't go everywhere, so why not consider the health angle of various destinations. A week in Paris will tempt you with all those five-star restaurants and their cream and butter sauces. A week in the South of France, on the other hand, will introduce you to the mouth-watering delights of Mediterranean cuisine that packs lots of fun and flavor without the fat.

Closer to home, old-fashioned health spas were places of deprivation and discomfort. Today they pamper their guests with engaging daily activities, facials and massages, and wonderfully creative approaches to low-fat cuisine fit for kings and queens.

LIFESTYLE: DON'T LEAVE HOME WITHOUT IT

There are certain things you just take for granted. You don't think about doing them, they're just part of your life. You brush your teeth every single day. You bathe at least once a day. You have a string of rituals that have become integral in your life that are done "for your own good," as your parents told you and you told your children.

A long time ago you had to be reminded to brush your teeth and to wash behind your ears. Today such activities are a part of life. Would you leave home without your toothbrush? Of course not. So why leave home without your commitment to diet and exercise?

During the first few months of modifying your lifestyle, you no doubt will wish you could forget all about getting your daily exercise or cutting back on fat and cholesterol. It takes time to form new habits, whether good or bad.

But once that habit is formed, it becomes second nature. Try going a day or two without brushing your teeth. It'll drive you nuts. You'll *want* to brush! In time, you'll feel the same way about diet and exercise.

Exercise, especially, becomes addictive. After several months of regular activity, you'll look forward to your workouts. You'll *miss* exercise if you can't do it.

In 1989 I broke five ribs while water skiing, attempting a trick to impress my kids. The doctor advised no strenuous exercise for six weeks. I hated it, and couldn't wait for those ribs to heal so I could get back to my sweaty workouts that make me feel so good for the rest of the day. I actually went through a sort of withdrawal, with irritable feelings and general sluggishness. I've become addicted to exercise, and I plan to exercise for the rest of my life whether at home or on the road.

The same goes for my diet. Gone are the days when I'd drool over greasy french fries and barbecued ribs. In fact, when I do eat some fatty foods, I feel queasy. I've grown to prefer broiled foods over those that are fried. To me, skim milk is the way milk should taste; whole milk tastes greasy and not at all refreshing. Again, it's a matter of what one becomes accustomed to.

Sure, it'll take some time, but by this time next year you'll no more pack your luggage without your healthy habits than without your toothbrush. Have a nice trip!

CHAPTER 18

The Art of the Second Chance: A Few Final Words of Encouragement

You, I, and many others have been given a second chance in life. The question now is what are you going to do with it? Actually you have quite a few options.

Of course you can ignore everything your doctors and I have to say. But the mere fact that you've read through the book this far indicates that you won't take that approach.

Next, you can grudgingly make a few lifestyle modifications. That's better than nothing, but without a real commitment it's likely you'll slip back into your old ways after a few months. It's rather like controlling alcoholism. The recovering alcoholic must make the admission that he or she is, indeed, an alcoholic and that it will take day-to-day effort to avoid taking even one more drink.

We've had a closer look at our own mortality than other living mortals. It's scary. One tendency, quite a human reaction, is to cover up the memory in our minds. But that reaction can be dangerous. I admire the Jewish people who refuse to allow the memory of the Holocaust to fade. Only by keeping it in our consciousness, they maintain, can we prevent it from happening again.

Don't dwell on your heart disease and mortality to the point of morbid obsession. But don't allow yourself to become lulled into a state of complacency that might argue that it can't happen again. It can. But it doesn't have to.

I'd like to leave you with one, very positive, analogy for your recovery. Let's compare your heart health with your financial health. Let's say that you're threatened with financial failure. You might lose your house and all your savings. You might face bankruptcy.

Now let's say that a group of respected financial analysts review your situation and come up with a solution that could not only solve your monetary problems but also make you a millionaire in the process. They assure you that it's almost a sure thing. But if you don't take the steps they advise, you'll surely go down the path to financial ruin.

What would you do? Go down the tubes? Or become a millionaire? Doubtless you're thinking that the choice is obvious. Nobody would choose to go broke when they have a chance to become wealthy. Right?

Well, you have a very similar choice to make. Where do you think we get the expression, "I feel like a million dollars"? You can, indeed, go from a state of health crisis to a state of exuberant, exultant good health. Your choice.

Do I exaggerate? When I sent the manuscript of this book out for critical review by a number of top physicians and health professionals, I thought that might be the one criticism. I knew I had my scientific facts in order, but I wondered whether they might feel that I overstated the promise of going beyond mere recovery to a potential of literally erasing heart disease from one's life.

I was delighted to hear that they supported my views. We have the data and experience to back up the promise in *those who really want to deliver it for themselves.* I emphasize those words quite deliberately. You've got to want to make it happen. And only you can deliver the goods. Your doctors and others can help, but it's ultimately your choice.

I'm behind you 100 percent. I wish I was there with you right now to give you a big hug, look you straight in the eyes, and say, "God bless you, you can do it!"

I'd love to hear from you. If you feel like writing you can reach me at P.O. Box 2039, Venice, CA 90294.

Index